HIGH-FUNCTIONING INDIVIDUALS WITH AUTISM

CURRENT ISSUES IN AUTISM

Series Editors: Eric Schopler and Gary B. Mesibov

University of North Carolina School of Medicine
Chapel Hill, North Carolina

AUTISM IN ADOLESCENTS AND ADULTS
Edited by Eric Schopler and Gary B. Mesibov

COMMUNICATION PROBLEMS IN AUTISM
Edited by Eric Schopler and Gary B. Mesibov

DIAGNOSIS AND ASSESSMENT IN AUTISM
Edited by Eric Schopler and Gary B. Mesibov

THE EFFECTS OF AUTISM ON THE FAMILY
Edited by Eric Schopler and Gary B. Mesibov

HIGH-FUNCTIONING INDIVIDUALS WITH AUTISM
Edited by Eric Schopler and Gary B. Mesibov

NEUROBIOLOGICAL ISSUES IN AUTISM
Edited by Eric Schopler and Gary B. Mesibov

SOCIAL BEHAVIOR IN AUTISM
Edited by Eric Schopler and Gary B. Mesibov

HIGH-FUNCTIONING INDIVIDUALS WITH AUTISM

Edited by
Eric Schopler
and
Gary B. Mesibov

University of North Carolina School of Medicine
Chapel Hill, North Carolina

PLENUM PRESS • NEW YORK AND LONDON

Library of Congress Cataloging-in-Publication Data

High-functioning individuals with autism / edited by Eric Schopler and Gary B. Mesibov.
p. cm. -- (Current issues in autism)
Includes bibliographical references and index.
ISBN 0-306-44064-4
1. Autism. I. Schopler, Eric. II. Mesibov, Gary B. III. Series.
[DNLM: 1. Autism. WM 203.5 H638]
RC553.A88H54 1992
616.89'82--dc20
DNLM/DLC
for Library of Congress 92-3458
CIP

ISBN 0-306-44064-4

A Division of Plenum Publishing Corporation
233 Spring Street, New York, N.Y. 10013

Printed in the United States of America

To the families seeking
more information on high-functioning autism,
with the hope that this volume
will be a valuable source of information and support

Contributors

MARY S. AKERLEY, 10609 Glenwild Road, Silver Spring, Maryland 20901

CHRISTIANE A. M. BALTAXE, Department of Psychiatry and Biobehavioral Sciences, UCLA School of Medicine, Los Angeles, California 90024

ANNE CARPENTER, 2200 Fuller Road 705-B, Ann Arbor, Michigan 48105

MARGARET A. DEWEY, 2301 Woodside Road, Ann Arbor, Michigan 48104

TEMPLE GRANDIN, Department of Animal Science, Colorado State University, Fort Collins, Colorado 80523

R. PETER HOBSON, Developmental Psychopathology Research Unit, Tavistock Clinic and University College, London NW3 5BA, England

KATHY LISSNER, 3649 Dunnica, St. Louis, Missouri 63116

CATHERINE LORD, Greensboro-High Point TEACCH Center, 2415 Penny Road, High Point, North Carolina 27265

GARY B. MESIBOV, Division TEACCH, Department of Psychiatry, The University of North Carolina at Chapel Hill, Chapel Hill, North Carolina 27599-7180

NANCY J. MINSHEW, Western Psychiatric Institute and Clinic, University of Pittsburgh School of Medicine, Pittsburgh, Pennsylvania 15213

SUSAN MORENO, MAAP, P.O. Box 524, Crown Point, Indiana 46307

NEIL OFFEN, 700 Bolinwood Drive, Chapel Hill, North Carolina 27514

CLARA PARK, 29 Hoxsey Street, Williamstown, Massachusetts 02167

THERESE MARIE RONAN, 9307 Slater, Overland Park, Kansas 66212

JUDITH M. RUMSEY, Child Psychiatry Branch and Child and Adolescent Disorders Research Branch, National Institute of Mental Health, Bethesda, Maryland 20892

ERIC SCHOPLER, Division TEACCH, Department of Psychiatry, The University of North Carolina at Chapel Hill, Chapel Hill, North Carolina 27599-7180

JAMES Q. SIMMONS III, Department of Psychiatry and Biobehavioral Sciences, UCLA School of Medicine, Los Angeles, California 90024

JIM SINCLAIR, P.O. Box 1545, Lawrence, Kansas 66044

RUTH C. SULLIVAN, Autism Services Center, P.O. Box 507, Huntington, West Virginia 25710-0507

CONSTANCE V. TORISKY, 738 Greenleaf Drive, Monroeville, Pennsylvania 15146

LUKE Y. TSAI, Child and Adolescent Psychiatry Service, Department of Psychiatry, University of Michigan Medical Center, Ann Arbor, Michigan 48109-0390

MARY E. VAN BOURGONDIEN, Division TEACCH, Department of Psychiatry, The University of North Carolina at Chapel Hill, Chapel Hill, North Carolina 27599-7180

ANDRE VENTER, Department of Pediatrics, University of the Witwatersrand, Baragwanath Hospital, Post Office Bertsham 2013, Johannesburg, Republic of South Africa

LORNA WING, MRC Social Psychiatry Unit, Institute of Psychiatry, University of London, London SE5 8AF, England

AMY V. WOODS, Division TEACCH, Department of Psychiatry, The University of North Carolina at Chapel Hill, Chapel Hill, North Carolina 27599-7180

Preface

Division TEACCH, located in the School of Medicine at The University of North Carolina at Chapel Hill, was one of the first—and remains one of the most comprehensive—programs in the world assisting people with autism and their families. As a comprehensive, lifelong diagnostic and treatment program, Division TEACCH treats a wide variety of clients of all ages. Those in TEACCH, therefore, are acutely aware of the similarities among clients who are described as having autism and equally aware of the differences within this group.

Of our over 2,000 clients with autism in North Carolina, approximately 30% would be classified as high functioning. Although those in this group evidence many of the difficulties typical of people with autism, their superior language skills and greater ability to conceptualize add unique challenges. It is important for parents and professionals working with high-functioning people with autism to recognize and respond to these. This book is designed to facilitate that process.

As were the preceding books in our series, *Current Issues in Autism,* this volume is based on one of the TEACCH conferences held in Chapel Hill each May. The books are not simply published proceedings of the conference papers. Instead, conference participants are asked to develop full chapters around their presentations. Other international experts whose work is beyond the scope of each conference but related to the major themes are asked to contribute chapters as well. These volumes provide the most up-to-date information on research and professional practice available on the most important issues in autism.

This volume is designed to advance our understanding of high-functioning people with autism. Current diagnostic and treatment approaches are presented, along with cogent analyses of the current conceptions about the neurological processes involved. Personal perspectives from parents and high-functioning clients add depth and a perspective not often found in professional books. These are included for those readers who have not yet had firsthand experience with the challenges and issues particular to high-level autism. They are included also because we found them to be both inspirational and a joy to read. We expect this volume to be of interest to students, professionals, and parents concerned with understanding and assisting individuals with autism.

Eric Schopler
Gary B. Mesibov

Acknowledgments

We are indebted to many people for their cooperation and generous assistance in the preparation of this volume. It is our great pleasure to acknowledge each of them. Our thanks go to Helen Garrison, who efficiently coordinated the conference that was the starting point for the book. Her meticulous attention to detail in organizing these major activities is greatly admired and appreciated. Our secretarial staff, including Vickie Weaver and Jeanette Fergerson, handled the many typing and administrative chores associated with a project of this scope with consistent good humor, cooperation, and competence. John Swetnam carefully reviewed each chapter, providing superb editorial and technical assistance. His thoroughness and care are evident throughout the book.

We also want to thank our many TEACCH colleagues, who are too numerous to name, for their ongoing help, assistance, and cooperation. Their insights and understanding of people with autism are a continuing source of information and inspiration to us. As with all of our efforts in the TEACCH program, this book would not have been possible without the assistance of the families of people with autism in North Carolina. We owe a special debt for this volume to those high-functioning individuals and their families whose cooperation and participation in our program have taught us what we know about this important topic. Finally, The University of North Carolina at Chapel Hill School of Medicine and the North Carolina State Legislature make all our work possible through their continued support.

Contents

Part I: Overview

Chapter 3

Chapter 4

Chapter 5

Chapter 14

Overview

1

Introduction to High-Functioning Individuals with Autism

GARY B. MESIBOV and ERIC SCHOPLER

INTRODUCTION

When Kanner (1943) first described autism, he recognized that individuals with this disability could be high-functioning in terms of their language and intellectual skills. Not only did Kanner recognize this possibility, he believed that all people with autism were within the normal range of intelligence with the potential for average language skills. The 11 children in Kanner's original sample were, in fact, above average in intelligence. As the investigation and treatment of autism progressed, however, this high-functioning group did not get the same attention as the more common clients with autism who were functioning intellectually in the retarded range with severe communication handicaps.

In the 1950s and 1960s, the focus was on this majority of the population with autism. Behavioral interventions were emphasized, replacing many of the psychoanalytic approaches that were in vogue earlier. As the most frequent intervention practice, specific responses were elicited in mentally retarded clients with autism. Applying reinforcement contingencies in different settings became the main topic of inquiry, and demonstrating the effectiveness of these contingencies was the focus of most professional efforts.

Everard (1976) reminded the field that a high-functioning group existed, with slightly different needs and behaviors than more typical children with autism. Levy (1986) supported this notion, arguing for specific strengths, needs, and discrepancies from normal functioning that could be identified in high-functioning children

---

GARY B. MESIBOV and ERIC SCHOPLER • Division TEACCH, Department of Psychiatry, The University of North Carolina at Chapel Hill, Chapel Hill, North Carolina 27599-7180.

High-Functioning Individuals with Autism, edited by Eric Schopler and Gary B. Mesibov. Plenum Press, New York, 1992.

with autism. Tsai and Scott-Miller (1988) called for clearer diagnostic criteria for high-functioning autism, suggesting the following identifying characteristics for this group: near-normal cognitive development, IQ above 60, academic capability, near-normal communication, nearly independent life skills, and positive social orientation. The movie *Rain Man* has, of course, stimulated considerable interest and awareness of this group among the general public. It is our unique intent with this volume to provide both the best of current knowledge about high-functioning autism and a sense of the subjective experience of coping with it. This is accomplished by presenting chapters by international experts in the field and personal essays by both high-functioning people with autism and the parents of such people.

OVERVIEW

Part I of this volume is an overview of significant issues. Luke Tsai begins with a discussion of important diagnostic issues. He reviews the classification of high-functioning autism in DSM-III and DSM-III-R, highlighting the changes that have occurred. He also reviews the international classification system (ICD-10) and how it relates to diagnostic concepts in the United States. Tsai offers clinical descriptions helpful in analyzing the disorder and describes how high-functioning autism differs from the related disorders of Asperger syndrome, schizoid disorder of childhood, learning disabilities, elective mutism, developmental disorders of receptive language, obsessive–compulsive disorders, and Tourette syndrome. This chapter provides an excellent overview of high-functioning autism and current controversies in the classification of it and related disorders.

Judith Rumsey follows with a review of neuropsychological studies. She argues that the neuropsychological profile of high-functioning clients with autism offers an opportunity to understand the effects of autism independent of cognitive deficiencies. Her careful review of the literature examines the primary neuropsychological functions: general intelligence, attention, memory and learning, language, sequential processing, and social deficits. Rumsey also examines claims of exceptional abilities in many high-functioning individuals with autism and concludes that cognitive deficits are still seen in these high-functioning clients, even though their overall IQ scores are within the average range. These deficits include difficulties with social and context-relevant information (both verbal and nonverbal), wandering attention, and memory difficulties with the encoding of information. Rumsey compares these deficits in autism with those in other developmental disabilities.

Nancy Minshew's chapter examines neurological localization in autism, reviewing brainstem, cerebellar, limbic, and cortical theories of dysfunction in autism. While acknowledging many possible interpretations of these complex data, she concludes that autism represents a diffuse deficit in complex information processing rather than a deficit in the acquisition of information. The neurobiological defect, according to Minshew, is in the development of the neural network responsible for complex information processing.

This overview section also contains parental and client perceptions. Susan Moreno, a parent of a high-functioning woman with autism and editor of the newsletter "More Able Autistic People" (MAAP), describes with humor and insight the parent perspective as experienced by her, her husband, and the parents she contacts through MAAP. Her poignant views of high-functioning autistic people and their families highlight important problems and potential solutions. Presently a college student educated in regular public school classrooms, Moreno's daughter Beth experienced many of the triumphs and tragedies associated with autism at her level of functioning. The chapter provides a fascinating view of how families struggle with high-functioning autism.

Temple Grandin is the most publicized adult with autism in the United States. Her dramatic success as a designer of livestock equipment has demonstrated how the strengths of people with autism can overcome many of their deficits. Her descriptions of autism, and especially the frustration accompanying her deficits, are powerful. Grandin's chapter will help parents and professionals understand autism in new and stimulating ways. Grandin has sufficient insight into her behaviors to describe what autism feels like. Her descriptions of language difficulties, auditory problems, tactile problems, and chronic anxiety communicate effectively with those lacking firsthand experience with these difficulties.

SOCIAL ISSUES

The topic of Part II is social issues in high-functioning autism. Chapters by Lorna Wing, Gary Mesibov, and Peter Hobson explore the idiosyncrasies of high-functioning people and what they suggest about cause and treatment. Subtle nuances of social interactions are described, with an emphasis on the difficulties these clients experience in social situations. Ways of assisting these clients are also discussed.

Wing explores the manifestations of social problems in high-functioning individuals with autism. She describes the primary reasons for the social deficits: affective and cognitive abnormalities, rigidity and repetitiveness of thoughts, and lack of understanding of other people's ideas and feelings. These deficits make social interactions difficult, even though social interest and emotional feelings are present in people with autism.

Wing categorizes high-functioning people with autism by their specific types of social problems: aloof and indifferent, socially passive, and active but odd. She argues that each of these three groups has different educational and treatment planning needs. Her data suggest that they also have different outcomes.

Mesibov reviews treatment strategies with high-functioning clients and proposes a combination of individual counseling and social-group learning opportunities. He believes that by learning about their autistic clients' perspectives of the world, counselors can help these clients to establish rapport and build a sense of trust so that individual counseling can help them organize their thinking, understand relationships between events, and cope with everyday problems.

Mesibov advocates social skills group training to provide opportunities for people with autism to develop their social abilities through real-life practice. Groups are designed to make social interaction more interesting by providing individualized social opportunities in relevant community contacts. Understanding social expectations and practicing appropriate social behaviors are major goals of this group approach.

Hobson examines social perception in high-functioning autism, beginning with an outline of perceptually grounded prerequisites for personal relatedness. Of particular relevance are the prerequisites for recognizing emotions in others. Hobson carefully analyzes the normal developmental process, delineating areas of difficulty for children with autism. Hobson views autism as a deficient concept of persons; social and affective recognition are impaired, making social judgments and decisions extremely difficult and unreliable. There are problems not only in the ability to understand and recognize emotion, but also in the perception of aspects such as age and sex. Broader concepts such as self-awareness are also impaired.

EDUCATIONAL ISSUES

The third part of the book describes educational factors in high-functioning autism. Cathy Lord and Andre Venter begin with a comprehensive summary of the long-term follow-up literature. They nicely summarize what is known about outcomes, emphasizing the predictive validity of cognitive measures. Lord and Venter also provide thoughtful ideas and new perspectives.

Christiane Baltaxe and James Simmons review language ability in high-functioning autism by comparing autism with related disorders. Their careful studies indicate that many differences in language behavior among the disorders disappear when cognitive level is held constant. Baltaxe and Simmons conclude—along with Tanguay (in press)—that a larger, more inclusive diagnostic category of "social communication spectrum disorder" might be a fruitful way to unify these groups. They argue for greater collaboration between communication specialists and psychiatrists so that both language and behavioral problems can be fully understood and treated.

Mary Van Bourgondien and Amy Woods close this section with a review of the key factors in successful vocational placements of high-functioning people with autism. These authors' extensive experience and understanding of important issues is evident in their thoughtful analysis of employment issues. They explore creative vocational options for high-functioning people with autism: the job-coach model, enclaves, mobile crews, and small businesses. Their description of the exciting new Carolina Living and Learning Center will be especially interesting to many readers.

Van Bourgondien and Woods conclude with an excellent discussion of how to prepare a high-functioning person with autism for successful community and vocational living.

PARENTAL ISSUES AND PERSONAL ACCOUNTS

In the first chapter of Part IV, parents of high-functioning people with autism describe their concerns and experiences through individual essays on topics of their own choosing. Although the topics vary from parent to parent, there is a common thread in these essays of determination, commitment, and resilience in the face of relentless challenges. As professionals, we are always inspired by the humor and resourcefulness that parents of handicapped children are able to combine.

Ruth Sullivan begins the chapter with a description of her son's involvement in the filming of *Rain Man*. With the film as her focus, she describes how society's ignorance about autism imposes major hardships on families. Many of the difficult experiences she describes will be familiar to parents. *Rain Man*, for Sullivan, was an opportunity to inform the public about her fascinating experiences and compelling needs. One of the most effective parent advocates for autism in this country, Sullivan's thoughts on educating the public are practical and thought provoking.

Clara Park writes with her usual insight and clarity about her daughter's art ability. The development of Jessy Park's ability to draw, one of the savant skills sometimes found in high-functioning people with autism, provides insight into this intriguing phenomenon. We learn how this savant skill is not totally intuitive; several gifted teachers—including Clara herself—played important roles in helping Jessy. Clara Park's perceptiveness allows rare insights into autism as well as this savant skill. Jessy's ability to paint, her attitude toward her own talent, her selection of subject matter, and her motivation are all delightfully presented.

Connie Torisky describes a familiar problem in high-functioning autism: her son's sensitivity to criticism. Parents and professionals are familiar with the paradox that autistic children are in greater need of assistance than their normal peers but often less willing to accept constructive suggestions. Torisky's discussion of all sides of this issue is interesting and enlightening. Her familiar examples offer good suggestions and provide important guidelines.

Even children with autism grow up and leave the nest. The problem of encouraging independence during the delicate separation period is thoughtfully discussed by Mary Akerley. She describes the difficult transitions made by her son Ed with poignant anecdotes. One of the most difficult issues confronting parents of high-functioning children with autism is whether or not their child should have a driver's license. Akerley's experience with this question is especially thought provoking.

Autism is an international phenomenon, although each culture copes differently. Neil Offen, an American parent, first learned about his son's problems while the family was living in France. Offen discusses their problems in getting information and a diagnosis in a foreign country. Although some might argue that many families fare no better in their own country, most will agree that the challenges presented here are different.

Margaret Dewey closes this chapter of parent essays by describing eccentricity in high-functioning autistic people. Using many fascinating examples, Dewey captures the charm and uniqueness that characterize this group. Although sometimes their limitations can be frustrating and irritating, we are also charmed by their appealing simplicity and straightforwardness. This is a fitting essay to end this chapter, reminding us of how enjoyable people with autism can be and how much they enrich our lives.

Taken together, these parental essays represent years of hard-earned experiences and astute observations. Although never requesting their special role and having little training to meet their responsibilities, these parents have accepted the challenge of a child with autism and directed this potential tragedy into something useful and productive. While reading about their experiences, one has to admire their insights and ingenuity.

The last chapter of this volume has people with autism writing about themselves. It is fitting that they should have the final word. Here we see how people with autism struggle to comprehend a world that does not usually make sense. These essays provide insights into how individuals with autism understand and interpret their experiences; they are a rare opportunity to see the world from the perspective of people with autism.

Anne Carpenter begins the chapter by tracing her personal development. Carpenter calmly, directly, and unemotionally describes the many failures she experienced while growing up. An engaging young woman, Anne is now mature, personable, and competent. Receiving the diagnosis of autism, interestingly enough, was her turning point; it explained why she did things and her inability to meet certain demands. She still struggles today with finding appropriate programs and services, but with new optimism and feelings of competence.

Jim Sinclair was diagnosed as gifted before anyone thought about autism. He continues to function at an extremely high level intellectually. Jim is a superb writer who provides rare insights into how people with autism think and understand. He sees autism as a difficulty in understanding and presents many excellent examples of how this manifests itself in everyday life. Jim understands many subtle differences between himself and people without autism; his essay gives us a rare personal glimpse of these differences.

Therese Ronan lives in the Midwest. Honest, simple, and straightforward, she has a fulfilling and dignified life in spite of her handicap. Like many high-functioning people with autism, she describes her experiences directly and without embellishment. Many will find her honesty appealing and informative.

The final view of autism is provided by Kathy Lissner. A child of the 1960s in many ways, Kathy is aware of civil rights issues and the need to assert oneself to achieve full citizenship. She is typical of people with autism because she frequently behaves in strange and unpredictable ways. Her uniqueness, however, is her insight into her behaviors and her ability to describe them. Kathy's descriptions of her own idiosyncrasies are clear and intriguing. This essay provides new insights into the atypical behaviors often associated with autism.

Taken together, the chapters in this book are clear, thoughtful, and comprehensive. They provide a description of high-functioning people with autism and a state-of-the-art understanding of what is known about this group. Treatment approaches are described and discussed, and personal accounts by parents and clients add a fascinating perspective rarely available in books of this kind. Readers interested in high-functioning autism will find much to think about in these pages.

REFERENCES

Everard, M. P. (1976, July). *Mildly autistic young people and their problems.* Paper presented at the International Symposium on Autism, St. Gallen, Switzerland.

Kanner, L. (1943). Autistic disturbances of affective contact. *Nervous Child, 2,* 217–250.

Levy, S. (1986). *Identifying high-functioning children with autism.* Bloomington, IN: Indiana Resource Center for Autism.

Tanguay, P. (in press). Infantile autism and social communication spectrum disorders. *Journal of Child and Adolescent Psychiatry.*

Tsai, L., & Scott-Miller, D. (1988). Higher-functioning autistic disorder. *Focus on Autistic Behavior, 2,* 1–8.

2

Diagnostic Issues in High-Functioning Autism

LUKE Y. TSAI

INTRODUCTION

Ever since Kanner (1943) published his first description of autism, views of its etiology and nature have evolved and changed. During the past four decades, in spite of the significant advances in the understanding of autism, disagreements over its validity and definition have never ceased. Lay people are confused by changes of the diagnostic terms and criteria for autism; they worry that different authorities are talking about different disorders when they talk about autistic people. This is particularly true in the borderline cases with near-normal functioning (i.e., high-functioning autism).

> Our son, age 8½, has been diagnosed by Dr. O. as having higher-functioning autistic disorder, but at least three other physicians disagree with him. This really leaves us frustrated and confused.

This extract from a mother's letter shows that parents are concerned whether it is ever possible that someday autism can be diagnosed reliably. Their worries are both understandable and not unwarranted.

It is not unusual that an individual with a less obvious form may be labeled "autistic" at one center and something else at another. For the present, there is no readily recognizable separate point between true autism and other disorders that show autisticlike features. It is quite obvious that there is the issue of boundaries of autism. In fact, recently Rutter and Schopler (1987) pointed out that there remain five controversial areas with respect to the boundaries of autism as a valid diagnostic entity: (1) autisticlike syndromes in children with severe mental retardation;

LUKE Y. TSAI • Child and Adolescent Psychiatry Service, Department of Psychiatry, University of Michigan Medical Center, Ann Arbor, Michigan 48109-0390.

High-Functioning Individuals with Autism, edited by Eric Schopler and Gary B. Mesibov. Plenum Press, New York, 1992.

(2) autisticlike disorders in people with normal intelligence; (3) later-onset autisticlike disorders following a prolonged period of normal development; (4) severe disorders arising in early or middle childhood characterized by grossly bizarre behavior; and (5) the overlap between autism and severe developmental disorders of receptive language. So long as the controversies continue, the concern of accurate diagnosis of high-functioning autism remains.

Any discussion of diagnosis must start with classification. Diagnostic classification is essential because it serves as a code for communication between clinicians. It provides a kind of language by which people can describe the disorders they investigate and treat (Rutter & Gould, 1985). Classification is necessary for the acquisition of knowledge and scientific progress in any field. Therefore, the first section of this chapter briefly discusses the changes and differences between earlier and contemporary diagnostic classifications of autism. For more detailed information on the classification of autism, the readers are referred to the recently published book *Diagnosis and Assessment in Autism* (Schopler & Mesibov, 1988). This section also discusses research problems caused by the earlier and current diagnostic systems. A new diagnostic system for Autism that is currently being proposed as part of the 10th edition of the World Health Organization's International Classification of Diseases (ICD-10), is presented. The future direction for the DSM-IV definition and classification of autism is proposed at the end of the section. The presentation and discussion of coming new classifications serve to prepare the readers for another major change of the conceptualization of autism.

In the section on review of studies of high-functioning autism, criteria of "high functioning" used by previous investigators are described. The external and internal diagnostic validity of high-functioning autism as defined by these studies is examined.

The next section of the chapter is concerned with the boundaries of high-functioning autism. Several disorders with various autisticlike features are described. Points that are helpful for differential diagnoses are offered.

The last major section of the chapter describes various systems that have been used by clinicians to qualify the severity of psychiatric disorders. An attempt by the Autism Society of America (ASA) to define high-functioning autism is described, and a working definition and diagnostic criteria for high-functioning autism are proposed.

DEFINITION AND CLASSIFICATION OF AUTISM

Changes and Differences in Definitions and Diagnostic Criteria of Autism

The term *autism* was first used by Kanner in 1943 to describe a group of 11 children with a previously unrecognized disorder. He noted a number of characteristic features in these children, such as an inability to develop relationships with people, extreme aloofness, a delay in speech development, noncommunicative use of speech after it developed, a lack of imagination, insistence on preserving sameness, repeated simple patterns of play activities, and islets of ability. He noted that these children had extreme autistic aloneness and an innate inability to form the usual biologically provided affective contact with people (Kanner, 1943). Despite all the variety of individual differences that appeared in the case description, Kanner believed that only two features were of diagnostic significance: "autistic aloneness" and "obsessive insistence on sameness." He adopted the term *early infantile autism* to describe the disorder and called attention to the fact that its symptoms were already evident in infancy.

During the next decade, clinicians in the United States and Europe reported cases with similar features (Bakwin, 1954; Despert, 1951; Van Krevelen, 1952). However, there was considerable controversy over the definition of the disorder because the name "autism" was ill-chosen. Confusion with Bleuler's (1911/1950) use of the same term to describe schizophrenia in adults led many clinicians to use "childhood schizophrenia" (American Psychiatric Association [APA], 1968; Bender, 1956), "borderline psychosis" (Ekstein & Wallerstein, 1954), "symbiotic psychosis" (Mahler, 1952), and "infantile psychosis" (Rutter & Lockyer, 1967) as interchangeable diagnoses. Each label had its roots in a particular view of the nature and causation of autism.

Rutter (1968) critically analyzed the existing empirical evidence and proposed four essential characteristics of autism: (1) a lack of social interest and responsiveness; (2) impaired language, ranging from absence of speech to peculiar speech patterns; (3) bizarre motor behavior, ranging from rigid and limited play patterns to more complex ritualistic and compulsive behavior; and (4) early onset, before 30 months of age. These features presented in nearly all autistic children; there were many other specific features, but they were unevenly distributed. These four essential features of autism were adopted by three sets of diagnosis-and-classification schemes that have been used widely by clinicians: the International Classification of Diseases, 9th Revision, Clinical Modification (ICD-9; U.S. Department of Health and Human Services [USDHHS], 1980); the *Diagnostic and Statistical Manual of Mental Disorders,* third edition (DSM-III) (APA, 1980), as well as the third edition, revised (DSM-III-R) (APA, 1987); and the immediate predecessor of the ASA, the National Society for Autistic Children (1978).

Although the ICD-9 and the DSM-III have similar definitions and diagnostic criteria for autism, there are apparent differences in their conceptions of autism. In ICD-9, autism is classified as a subtype of "psychoses with origin specific to childhood," whereas in the DSM-III and DSM-III-R systems autism is viewed as a "developmental disorder" and is grouped under the broad class of pervasive developmental disorders (PDDs). The PDDs are defined as a group of severe, early developmental disorders characterized by delays and distortion in the development of social skills, cognition, and communication. In the DSM-III, PDDs include (a) infantile autism (i.e., those with the onset before the age of 30 months), (b) childhood-onset pervasive developmental disorder (i.e., those in whom the disorder develops after the age of 30 months), (c) atypical pervasive developmental disorder, and (d) residual infantile autism (i.e., once was but no longer meets full criteria of infantile autism). Empirical data published after 1980, however, could not find any significant differences (except age of onset) between individuals with infantile autism and those with a diagnosis of childhood-onset pervasive developmental disorder. Therefore, in the DSM-III-R system, the childhood-onset PDD category was dropped. In addition, it was also found difficult to differentiate between atypical PDD and residual infantile autism. Therefore, the DSM-III-R PDDs work group decided to include only two categories, namely, autistic disorder and pervasive developmental disorder not otherwise specified (PDDNOS). Although the concept of PDDs is retained in DSM-III-R, the diagnostic criteria for autism have been revised considerably. The DSM-III criteria are descriptive, whereas the menulike scheme of DSM-III-R criteria requires the presence of a minimum number of criteria in each of the three cardinal features described above. The revised criteria are much more concrete, observable, and operational than those in DSM-III. The new criteria do not require raters to determine subjectively whether there is a "pervasive impairment" or a "gross deficit"; hence clinicians' hesitation to use the diagnosis of autism with older and higher-functioning autistic individuals has been removed.

On the other hand, the DSM-III-R definition has broadened the diagnostic concept of autism from the DSM-III, allowing for the gradation of behavior seen in autistic individuals. Thus the definition of autism (or autistic disorder) of the DSM-III-R system includes autism with (intellectually) higher-functioning persons (e.g., the severe form of Asperger syndrome; this will be described later) at one end, followed by Kanner autism cases with mild to moderate mental retardation, and then with lower-functioning, severely and profoundly retarded individuals (which may even include patients with a severe form of Rett syndrome) at the other end.

Reliability and Sensitivity of DSM-III and DSM-III-R

There had been concern that the new DSM-III-R criteria would identify many more cases of autistic disorder than were previously identified with the DSM-III category of infantile autism. In the DSM-III-R field trial of pervasive developmental disorders, the autistic disorder with the DSM-III-R criteria was found to be significantly higher than the prevalence of infantile autism with the DSM-III criteria (54% versus 41%; Spitzer & Siegel, personal communication). Volkmar, Bregman, Cohen, and Cicchetti (1988) examined the reliability, sensitivity, and specificity of DSM-III and DSM-III-R criteria for autism in relation to each other and to clinical diagnoses in 114 children and adults (52 diagnosed by clinicians' best judgment as autistic, and 62 as nonautistic but developmentally disordered). The reliability of specific criteria was found to be generally high. Although DSM-III criteria were highly specific, they were less sensitive; the reverse was true for DSM-III-R. The authors conclude that the diagnostic concept of autism in DSM-III-R has been substantially broadened.

A recent study of a group of lower-functioning (mean Full Scale IQ, 33.5; SD, 20.7) autistic adolescents (mean age, 14 years 11 months), using DSM-III criteria only, determined that 25 of the 39 adolescents (64%) were diagnosed as autistic, while 36 of the 39 (92%) were diagnosed as autistic using the DSM-III-R (Factor, Freeman, & Kardash, 1989). There is another study that compared the DSM-III and DSM-III-R diagnoses of 112 developmentally disordered preschool children (Hertzig, Snow, New, & Shapiro, 1990); nearly twice as many cases (58) were diagnosed as having autistic disorder by DSM-III-R criteria as were diagnosed as infantile autism (31) by DSM-III. This particular study noted that the DSM-III-R criteria have broadened the concept of autism to include children who, although socially impaired, are not pervasively unresponsive to others.

On the other hand, the new category of PDDNOS refers to individuals who have some of the characteristics of PDD but not enough to qualify for a diagnosis of autistic disorder. The PDDNOS of DSM-III-R is more or less equivalent to the atypical PDD plus the residual infantile autism of DSM-III. PDDNOS refers to the whole spectrum of atypical autism, as well as the nonautistic forms of PDDs, including a form of Asperger syndrome, a mild form of Rett syndrome, disintegrative disorder, and so forth (Figure 2-1).

Autistic Continuum

The full range of clinical features of typical autism and atypical autism described in both DSM-III and DSM-III-R is more or less equivalent to the "autistic continuum" as proposed by Wing and Gould (1979). According to Wing and

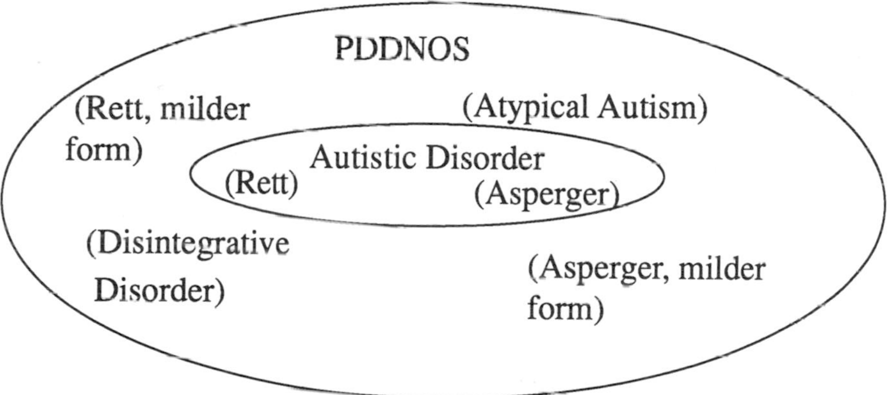

Fig. 2-1. DSM-III-R pervasive developmental disorders.

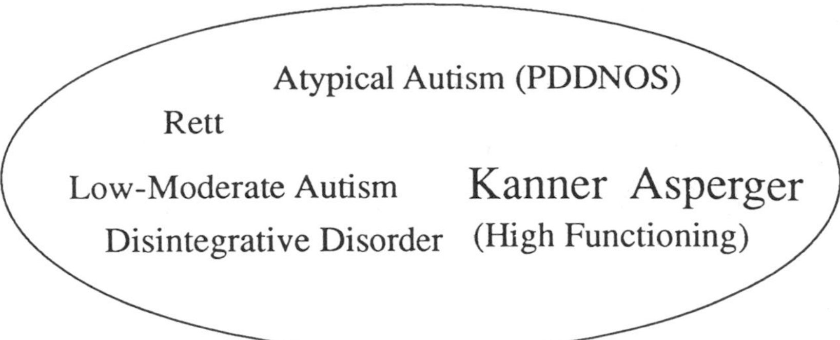

Fig. 2-2. Autistic continuum.

Gould, Kanner autism is viewed as a part of a "continuum" of autistic disorder. The central problem of the continuum is an intrinsic impairment in development of the ability to engage in reciprocal social interaction. The manifestations of the social and other problems of the continuum vary widely in type and severity. Wing and Gould also emphasize that the term *continuum* represents a concept of considerable complexity, rather than simply a straight line from severe to mild. Thus, Wing and Gould's autistic continuum has an even broader definition and set of diagnostic criteria of autism. It includes the autistic disorder of DSM-III-R at one end of the continuum, and has the PDDNOS at the other end (Figure 2-2).

Research Problems of the Existing Classifications

The DSM-III, DSM-III-R, and autistic-continuum diagnostic systems can be considered as based on a "lumpers" approach. This approach, no doubt, would net more individuals who otherwise might be given other mental disorder diagnoses, and hence would never be included in any study of autism. Because of the much-broadened definition of autism, clinicians would have very little difficulty reaching diagnostic agreement except in some borderline cases. However, this approach also includes too heterogeneous a group of individuals, and hence is problematic for the study of external validity (i.e., to what extent does autism differ from other disorders with autisticlike symptoms on variables that are external to the diagnostic criteria, such as family history of psychopathology, markers of etiology, clinical course, outcome, or response to treatment or treatment needs?). In other words, this approach is likely to lead to all the different groups being bundled together in a way that will lose crucial diagnostic distinctions. Furthermore, such an approach also produces very poor replication of research findings. Hence scientific data that could lead to further understanding of etiology, pathogenesis, and outcomes of autism could hardly be generated, due to the inclusion of a very heterogeneous group of subjects.

On the other hand, these diagnostic systems also allow for the inclusion of all autisticlike conditions (e.g., milder forms of Asperger syndrome, milder forms of Rett syndrome). It is quite confusing to see that some patients with Rett syndrome or Asperger syndrome are given a diagnosis of "autistic disorder," while other individuals having the same disorder (except a milder form) are diagnosed as having PDDNOS. Thus, the phenomenologic and etiologic heterogeneity of all the various syndromes contained in the PDDs presents an obstacle for the study of autism. What is needed is a system that can break down symptom clusters into smaller, homogeneous, and meaningful subgroups (i.e., a "splitters" approach). Such a system would enhance and ensure both reliability and validity of mental disorders under study. The ICD-10 diagnostic classification currently being proposed takes exactly such an approach.

ICD-10 Definition and Diagnostic Criteria for Autism

The draft of the ICD-10 definition of autism shows that it has also adopted the diagnostic term of pervasive developmental disorders. In the ICD-10 system, PDDs include (a) childhood autism, (b) atypical autism, (c) Asperger syndrome, (d) Rett syndrome, (e) childhood disintegrative disorders, (f) overactive disorders associated with mental retardation and stereotyped movements, (g) other pervasive disorders, and (h) unspecified pervasive disorder (Figure 2-3). The ICD-10 definition of PDDs emphasizes that "childhood autism" is a distinct subgroup of PDDs. It is obvious that the conception of PDDs in ICD-10 is a "splitters" approach. This approach believes that there is taxonomic validity of each subtype of PDDs. It

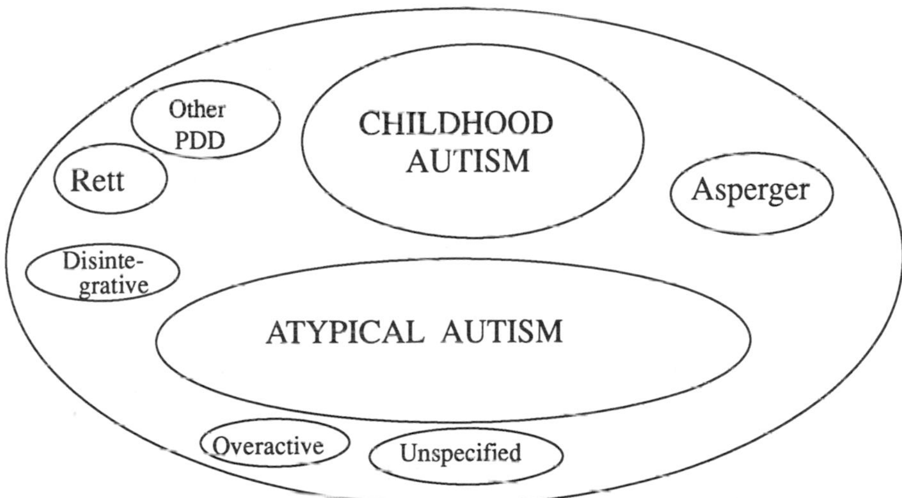

Fig. 2-3. ICD-10 pervasive developmental disorders.

would allow the study of both internal and external validities of each subtype of PDDs. It also would allow focal presentation and discussion of a disorder such as this book intends to accomplish.

The ICD-10 system defines childhood autism as "a type of pervasive developmental disorder that is defined by the presence of abnormal and/or impaired development that is manifest before the age of three years; and by the characteristic type of abnormal functioning in all three areas of social interaction, communication, and restricted, repetitive behavior." The ICD-10 system further defines the following *research diagnostic criteria* for childhood autism:

A. Presence of abnormal/impaired development from before the age of 3 years
   Usually there is no period of unequivocally normal development, but when present, the period of normality does not extend beyond age 3 years. Delay and/or abnormal patterns of functioning before 3 years (whether or not recognized as such at the time) in at least one out of the following areas is required:
   1. receptive and/or expressive language as used in social communication
   2. the development of selective social attachments and/or of reciprocal social interaction
   3. functional and/or symbolic play
B. Qualitative impairments in reciprocal social interaction
   Diagnosis requires demonstrable abnormalities in at least three out of the following five areas:
   1. failure to use eye-to-eye gaze, facial expression, body posture and gesture adequately to regulate social interaction
   2. failure to develop (in a manner appropriate to mental age, and despite ample opportunities) peer relationships that involve a mutual sharing of interests, activities, and emotions
   3. rarely seeking and using other people for comfort and affection at times of stress or distress and/or offering comfort and affection to others when they are showing distress or unhappiness
   4. lack of shared enjoyment in terms of vicarious pleasure in other people's happiness and/or a spontaneous seeking to share their own enjoyment through joint involvement with others
   5. a lack of socioemotional reciprocity, as shown by an impaired or deviant response to other people's emotions; and/or lack of modulation of behavior according to social context and communicative behaviors
C. Qualitative impairments in communication
   Diagnosis requires demonstrable abnormalities in at least two out of the following five areas:
   1. a delay in, or total lack of development of spoken language that is not accompanied by an attempt to compensate through the use of gesture or mime as alternative modes of communication (often preceded by a lack of communicative babbling)

2. relative failure to initiative or sustain conversational interchange (at whatever level language skills are present) in which there is reciprocal to-and-from responsiveness to the communications of the other person
3. stereotyped and repetitive use of language and/or idiosyncratic use of words or phrases
4. abnormalities in pitch, stress, rate, rhythm, and intonation of speech
5. a lack of varied spontaneous make-believe play, or (when young) in social imitative play

D. Restricted, repetitive, and stereotyped patterns of behavior, interests, and activities
Diagnosis requires demonstrable abnormalities in at least two out of the following six areas:
1. an encompassing preoccupation with stereotyped and restricted patterns of interest
2. specific attachments to unusual objects
3. apparently compulsive adherence to specific, nonfunctional routines or rituals
4. stereotyped and repetitive motor mannerisms that involve either hand/finger flapping or twisting, or complex whole body movements
5. preoccupations with part-objects or nonfunctional elements of play materials (such as their odor, the feel of their surface, or the noise/vibration that they generate)
6. distress over changes in small, nonfunctional details of the environment

E. The clinical picture is not attributable to the other varieties of pervasive developmental disorder; specific developmental disorder of receptive language with secondary socioemotional problems; reactive attachment disorder or disinhibited attachment disorder; mental retardation with some associated emotional/behavioral disorder; schizophrenia of unusually early onset; Rett's syndrome.

It should be pointed out here that the proposed ICD-10 diagnostic criteria for PDDs are not based on any systematically collected data. Therefore, it is expected that the new criteria of ICD-10 will not satisfy everyone, and will no doubt also be revised when an improved understanding of autism is gained. Nonetheless, further research of refinement of the criteria would assure more reliable diagnoses of autism. It is hoped that refinement of the criteria would not only assure more reliable diagnoses, but also provide further support of the taxonomic validity of autism.

Where Should the DSM-IV Go?

The United States is under a treaty obligation with the WHO to maintain a coding and terminological consistency with the ICD. The APA has already appointed several committees to develop DSM-IV and to publish it in 1993. It is quite certain that the DSM-IV will continue to adopt the concept that autism/autistic disorder is a subtype of PDDs. However, it is uncertain at the present time which approach (i.e., "lumpers" or "splitters") the DSM-IV will take to subclassify the PDDs. I agree that the DSM-IV should continue the use of pervasive developmental disorders as the major diagnostic category; however, the subclassification of PDDs should follow what is currently being proposed for the ICD-10. There are several reasons for such a position. First, it is quite clear that there is heterogeneity within PDDs. Second, on the basis of available empirical data, it would be unsatisfactory to bury these subgroups in an undifferentiated fashion such as the approach adopted by the DSM-III-R and the "autistic continuum." If we are to learn more about autism and autism-related disorders, it is critical that the conditions be identified so as to enable them to be studied reliably. Third, every attempt should be made to achieve compatibility with ICD-10 so that a common language will be used throughout the word. However, I feel that the diagnostic term "autistic disorder" should be used in DSM-IV instead of the proposed ICD-10 category of "childhood autism," because this disorder does not occur only in children.

WHAT IS HIGH-FUNCTIONING AUTISM?

Clinical Description of People with High-Functioning Autism

Since autism/autistic disorder is being viewed by the contemporary clinicians and researchers as a neurobiological disorder, the best way to present high-functioning autism is to describe the clinical entities first. This is similar to the idea that medical students start to learn by seeing patients, and then categorization occurs. After that, sections dealing with definition and diagnostic criteria become more meaningful.

Social Relationships

In the study of 19 "normally intelligent" autistic children (mean age, 8 years 5 months), Bartak and Rutter (1976) noted that these children all showed serious impairment in the development of social relationships, especially with other children. None of the autistic children had made personal friends, and all functioned poorly in a group play situation. Almost all had shown lack of eye contact in early childhood. About one-quarter of the children had not been cuddly as babies. Deviant social responses (e.g., touching adults) were also observed in about a quarter of the children. Approximately three-quarters of them showed disturbances when visiting the houses of family friends and when taken to hotels or guest houses. About one-half of these children showed disruptive or embarrassing behaviors in public places such as shops or theaters; however, they usually showed good behavior in buses or trains.

Speech and Language

Speech disorders reported in high-functioning autistic persons include disorders of speech sound discrimination, analysis, and synthesis; delayed mastery of constructions involving pronouns, negatives, interrogatives, and comparative, spatial, and temporal relationships; and difficulty producing speech, resulting in monotonic delivery and unusual pronunciation (Shea & Mesibov, 1985).

Bartak and Rutter (1976) noted that high-functioning autistic children were late in speaking; the mean age of first use of phrases to communicate was 4 years 8 months. Echolalia was noted in all subjects who could speak. Most of the speaking children (85%) had also shown pronominal reversal. There was a strong tendency for these children (about 90%) to have shown undersensitivity to noise. About 80% of them had been thought to be deaf at some time.

Rumsey, Rapoport, and Sceery (1985) reported that the speech of high-functioning autistic men was often monotonous and lacked normal intonational contours. They tended to repeat words or phrases within a sentence and often were unable to move on to the next word, giving their speech a stammering quality. Several of these men mumbled to themselves when with others or talked to themselves when alone. Poverty of speech and stereotyped speech were also seen in some of these men.

Even when gross language impairments have receded or were never present, high-functioning autistic individuals show impairments on tasks that require verbal abstraction and social reasoning. Many of them are unable to understand the shifting meaning of words in changing situations. They tend to persevere in their first impression rather than discarding it to test other meanings. They generally are not able to discuss their feelings or attend to the feelings or social cues of others.

Some high-functioning autistic persons also tend to talk too much when they are exceedingly interested in a topic. They concentrate on what they are trying to say and do not consider that listeners may not share their enthusiasm. Often it is difficult ti interrupt such a monologue or to change the conversation course through comments by others. The to-and-fro of normal conversation usually is missing. Generally speaking, autistic persons are poor listeners. Often they seem to be completely unaware of the fact that other people are trying to talk to them (Dewey & Everard, 1974). Their conversations are often superficial, repetitive, or esoteric in content. Irrelevant speech is also a common feature among these individuals.

Ritualistic or Compulsive Behaviors

Bartak and Rutter (1976) noted that approximately one-third of high-functioning autistic children exhibited attachment to odd objects, and slightly less than one-half of them showed resistance to environmental changes and exhibited stereotyped movements. These children also displayed a fairly high frequency of ritualistic behaviors (68%), difficult adaptation to new situations (74%), and quasi-obsessive behaviors (84%). Unusual play activities such as repeating dialogue from radio and television, continually talking about and playing with a single toy, or repetitively writing or drawing numbers, words, maps and so forth have often been observed in high-functioning autistic children (Shea & Mesibov, 1985).

Some investigators (Mesibov & Shea, 1980) described that ritualistic and compulsive behaviors were most intense during middle childhood, and that these behaviors tended to decrease during adolescence and adulthood. However, Rumsey *et al.* (1985) reported that stereotyped, repetitive movements were highly prevalent (78%) and were directly observable among the autistic men they studied. These men seemed to suppress their movements intentionally in social situations, and some appeared embarrassed when seen engaging in such movements. When parental reports were included, all the autistic men continued to show some stereotyped movements. Some parents reported that, in some instances, such movements occurred in response to stress or emotional upset. The movements most frequently involved the hands or arms with individual finger movements, rotating movements of the hand, arm flapping, and shaking of the hands or arms. Rhythmic movements of whole body rocking and pacing were also noted. Other motor symptoms included compulsions and hyperactivity.

Affect, Anxiety, and Thought Processes

Bartak and Rutter (1976) reported that slightly more than a third of young high-functioning autistic children showed flat affect. DeMyer (1982) noted that emotional control remained a problem among the grade-school high-functioning autistic children; they lost their tempers easily or tended to plunge into despair over trivial things. During middle or later childhood, some of the autistic men in the study of Rumsey *et al.* (1985) showed flattening, monotonous intonation, restricted facial expression, and little body movement. Chronic, generalized anxiety was noted in about half of them. About half of the subjects' parents reported infrequent temper outbursts, stimulated by frustration and inability to cope with environmental changes and demands. The incidents involved outward aggression, destruction of property, and in some cases stereotyped arm or hand flapping. Approximately three fourths of these autistic men were concrete in their thinking. They also exhibited perseverative, impoverished, circumstantial, and obsessional thinking. While some parents reported their autistic children as having immature beliefs and naïveté, none was reported as incoherent, delusional, or having hallucinations.

BOUNDARIES OF HIGH-FUNCTIONING AUTISM

One of the frequently expressed concerns of parents of high-functioning autistic children is the professionals' inability to provide consistent diagnostic opinions. A mother recently wrote to me, "Although I felt that my son displayed autisticlike behavior from a very early age, I was rebuffed by pediatricians and neurologists whenever I mentioned the word *autism*. I was told repeatedly, 'But he can't be autistic—look at how bright he is!' Although I do not have a medical background, I felt sure that there must be gradations of autism, just as there are for any medical disorder." Many high-functioning autistic children have been missed in the early diagnostic process due to professionals' lack of awareness of high-functioning autism. It is not uncommon that many of these youngsters are identified sometime after they enter school. Many parents feel frustration and anger about the intervention time lost.

Another concern is that many school systems either refuse to identify students as high-functioning autistics or misdiagnose them as "learning disabled" or "emotionally disturbed/impaired." The following sections will discuss four controversial areas: (1) differences between giftedness and high-functioning autism; (2) autisticlike disorders in individuals of normal intelligence; (3) the overlap between autism and severe developmental disorders of receptive language; and (4) the overlap between autism and severe mental disorders arising in early or middle childhood characterized by grossly bizarre behaviors.

Giftedness

Many higher-functioning autistic individuals have particular islands of ability such as unusual memory, including map memorizing and repeating verbatim the contents of a newspaper; phonologically accurate word decoding (e.g., the child may show an early interest and ability to recognize and sound out written verbal material, even before the age of 3 years); lightning-fast calculating and mathematical ability, including calendar calculating (i.e., the ability to identify on which day of the week a particular day on the calendar will fall); artistic talents; musical skills (e.g., the child may hear a song once and be able to reproduce it perfectly, play it on different instruments, or transpose it into different keys); and extrasensory perception, including finding embedded figures or assembling a difficult jigsaw puzzle (perhaps with the picture side down).

Early diagnosis of young high-functioning autistic children is particularly difficult. Many professionals hesitate to make autism diagnoses in these individuals, who appear to possess some "gifted talents." Parents of these young children also tend to have difficulty thinking of their children as having "developmental disorder." These individuals usually would be identified only sometime after they enter school. Experienced teachers usually have little problem differentiating these students from truly gifted students because these isolated areas of exceptional performance are quite incongruous with the autistic students' otherwise impaired level of social and communicative functionings.

On the other hand, it is commonly recognized that gifted individuals possess three traits: above-average general abilities, high levels of task commitment, and high levels of creativity. Gifted people usually have demonstrated leadership ability and are capable of high performance (Renzulli, 1978). However, no single trait makes "giftedness." Rather, it is the "equal interaction" among the three traits that results in the creative/productive accomplishment. It is the "equal interaction" of the three traits and "creative/productive performance" that separates giftedness from high-functioning autism.

Autisticlike Disorders in Individuals of Normal Intelligence

Asperger Syndrome

Asperger syndrome (AS) was first described in 1944 by Hans Asperger, an Austrian physician. Asperger (1944) regarded the syndrome as a personality disorder that he termed "autistic psychopathy." According to his observation, AS individuals usually began to speak at the expected age, as in normal children. A full command of grammar was acquired sooner or later, but there might be difficulty in using pronouns correctly. The content of speech was usually abnormal and pedantic, and consisted of lengthy disquisitions on favorite subjects. Often a word or phrase was repeated over and over again in a stereotyped fashion. The other features he described were the impairment of two-way social interactions, totally ignoring demands of the environment, repetitive and stereotyped play, and isolated areas of interests. He believed that the condition was never recognized in infancy, and that those with the syndrome had excellent ability of logical abstract thinking and were capable of originality and creativity in chosen fields.

Wing (1981), however, modified these observations and described that half her sample of 34 cases had been slow to talk, that careful questioning often elicited a history of a lack of communication behaviors in infancy, and that the apparent originality and special abilities were best explained by reliance on rote memory skills. Wing (1981) has since suggested that AS be considered part of the "autistic continuum." She believes that AS is possibly a mild variant of autism in relatively bright children. This view of AS has received support from several prominent researchers in the field of autism research (Gillberg, 1985; Rutter & Schopler, 1987; Schopler, 1985; Szatmari, Bartolucci, & Bremner, 1989a; Szatmari, Bremner, & Nagy, 1989b; Szatmari, Tuff, Finlayson, & Bartolucci, 1990).

Recently Szatmari and colleagues (Szatmari, Bartolucci, & Bremner, 1989; Szatmari, Bremner, & Nagy, 1989; Szatmari *et al.*, 1990) identified 28 children and adolescents who did not meet the DSM-III criteria for infantile autism but met the following adapted Wing's criteria for AS: (a) solitary child; (b) impaired two-way social interactions; (c) odd patterns of speech, impaired nonverbal communication, or an interest in repetitive activities; and (d) onset in the preschool years. When the DSM-III-R criteria were applied to the 28 AS subjects, 14 of them also met the criteria for autistic disorder. This finding confirms the notion that the development of DSM-III-R criteria for the autistic disorder had a significant influence from Wing's concept of an autistic continuum. This finding also indicates that to study the specificity of AS, autistic disorder as defined by the DSM-III-R criteria cannot be used as a "gold standard." Nonetheless, the authors find that the sex ratio, family history, presence of neurologic disease (Szatmari, Bremner, & Nagy, 1989), and cognitive deficits (Szatmari *et al.*, 1990) in some AS cases are similar to those in infantile autism. However, the authors also find that the autistic subjects spent more time in special education classes but developed fewer accessory psychiatric symptoms than the AS children (Szatmari, Bartolucci, & Bremner, 1989). The authors conclude that AS should be considered a mild form of high-functioning autism, as there is only a weak "external validity" of AS as compared with autism.

Asperger (1979) disagrees that AS is a variant of autism. He maintains that the two conditions are differentiated by age of onset, speech delay, clinical features, and prognosis. This view has gained some support from Rutter, who recently reassessed this issue and wrote to the DSM-IV Advisors on Pervasive Developmental Disorders stating, "My own clinical research has been concerned with Asperger syndrome, and I do think that there might be enough valid data at this point to support this as a valid subtype." He continued: "Our data suggests that children with autism and Asperger syndrome differ on both early history and outcome. It is this difference on outcome, it seems to me, that would justify the specification of an Asperger syndrome subgroup in ICD-10" (Rutter, 1989, personal communication).

It is quite obvious that much more research is needed before a conclusion can be made. I take a cautious approach that calls for adopting AS as a subgroup of PDDs. It is hoped that future data collection based on such a concept will provide further information for a final study of taxonomy of AS.

Schizoid Disorder of Childhood

Wolff and colleagues (Wolff & Barlow, 1979; Wolff & Chick, 1980) classified a group of adolescents as "schizoid personality," many if not all of whom have the clinical features that would be diagnosed by others as Asperger syndrome. On the other hand, Wolff and Barlow (1979) argued that Asperger syndrome should be classified as schizoid personality. This latter term is defined so loosely that it could include more able (i.e., higher functioning) but withdrawn autistic people. It remains unclear whether such cases represent subclinical varieties of autism or some very different condition (Rutter & Schopler, 1987).

Atypical Autism

The inclusion of "atypical autism" as another subtype of PDDs in the ICD-10 classification implies that there are individuals whose disorder appears to lie along the same phenomenological continuum as childhood autism. The draft of ICD-10 describes atypical autism as "a type of PDD that differs from autism in terms of either age of onset or of failing to fulfill all three sets of diagnostic criteria." Atypical autism occurs most often in profoundly retarded people; it also has been noted in individuals with a severe specific developmental disorder of receptive language, some of whom show social, emotional, and/or behavioral symptoms that overlap with childhood autism. Individuals with atypical autism may be more common than those with childhood autism, though they are less frequently studied. The validity of this diagnostic entity and its relationship to childhood autism and other PDDs remains unclear. It is highly possible that there is great heterogeneity, and it may be further divided into smaller groups in the future.

Severe Learning Disability and Developmental Learning Disability of the Right Cerebral Hemisphere

Schopler (1985) called attention to the overlap of learning disabilities (LD), higher-level autism, and Asperger syndrome. The recent publication of a new definition of learning disabilities that includes significant difficulties in "social skills" (Interagency Committee on Learning Disabilities, 1987, p. 222) would certainly cause more controversy over the boundary between learning disabilities and high-functioning autism. The group of children included in the category of LD is very heterogeneous; there are many subgroups of LD that are readily distinguishable from autism. However, in recent years an additional subgroup of children has been detected. The problems of these children encompass both academic and social spheres, and often present through channels of pediatric neurology or educational psychology. These children usually have at least average intelligence but generally have some academic failure, particularly in arithmetic. Examination usually reveals neurologic and neuropsychological signs consistent with right hemisphere dysfunction. Most of these children avoid eye contact and lack the gesture and prosody that normally accompany and accentuate speech. They exhibit monotonic and/or exaggerated speech patterns. They also show serious difficulties with interpersonal relationships; an idiosyncratic, concrete, and perseverative style of responding; and deficient processing of nonverbal, visuospatial stimuli. Some of them cannot express their feelings, but appear to be sensitive and aware of the emotions of others. Weintraub and Mesulam (1983) classified the problems as "developmental learning disabilities of the right hemisphere." Baron (1987) described these children as having socioemotional learning disabilities.

Unfortunately, the DSM-III classifications were not applied to the children included in the few recent studies (Baron, 1987; Weintraub & Mesulam, 1983). It is unclear whether these children would meet the diagnostic criteria of autism or atypical autism. Baron (1987), however, felt that these children with socioemotional LD might in fact be in the continuum of Asperger syndrome. If these children met criteria for autism, then the findings would support the notion that even in higher-functioining autism, evidence of brain organicity is a fairly frequent presentation. The findings would also suggest that there are at least two types of high-functioning autism, based on brain pathology: one type with predominantly left hemisphere involvement, the other with right hemisphere involvement. Further research is needed in order to substantiate this notion.

On the other hand, Shea and Mesibov (1985) recently proposed that autism should be viewed as "a severe, pervasive learning disability" (p. 433). They believe there are individuals who share characteristics of both high-functioning autism and severe LD. They, however, also recognize that many children with a severe LD can be ruled out from having high-functioning autism based on the quality of their interpersonal relationships and the appropriateness of their play interests. The current definition of LD, as proposed by either the National Joint Committee for Learning Disabilities (see Shea & Mesibov, 1985) or the Interagency Committee on Learning Disabilities (1987), is a vague and broad concept that includes a heterogeneous group of children. It is no surprise that some higher-functioning autistic children could also be placed in the LD group. Such a diagnostic category (LD) does not have taxonomic validity; hence it is not useful for study of developmental disorders.

Elective Mutism

Many verbal and higher-functioning autistic people speak more in a familiar than in a new or strange environment. Some higher-functioning autistic persons become mute when they don't know how to respond or answer certain questions. It is not clear whether there is an underlying anxiety disorder, or this is just a part of the autistic disorder (i.e., difficulty in adjusting to new situations). This behavior, however, may cause a diagnostic difficulty with elective mutism.

In elective mutism, the child refuses to speak in almost all social situations, despite the ability to comprehend spoken language and to speak. The child may communicate by gestures, nodding or shaking the head, or in some cases by monosyllabic or short, monotone utterances. The same child talks normally at home with family members; autistic people retain their characteristic language and speech abnormalities in all situations. Thus, the whole pattern of behavior is markedly different in the two conditions.

Developmental Disorder of Receptive Language

Bartak, Rutter, and Cox (1975) noted that most children with specific developmental receptive language disorder differed sharply from autistic children in linguistic,cognitive, and behavioral features. Social behavior might be immature, but children with a specific developmental receptive language disorder were eager to communicate in whatever ways they could; they also interacted with age peers and developed pretend play. However, the same study also found that there was a small group with mixed features. A further follow-up by Cantwell, Baker, Rutter, and Mawhood (1989) showed that as they got older, some children with specific developmental receptive language disorders exhibited severe behavioral and social difficulties, even though the two groups tended to remain distinctive.

Recently, Courchesne and colleagues (Courchesne, Lincoln, Yeung-Courchesne, Elmasian, & Grillon, 1989) studied event-related brain potential (ERP) in nonretarded autistic children, children with a receptive developmental language disorder, and normal children. Two ERP components, Nc and P3b, were specifically studied. Nc and P3b are endogenous responses in the ERP; they represent neurophysiological activities that are generated by purely internal, consciously initiated attentional and cognitive mechanisms and can be triggered by events that are attention getting or important to the person being recorded, even if the event is the omission of an expected stimulus (Courchesne *et al.*, 1989). Nc and auditory P3b responses of the autistic and the language-disorder subjects differed strikingly from each other. Nc responses of the language-disorder subjects were within normal limits, whereas in the autistic group there was actually a positive potential over the frontal scalp, where the negative Nc potential normally resides. The auditory P3b was very much smaller in the autistic group than normal, but in the language-disorder group it was larger than normal. These findings show that high-functioning autism may be differentiated from receptive developmental language disorder using quantitative neurophysiological measures. The findings also take us one step closer toward unveiling the myth of high-functioning autism.

Severe Disorders in Early or Middle Childhood

Obsessive–Compulsive Disorder

As described earlier, stereotyped and repetitive movements are highly prevalent among high-functioning autistic people. Some of the movements have obvious similarities to that seen in an obsessive–compulsive disorder (OCD). However, in a classic OCD, the developmental history is usually within normal limit. People with an OCD struggle against their compulsions, often develop a dysphoric mood, and become irritable, tense, and depressed. Although their symptoms may interfere with their usual social activities or relationships with others, individuals with an OCD almost always develop and maintain an interest in their environment and do not have deviant social skills in terms of relating with other people.

Due to problems in communicating with other people, as well as in showing appropriate affect, autistic individuals do not appear to be resisting their compulsions or manifesting distress. Thus, clinicians usually are reluctant to add a diagnosis of OCD to a person with autism. However, it is conceivable that some higher-functioning autistic people's quasi-obsessive behaviors reflect true symptoms of a coexisting OCD. Recently, I interviewed a high-functioning verbal autistic woman who throughout the interview never complained about any obsessive–compulsive symptoms. However, when she was questioned about such symptoms, she reported that every evening she "had to" check her doors and stove many times. Even when she was quite sure that she did not use the stove at all that day, she still had to check repeatedly. She stated, "It was crazy to do those things." She was quite "upset" by her "inability" to control such behaviors. Yet, despite being bothered by such symptoms for several years, she never discussed her OCD symptoms with any other person, nor did she ever seek any treatment.

Tourette Syndrome

Compulsive and ritualistic behaviors (e.g., keeping objects neatly arranged and routines unchanged; compulsive touching of people and things nearby; compulsive shouting and swearing; echoing of words, sounds, and actions) occurring in Tourette syndrome (or the syndrome of chronic multiple tics) resemble some phenomena occurring in autism. Sometimes, separating symptoms of Tourette syndrome from that of autism can be difficult. A careful examination of the total behavior pattern and developmental history is the key to differentiating the two disorders. Individuals with Tourette syndrome usually do not have significantly delayed and deviant language and speech development. Their tics often have a waxing and waning pattern. They often are aware of their handicap; they are frightened and are distressed because they do not feel that they can control it.

Several recently published papers have described the development of Tourette syndrome in autistic individuals (Barabas & Matthews, 1983; Burd, Fisher, Karbeshian, & Arnold, 1987; Kerbeshian & Burd, 1986; Realmuto & Main, 1982). I have also seen a few such cases. It is, however, unclear how frequently the two disorders might occur coincidentally. It is also uncertain how this finding might be linked to the etiology of the two disorders. This remains one of many areas requiring further investigation.

Schizophrenia in Childhood and Adolescence

The relationship between autism and schizophrenia has long been the subject of controversy. There were isolated reports of children originally diagnosed as having autism who later exhibited "schizophrenic symptomatology" (Howells & Guirguis, 1984; Petty, Ornitz, Michelman, & Zimmerman, 1984). The notion of continuity of autism in childhood and schizophrenia in adulthood was created mainly on the basis of the severity of the disorders and some general similarities in behavioral impairment and long-term outcome (Volkmar *et al.*, 1988). Rutter and Schopler (1987), however, question what weight to attach to these reports, as the systematic studies of autistic individuals have not found this transition. They suspect that the "supposed autism-to-schizophrenia change reflects a broader concept of autism or of schizophrenia or a difference in the interpretation of the odd thinking that is quite common in older autistic individuals" (p. 176).

Most autistic individuals do manifest prodromal or residual symptoms of schizophrenia such as social isolation, impairment in self-care functioning, inappropriate affect, and so on. Many high-functioning autistic people exhibit illogical thinking, incoherence, and poverty in content of speech. Their lack of nonverbal communication may be seen as exhibiting blunt affect. Autistic people's inappropriate laughing or weeping due to inability to comprehend the meaning of events may be interpreted as labile or abnormal affect. Some high-functioning, verbal autistic persons have strange beliefs (e.g., some may believe there is no air in other states), idiosyncratic interests (e.g., spending an enormous amount of time studying dinosaurs), or sensory experiences (e.g., seeing other people's faces in the air when alone in the room) bordering on delusions or hallucinations.

These symptoms, however, are qualitatively different than those shown in schizophrenic patients. These "schizophrenic symptoms" may be caused by underdevelopment of cognitive and language/speech functions in autistic individuals, whereas the symptoms in schizophrenic patients are a deviance of previously relatively normal cognitive and language/speech development. Autistic persons tend to answer "yes" to questions they do not understand, or to interpret literally meanings of words. An inexperienced interviewer may record the presence of delusions or hallucinations in these people (e.g., an autistic adolescent answered "yes" when asked about "hearing voices when alone in his room," but did not explain that he could hear his mother talking to him in the next room). Often, an autistic person may talk or laugh to himself or herself while looking at something the observer cannot identify, or while having some funny thoughts he or she doesn't know how to share with the observer. This tends to be interpreted as "listening to voices" or "seeing visions." Some autistic adolescents or adults continue to have childish fantasies of being an inanimate object, an animal, or a character of a fairy tale. This may be mistaken for "delusions" by someone lacking experience of working with higher-functioning autistic people. Many verbal and talkative autistic persons tend to make irrelevant remarks or to talk too much when they are exceedingly interested in a topic; this may be interpreted as having a "thought disorder."

Nevertheless, individuals with schizophrenia can be differentiated from high-functioning autistic people on the basis of such factors as age of onset, developmental history, clinical features, and family history. Almost all autistic people have an onset before 5 years of age, whereas the onset of schizophrenia in childhood is most often during the preadolescent or adolescent period (Rutter, 1977). Eggers (1978) reported that the early development in slightly half the schizophrenic children was unremarkable. While there is no evidence that schizophrenic children diagnosed by DSM-III-R criteria manifest severe developmental deficits, all autistic people, including those with a higher-functioning disorder, have a history of pervasive developmental disorder. There is an increased incidence of schizophrenia in the families of children with schizophrenia, but not of autistic persons (Kolvin, Ounsted, Humphrey, & McNay, 1971). A recent study of patterns involving intellectual functioning (WISC-R factor scores) by Asarnow, Tanguay, Bott, & Freeman (1987) found that schizophrenic and autistic children did not significantly differ on the verbal and perceptual organization factors, but that the schizophrenic children had significantly lower scores on the freedom-from-distraction factor (including attention, short-term memory, visual–motor coordination, speed of responding, and mental arithmetic) than the nonretarded (higher functioning) autistic children. The only subtest on which the autistic children scored significantly lower than the schizophrenic children was the comprehension subtest.

EXISTING DEFINITION AND DIAGNOSTIC CRITERIA FOR HIGH-FUNCTIONING AUTISM

At the present time, both the ICD-9 and the DSM-III-R systems have not established any definition or diagnostic criteria for high-functioning autism. Although no professional consensus has yet been developed on the severity boundary of autism, a cognitive level as determined by a valid and individually administered IQ test has been used by investigators in the field of autism research. Bartak and Rutter (1976) reported that autistic children with Performance IQs above 70 exhibited different behaviors and patterns of skills on cognitive tests than those with IQs below 70. Since then, investigators in the field of autism research have chosen Performance IQs above 70 (Freeman, Lucas, Forness, & Ritvo, 1985); Full Scale IQs above 80 (Rumsey *et al.*, 1985); Full Scale IQs above 70 (Asarnow *et al.*, 1987; Van Bourgondien & Mesibov, 1987); Full Scale IQs above 65 (Gillberg, Steffenburg, & Jakobsson, 1987); or Full Scale IQs above 60 (Gaffney & Tsai, 1987) as the cognitive criterion for high-functioning autism. A question that awaits to be answered is how good the external validity is of the high-functioning autism that is defined solely by the IQ criterion.

COMPARISON BETWEEN HIGH-IQ AUTISM AND LOW-IQ AUTISM

There are only a few studies that have systematically compared high-IQ autistic individuals with low-IQ autistic individuals. DeMyer, Barton, DeMyer, Norton, Allen, and Steele (1973) reported a follow-up study of autism in which children were placed in subcategories of "high autism" (defined as having a mixture of noncommunicative and communicative speech and some intellectual or perceptual–motor activity that was near chronological age in complexity), "middle autism" (defined as having little communicative speech beyond infrequent communicative words, but at least one intellectual or perceptual–motor activity that approximated age level), or "low autism" (defined as for middle autism, except that the intellectual and perceptual–motor performances were globally retarded). The mean full-scale IQ of the high-autism group at initial evaluation was 61; the middle-autism group, 44; and the low-autism group, 30. At follow-up, the high-autism group showed an upward change of IQ scores, especially on Verbal IQ, whereas the middle- and low-autism groups tended to have an IQ (especially Performance IQ) change in the downward direction. The high-autism group had a greater reduction of autistic symptoms than that of the middle and low groups. More children from the high-autistic group (14%) functioned educationally like normal children at follow-up than children from the middle-autistic group (10%) and the low-autistic group (0%).

Bartak and Rutter (1976) found that significantly more of the mentally retarded (defined as having a nonverbal IQ below 70) autistic children had deviant social development, as well as deviant social responses as compared to the normally intelligent autistic children. The retarded group displayed more severe retardation in language development; more self-injurious behaviors and stereotyped hand and finger movements; greater difficulty with environmental changes; a higher rate of seizure disorders; and more individuals with a "poor" outcome. Bartak and Rutter (1976) suggested that "there may be differences in the origin of autism according to the presence or absence of mental retardation" (p. 119).

Freeman, Ritvo, Schroth, Tonick, Guthrie, and Wake (1981) studied the behavioral characteristics of high- and low-IQ (i.e., with Performance IQs above and below 70, respectively) autistic children aged 30 to 60 months. In this study, the high-IQ autistic group was not compared directly with the low-IQ autistic group; the high-IQ autistic group was compared with the normal children, and the low-IQ autistic group was compared with the mentally retarded children. Nonetheless, the authors commented that "the present results also confirm the clinical observations of Bartak and Rutter, who reported that high-IQ and low-IQ autistic children tended to exhibit different behaviors" (p. 28).

As diagnostic categories, both high-functioning autism and low-functioning autism (as defined by both IQ and DSM-III-R criteria) seem to have good internal validity (i.e., two clinicians can agree on the diagnosis for an individual). There is some evidence of external validity in terms of differences between the two subtypes of autism (e.g., outcome differences); however, the evidence is only suggestive.

On the other hand, in a review of follow-up studies of autism, Lotter (1978) agreed with Rutter (1970) and concluded that "a high nonverbal score with no subsequent language development is of no predictive value, whereas if language subsequently does develop, the nonverbal score is a useful guide to later general IQ scores" (Lotter, 1978, p. 483). Lotter also commented that "some combination of speech and IQ may be a more useful predictor than either separately" (p. 483).

These research findings lend some support of the validity of subtyping autism based on cognitive functioning level. Further study should focus on establishing diagnostic criteria that include other aspects of human functioning, such as social and communicative functionings.

ESTABLISHING A NEW DEFINITION AND DIAGNOSTIC CRITERIA FOR HIGH-FUNCTIONING AUTISM

Existing Definition of Functioning Level

Although the DSM-III-R has provided specific criteria for levels of severity for several childhood psychiatric disorders, the autistic disorder has not been provided with such criteria. For all the disorders without such criteria, the DSM-III-R recommends the following guidelines (APA, 1987, p. 24) for clinicians to indicate the severity of a certain disorder: (a) *Mild*—few symptoms, with minor impairment in occupational functioning or in usual social activities or relationships with others;

(b) *Moderate*—symptoms or functional impairment between "mild" and "severe", and (c) *Severe*—Several symptoms with marked impairment of occupational functioning or of usual social activities or relationships with others.

There are some clinicians who use such as system to describe the severity of their autistic patients. Data collected based on such a system, however would be prone to being criticized as biased because the system relies on clinicians' subjective judgment. Therefore, this descriptive system of measuring severity has never been used by any investigator for the study of high-functioning autism.

The DSM-III-R diagnostic system also allows the clinician to indicate his or her overall judgment of a person's psychological, social, and occupational functioning on a scale of 1 to 90 points using the Global Assessment of Functioning (GAF) scale (APA, 1987, p. 12). A person who received a score of 60 is considered to have moderate to severe impairment of global functioning. A score from 61 to 70 indicates some mild symptoms with some difficulty in social, occupational, or school functioning, but a generally good level of overall functioning, with some meaningful interpersonal relationships. When symptoms are transient and expectable reactions to psychosocial stressors, a score between 70 and 81 is given to indicate a slight impairment in social, occupational, or school functioning. A score from 81 to 90 indicates minimal symptoms with no more than everyday problems or concerns.

No one has yet published a paper on high-functioning autism based on the criteria of GAF scale. This is because the GAF scale depends on the clinician's subjective judgment of an individual's overall functioning; hence, quantitative and objective data cannot be obtained for any meaningful statistical analysis. On the other hand, due to the lifelong nature of the disorder, no autistic person could be given a score of 71 or more. There are only a few autistic individuals who may be considered as having a rating score between 60 and 71 (i.e., some mild symptoms). Virtually all autistic individuals would have a rating of 60 or below (i.e., moderate to serious symptoms). The GAF scale is developed mainly for assessment of non-autistic mental disorders, such as major affective disorders and anxiety disorders. Thus the GAF scale is a rather useless instrument for the study of high-functioning autism.

Autism Society of America Survey Study

To study the functioning level of autistic people reliably and effectively, there is an urgent need to develop an empirically based system that can be agreed upon by the majority of the investigators and clinicians in the field of autism. Recently, a committee has been organized by the Autism Society of America to work on the issue of definition and diagnostic criteria of high-functioning autism; I have been appointed as the chairperson. A preliminary survey questionnaire developed by this committee was sent to each of the Professional Advisory Board (PAB) members of the ASA, several internationally known professionals, and those who attended the "High-Functioning Individuals with Autism" conference held in May of 1989 at

Chapel Hill, North Carolina. Out of the 29 questionnaires sent out to the PAB members and other professionals, one could not be delivered due to a change of address; 13 other questionnaires were completed and returned. Thirty parents and 32 professionals attended the conference and also completed the questionnaire.

One of the survey questions asked, "Do you believe there is a need for greater clarity about what is high-functioning autism?" All the parents, 29 professionals, and 11 PAB members answered "yes"; 3 professionals and 2 PAB members said "no."

Another question asked, "What features do you consider critical in referring to an individual as 'higher functioning'? What are the specific criteria you believe are essential in developing a definition of high-functioning autism'?" The responses included:

1. "Cognitive development in normal to near-normal range"; "average or above-average intellectual potential"; "a properly administered IQ test should show a score of 65 or above"; "IQ greater than 70"; "progress in academics"; "some academic capabilities"; "has better overall scholastic ability"; "completing an education"; "unable to integrate abstract concepts"
2. "The ability to communicate through word, sign, etc., in a normal or near-normal range"; "often excellent vocabularies"; "disproportionate in pragmatic aspects of language use"; "expressive and/or receptive language skills should be present"; "communication at a language-discourse level, which may include oral and/or written language, or other symbol system"; "ability to think and communicate about remote events in time"; "spoken language can be used by parents and teachers as primary method for instruction as appropriate to age level or developmental level"; "has a level of awareness that usually goes with language skills"; "ability to give and follow instructions"; "ability to use reasoning and problem solving"
3. "Independence in life skills"; "level of adaptive functioning normal or near normal"; "ability to function with minimal/moderate guidance in chronological age-appropriate responsibilities in community settings"; ability to be self-sufficient in most grooming and self-care activities relative to chronological-age expectations"; "some vocational skills"; "ability to hold a long-term and satisfying job"
4. "Difficulties in social awareness, social relationships, and social interaction"; "disproportionate delay in social skills and social cognition (knowledge of other's beliefs, intentions, etc.)"; "positive social orientation and motivation, even though problems in appropriateness in following social conventions may remain"; "awareness of environment and self"; "is able to establish relationships"; "ability to form loving and satisfying relationships"
5. "Sustained interest in unusual, repetitive, and in-depth topics"; "special interests"

6. "Appropriate behavior"; "behavioral problems are usually mild, restricted to episodes"; "no severe self-injurious behavior"; "no apparent self-stress"; "ability to cope with stress"; "few overt stereotypic behaviors"; "less compulsive behavior"; "ability to feel emotions"

All in all, the diagnostic criteria for high-functioning autism as suggested by the respondents are descriptive. There is only one quantitative criterion being suggested—an IQ greater than 65 or 70. There remains the question of what the quantitative criteria on other developmental aspects should be. Moreover, several respondents commented that there is a lack of information regarding the recognition of preschool-aged higher-functioning autistic children.

The committee is well aware that the ASA's final position on the issue of high-functioning autism will have a long-lived and major impact on health care systems, educational services, and scientific researches that deal with autistic people. Therefore, the committee takes a cautious approach and continues to study this issue via empirical research.

It is important to point out that individuals who receive a diagnosis of high-functioning autism, based on whatever organization's criteria, still have as many problems in educational achievement, competitive employment, and social life as those who are diagnosed as retarded and autistic. If higher-functioning autistic persons are compared with their normal peers, "one is instantly aware of how different they are and the enormous effort they have to make to live in a world where no concessions are made and where they are expected to conform" (Everard, 1976, p. 2).

A Proposal of a New Definition and Diagnostic Criteria for High-Functioning Autism

On the basis of available knowledge, I view autism as a developmental disorder with a neurobiological cause and as the consequence of organic dysfunction. Such an approach is based on a medical model of classification. As biomedical research advances, the available empirical data of external validity suggests that autism should be broken down into smaller subgroups. At the moment, there is evidence indicating that within "childhood autism" there are at least two subgroups of patients, namely, high-functioning and low-functioning groups. This new conceptualization of autism leads to the recommendation that the DSM-IV classification of autism should consider further subtyping that would include a high-functioning autism subgroup as defined by the following proposed definition and diagnostic criteria.

Definition:

High-functioning autism is a subtype of pervasive developmental disorders. It is defined by the presence of *slightly* abnormal and/or *mildly* impaired development in the areas of social interaction and communication, as well as by the presence of restricted, repetitive behavior. The characteristic type of abnormal functioning is manifested before the age of 3 years. There is some difficulty in domestic, school, occupational, or social functioning, but there are some meaningful interpersonal relationships.

Diagnostic Criteria:

A. Criteria A, B, C, and D as described in the proposed ICD-10 definition and diagnostic criteria of childhood autism (see earlier section).
B. Nonverbal IQ of 70 or above on an individually administered standardized test.
C. Language comprehension, as assessed on a standardized test, that falls no lower than one standard deviation below the mean for children younger than the age of 8, or two standard deviations for children age 8 or older.
D. Expressive language skills, as assessed on a standardized test, that fall no lower than one standard deviation below the mean for children younger than the age of 8, or two standard deviations for children age 8 or older.
E. Social functioning, as assessed on a standardized test, that falls no lower than one standard deviations below the mean for children younger than the age of 8, or two standard deviations for children age 8 or older.
F. The clinical picture is not attributable to the other varieties of pervasive developmental disorders; specific developmental disorder of receptive language with secondary socioemotional problems; reactive attachment disorder or disinhibited attachment disorder; Asperger's syndrome; obsessive–compulsive disorders; Tourette syndrome; or schizophrenia of unusually early onset.

It is obvious that this definition and set of diagnostic criteria for autism is based on ICD-10 system. However, quantitative criteria have been added to identify high-functioning autistic individuals. It should be pointed out that at the present time there are very few standardized tests for measuring social functioning. Nevertheless, the Vineland Adaptive Behavior Scales (Sparrow, Balla, & Cicchetti, 1985) can be used to determine the social development of individuals from birth through 18 years of age. This particular scale, however, does not provide information regarding *deviant* social behaviors. Furthermore, the criteria above do not include school and/or job attainment because these criteria appear to be under cultural/environmental influence.

The presently opposed criteria obviously would exclude those individuals who are high functioning in visuospatial skills but are quite low in functioning in language and speech development. The criteria would also exclude those persons who are quite poor in motor/nonverbal performance but are relatively good in verbal communication and other language/speech-related tasks. As described earlier in the section on severe learning disabilities and developmental learning disabilities of the right cerebral hemisphere, there may be subtypes based only on brain pathologies.

The present criteria are developed to prevent the inclusion of such potentially heterogeneous groups of high-functioning autistic individuals. The goal of these criteria is to identify a homogeneous group of high-functioning autistic individuals who have fairly even brain hemispheric functions. When we gain more knowledge of this particular subgroup of high-functioning autistic people, our understanding of the other subgroups will be greatly enhanced.

It is not clear whether moderate- to low-functioning autism should be further divided into moderate-functioning autism and low-functioning autism. There are very few, if any, studies that specifically examine such an issue. It is conceivable that once the diagnostic validity of high-functioning autism is established, the direction of further research of autism would turn to subtyping the above two subgroups.

Finally, it should be pointed out that the present chapter has not dealt with "atypical autism." However, it can be expected that there are also subgroups with various functioning levels within this category.

CONCLUSION

There are some studies that conclude that, in some respects, higher-functioning autistic persons have a mild form of autism as compared to that manifested in retarded (i.e., lower-functioning) autistic people. As compared to the former group, the retarded group often has a greater language delay, their personal relationships are more severely disturbed, they display socially disruptive behavior more often, and they have a much poorer outcome in terms of educational placement and/or employment. On the other hand, higher-functioning autistic persons exhibit more pronominal reversal, undue sensitivity to noise, and rituals.

These findings have provided some external validity for the subtypes of autism based on IQ level. These findings also suggest the possibility that there may be differences in the origin of autism according to functioning level. It appears that there is evidence supporting the notion of subtyping autism according to functioning level; however, it remains unclear what criteria would yield the highest taxonomic validity and thus would justify the establishment of separate diagnostic categories. Nevertheless, such an approach promises to provide a well-tested route toward further unveiling of the myths of autism.

It is important to point out that it is not uncommon in medicine to find that conditions that were once thought to be homogeneous ultimately turn out to be heterogeneous, once knowledge on etiology becomes available (Rutter *et al.*, 1988). It is conceivable that the same would happen in high-functioning autism as defined by the definition and criteria in this chapter. It is expected that the new criteria will not satisfy everyone, and no doubt will be revised when further knowledge of high-functioning autism is gained. Nevertheless, the development of the present subclassification is another step that could facilitate our further understanding of autism. It would ensure adequate educational and vocational services (Tsai & Scott-Miller, 1988), as well as appropriate medical treatment for high-functioning autistic individuals.

REFERENCES

American Psychiatric Association. (1968). *Diagnostic and statistical manual of mental disorders* (2nd ed.). Washington, DC: Author.

American Psychiatric Association. (1980). *Diagnostic and statistical manual of mental disorders* (3rd ed.). Washington, DC: Author.

American Psychiatric Association. (1987). *Diagnostic and statistical manual of mental disorders* (3rd ed.–Revised). Washington, DC: Author.

Asarnow, R. F., Tanguay, P. E., Bott, L., & Freeman, B. J. (1987). Patterns of intellectual functioning in non-retarded autistic and schizophrenic children. *Journal of Child Psychology and Psychiatry, 28*(2), 273–280.

Asperger, H. (1944). Die "Autistischen psychopathen" im Kindesalter. *Archiv fur Psychiatrie und Nervenkrankheiten, 117,* 76–136.

Asperger, H. (1979). Problems of infantile autism. *Communication, 13,* 45–52.

Bakwin, H. (1954). Early infantile autism. *Pediatrics, 45,* 492–497.

Barabas, G., & Matthews, W. S. (1983). Coincident infantile autism and Tourette syndrome: A case report. *Journal of Developmental Pediatrics, 4,* 280–281.

Baron, I. S. (1987, February). *The childhood presentation of social–emotional learning disabilities: On the continuum of Asperger's syndrome.* Paper presented at the 15th annual International Neuropsychological Society meeting, Washington, DC.

Bartak, L., & Rutter, M. (1976). Differences between mentally retarded and normally intelligent autistic children. *Journal of Autism and Childhood Schizophrenia, 6,* 109–120.

Bartak, L., Rutter, M., & Cox, A. (1975). A comparative study of infantile autism and specific developmental receptive language disorder. I. The children. *British Journal of Psychiatry, 126,* 127–145.

Bender, L. (1956). Schizophrenia in childhood—its recognition, description, and treatment. *American Journal of Orthopsychiatry, 26,* 499-506.

Bleuler, E. (1950). *Dementia Praecox on the Group of Schizophrenias* (J. Zinkin, Trans.). New York: International University Press. (Original work published 1911)

Burd, L., Fisher, W. W., Kerbeshian, J., & Arnold, M. E. (1987). Is development of Tourette disorder a marker for improvement in patients with autism and other pervasive developmental disorders? *Journal of American Academy of Child and Adolescent Psychiatry, 26*(2), 162–165.

Cantwell, D., Baker, L., Rutter, M., & Mawhood, L. (1989). Infantile autism and developmental receptive dysphasia: A comparative follow-up into middle childhood. *Journal of Autism and Developmental Disorders, 19,* 19–31.

Courchesne, E., Lincoln, A. J., Yeung-Courchesne, R., Elmasian, R., & Grillon, C. (1989). Pathophysiologic findings in nonretarded autism and receptive developmental language disorder. *Journal of Autism and Developmental Disorders, 19,* 1–17.

DeMyer, M. K. (1982). Infantile autism: Patients and their families. *Current Problems in Pediatrics, 12*(4), 1–52.

DeMyer, M. K., Barton, S., DeMyer, W., Norton, J. A., Allen, J., & Steele, R. (1973). Prognosis in autism: A follow-up study. *Journal Of Autism and Childhood Schizophrenia, 3*(3), 199–246.

Despert, J. L. (1951). Some considerations relating to the genesis of autistic behavior in children. *American Journal of Orthopsychiatry, 21,* 335–350.

Dewey, M. A., & Everard, M. P. (1974). The near-normal autistic adolescent. *Journal of Autism and Childhood Schizophrenia, 4,* 347–356.

Eggers, C. (1978). Course and prognosis of childhood schizophrenia. *Journal of Autism and Childhood Schizophrenia, 8,* 21–36.

Ekstein, R., & Wallerstein, J. (1954). Observations on the psychology of borderline and psychotic children. *Psychoanalytic Study of the Child* (vol. 9). New York: International University Press.

Everard, M. P. (1976, July). *Mildly autistic young people and their problems.* Paper presented at the International Symposium on Autism, St. Gallen, Switzerland.

Freeman, B. J., Lucas, J. C., Forness, S. R., & Ritvo, E. R. (1985). Cognitive processing of high-functioning autistic children: Comparing the K-ABC and the WISC-R. *Journal of Psychoeducational Assessment, 4,* 357–362.

Gaffney, G. R., & Tsai, L. Y. (1987). Magnetic resonance imaging of high level autism. *Journal of Autism and Developmental Disorders, 17,* 433–438.

Gillberg, C. (1985). Asperger's syndrome and recurrent psychosis—a neuropsychiatric case study. *Journal of Autism and Developmental Disorders, 15,* 389–398.

Gillberg, C., Steffenburg, S., & Jakobsson, G. (1987). Neurobiological findings in 20 relatively gifted children with Kanner-type autism or Asperger's syndrome. *Developmental Medicine and Child Neurology, 29,* 641–649.

Factor, D. C., Freeman, N. L., & Kardash, A. (1989). A comparison of DSM-III and DSM-III-R criteria for autism. *Journal of Autism and Developmental Disorders, 19,* 637–640.

Freeman, B. J., Ritvo, E. R., Schroth, P. C., Tonick, I., Guthrie, D., & Wake, L. (1981). Behavioral characteristics of high- and low IQ autistic children. *American Journal of Psychiatry, 138,* 25–29.

Hertzig, M. E., Snow, M. E., New, E., & Shapiro, T. (1990). DSM-III and DSM-III-R diagnosis of autism and pervasive developmental disorder in nursery school children. *Journal of American Academy of Child and Adolescent Psychiatry, 29*(1), 123–126.

Howells, J. G., & Guirguis, W. R. (1984). Childhood schizophrenia 20 years later. *Archives of General Psychiatry, 41,* 123–128.

Interagency Committee on Learning Disabilities. (1987). Recommendations of the Committee. In *Learning disabilities: A report to the U.S. Congress* (pp. 219–232). Washington, DC: Department of Health and Human Services.

Kanner, L. (1943). Autistic disturbances of affective contact. *Nervous Child, 2,* 217–250.

Kerbeshian, J., & Burd, L. (1986). Asperger's syndrome and Tourette syndrome: The case of the pinball wizard. *British Journal of Psychiatry, 148,* 731–736.

Kolvin, I., Ounsted, C., Humphrey, M., & McNay, A. (1971). Studies in the childhood psychoses. II. The phenomenology of childhood psychoses. *British Journal of Psychiatry, 118,* 385–395.

Lotter, V. (1978). Follow-up studies. In M. Rutter & E. Schopler (Eds.), *Autism: A reappraisal of concepts and treatment* (pp. 475–495). New York: Plenum.

Mahler, M. (1952). On child psychosis and schizophrenia. Autistic and symbiotic psychoses. In *Psychoanalytic study of the child* (vol. 7). New York: International University Press.

Mesibov, G. B., & Shea, V. (1980, March). *Social and interpersonal problems of autistic adolescents and adults.* Paper presented at the meeting of the Southeastern Psychological Association, Washington, DC.

National Society for Autistic Children. (1978). National Society for Autistic Children definition of the syndrome of autism. *Journal of Autism and Developmental Disorders, 8,* 162–167.

Petty, L. K., Ornitz, E. M., Michelman, J. D., & Zimmerman, E. G. (1984). Autistic children who become schizophrenic. *Archives of General Psychiatry, 41,* 129–135.

Realmuto, G. M., & Main, B. (1982). Coincidence of Tourette's disorder and infantile autism. *Journal of Autism and Developmental Disorders, 12,* 367–372.

Renzulli, J. S. (1978, November). What makes giftedness? Reexamining a definition. *Phi Delta Kappan,* 180–184.

Rumsey, J. M., Rapoport, J. L., & Sceery, W. R. (1985). Autistic children as adults: Psychiatric, social and behavioral outcomes. *Journal of the American Academy of Child Psychiatry, 24,* 465–473.

Rutter, M. (1968). Concepts of autism: A review of research. *Journal of Child Psychology and Psychiatry, 9,* 1–25.

Rutter, M. (1970). Autistic children: Infancy to adulthood. *British Journal of Psychiatry, 2,* 435–450.

Rutter, M. (1977). Infantile autism and other child psychoses. In M. Rutter & L. Henson (Eds.)., *Child psychiatry: Modern approach* (pp. 717–747). Oxford: Blackwell.

Rutter, M., & Gould, M. (1985). Classification. In M. Rutter & L. Hersov (Eds.), *Child and adolescent psychiatry: Modern approach* (pp. 304–321). Oxford: Blackwell.

Rutter, M., LeCouteur, A., Lord, C., MacDonald, H., Rios, P., & Folstein, S. (1988). Diagnosis and subclassification of autism—concepts and instrument development. In E. Schopler & G. B. Mesibov (Eds.), *Diagnosis and assessment in autism* (pp. 239–259). New York: Plenum.

Rutter, M., & Lockyer, L. (1967). A five- to fifteen-year follow-up study of infantile psychosis. I. Description of sample. *British Journal of Psychiatry, 113,* 1169–1182.

Rutter, M., & Schopler, E. (1987). Autism and pervasive developmental disorders: Concept and diagnostic issues. *Journal of Autism and Developmental Disorders, 17,* 159–186.

Schopler, E. (1985). Editorial: convergence of learning disability, higher-level autism, and Asperger's syndrome. *Journal of Autism and Developmental Disorders, 15,* 359–360.

Schopler, E., & Mesibov, G. B. (Eds.). (1988). *Diagnosis and assessment in autism.* New York: Plenum.

Shea, V., & Mesibov, G. B. (1985). The relationship of learning disabilities and higher-level autism. *Journal of Autism and Developmental Disorders, 15,* 425–435.

Sparrow, S., Balla, D., & Cicchetti, D. (1985). *Vineland Adaptive Behavior Scales (classroom edition).* Circle Pines, MN: American Guidance Service.

Szatmari, P., Bartolucci, G., & Bremner, R. (1989). Asperger's syndrome and autism: Comparisons on early history and outcome. *Journal of Developmental Medicine and Child Neurology, 31,* 709–720.

Szatmari, P., Bremner, R., & Nagy, J. (1989). Asperger's syndrome: A review of clinical features. *Canadian Journal of Psychiatry, 34,* 554–560.

Szatmari, P., Tuff, L., Finlayson, M. A. J., & Bartolucci, G. (1990). Asperger's syndrome and autism: Neurocognitive aspects. *Journal of American Academy of Child and Adolescent Psychiatry, 29*(1), 130–136.

Tsai, L. Y., & Scott-Miller, D. (1988). Higher-functioning autistic disorder. *Focus on Autistic Behavior, 2*(6), 1–8.

U. S. Department of Health and Human Services. (1980). *International classification of disease, 9th revision, clinical modification.* Washington, DC: Author.

Van Bourgondien, M. E., & Mesibov, G. B. (1987). Humor in high-functioning autistic adults. *Journal of Autism and Developmental Disorders, 17,* 417–424.

Van Krevelen, D. A. (1952). Early infantile autism. *Acta Paedopsychiatrica, 91,* 81–97.

Volkmar, F. R., Bregman, J., Cohen, D. J., & Cicchetti, D. V. (1988). DSM-III and DSM-III-R diagnosis of autism. *American Journal of Psychiatry, 145,* 1404–1408.

Weintraub, S., & Mesulam, M. M. (1983). Developmental learning disabilities of the right hemisphere—emotional, interpersonal, and cognitive components. *Archives of Neurology, 40,* 463–468.

Wing, L. (1981). Asperger's syndrome: A clinical account. *Psychological Medicine, 11,* 115–129.

Wing, L., & Gould, J. (1979). Severe impairments of social interaction and associated abnormalities in children: Epidemiology and classification. *Journal of Autism and Developmental Disorders, 9,* 11–29.

Wolff, S., & Barlow, A. (1979). Schizoid personality in childhood: A comparative study of schizoid, autistic and normal children. *Journal of Child Psychology and Psychiatry, 20,* 19–46.

Wolff, S., & Chick, J. (1980). Schizoid personality in childhood: A controlled follow-up study. *Psychological Medicine, 10,* 85–100.

3

Neuropsychological Studies of High-Level Autism

JUDITH M. RUMSEY

INTRODUCTION

The study of nonretarded autistic persons is important, as it allows comparisons with normal age-matched controls and patients with focal brain lesions using tests with adequate norms, sensitivity to cerebral dysfunction, and localizing value. This allows us to address the question of the universality and specificity of cognitive deficits in autism.

High-functioning patients, especially those with average and higher IQs, offer an opportunity for testing the hypothesis that autism occurs without cognitive deficits. The existence of such patients has been cited as evidence that social-affective symptoms are primary, rather than secondary to cognitive deficits (Fein, Pennington, Markowitz, Braverman, & Waterhouse, 1986). Others have argued that cognitive deficits are basic and underlie many important handicaps in autism. "Of all psychiatric conditions, autism is the one in which there is the closest, and probably most direct, connection between cognitive deficits and social malfunction" (Rutter, 1987, p. 13).

Social impairments such as literalness, poor social comprehension, lack of empathy, lack of reciprocity, inappropriate social behavior, failure to appreciate subtle humor, and restricted behavioral repertoires—all observed in high-functioning autistic patients (Rutter, 1983)—may stem from a variety of deficits. These range from primary affective failures (such as a lack of social interest and affective flattening) to specific social-perceptual and social-cognitive deficits (such as an inability to read vocal or facial expression or to understand the complexities of

---

JUDITH M. RUMSEY • Child Psychiatry Branch and Child and Adolescent Disorders Research Branch, National Institute of Mental Health, Bethesda, Maryland 20892.

High-Functioning Individuals with Autism, edited by Eric Schopler and Gary B. Mesibov. Plenum Press, New York, 1992.

social interaction) to more general cognitive deficits (involving the integration of information and complex problem solving) to motor deficits. Motor/output deficits in vocal intonation and facial expression might preclude a patient from expressing felt emotion, leading others to misperceive him or her as unfeeling or aloof.

A neuropsychological approach can clarify the nature of the deficits and provide hypotheses concerning localization of dysfunction through analogies to patients with known lesions. However, such analogies are limited by the differential anatomical and behavioral effects of damage during brain development versus damage later in life (Goldman-Rakic & Rakic, 1984; Kolb, 1989). Developmental neuropathology, such as that seen in autism, may result in aberrant neural circuitry (Bauman & Kemper, 1985, 1987). Early postnatal damage may allow greater functional reorganization and recovery of cognitive function than later damage, though this principle may not apply universally.

For purposes of this chapter, *high-level autism* refers to the syndrome of infantile autism and its residual state—as defined by DSM-III or highly similar criteria—in the absence of mental retardation or severe language impairment. Absence of mental retardation is defined by an IQ (verbal or nonverbal) of 70 or higher on standard tests of general intelligence, a definition that stems from the close association between IQ and social-adaptive functioning in autism (Bartak & Rutter, 1976).

Studies of patients with IQs greater than 70 that use tests to assess cognitive, perceptual, sensory, and motor functioning—thought to implicate the involvement of various brain regions and systems—are included, while those not reporting IQs (including those reporting only mental ages, whose psychometric properties do not allow direct translation into IQ scores) are excluded. Because autism without mental retardation is rare, the samples are small. This poses a greater risk of false negative findings (type II error) than of false positive findings (type I error) (Altman, 1982).

Another weakness is the limited success in IQ matching of patients and controls. Several studies match only on Performance IQ, leaving potentially significant Verbal IQ differences. Some fail to report any measure of verbal or language functioning. Many begin with significant or nearly significant IQ differences, raising the possibility that differences in the dependent measures (particularly subtle differences) may be confounded with general intelligence.

The following questions are addressed: (a) What, if any, neuropsychological deficits are associated with high-level autism? (b) What similarities and dissimilarities in neuropsychological profiles exist across levels of cognitive functioning? (c) Do the neuropsychological deficits seen in high-level autism resemble those seen in other neurological, psychiatric, and developmental disorders, or are they specific to autism? Several neuropsychological domains and localization hypotheses are covered in an attempt to answer these questions.

GENERAL INTELLIGENCE

A consistent finding in autism is the uneven profile of abilities documented on various versions of the widely used Wechsler intelligence scales (WISC, WISC-R,

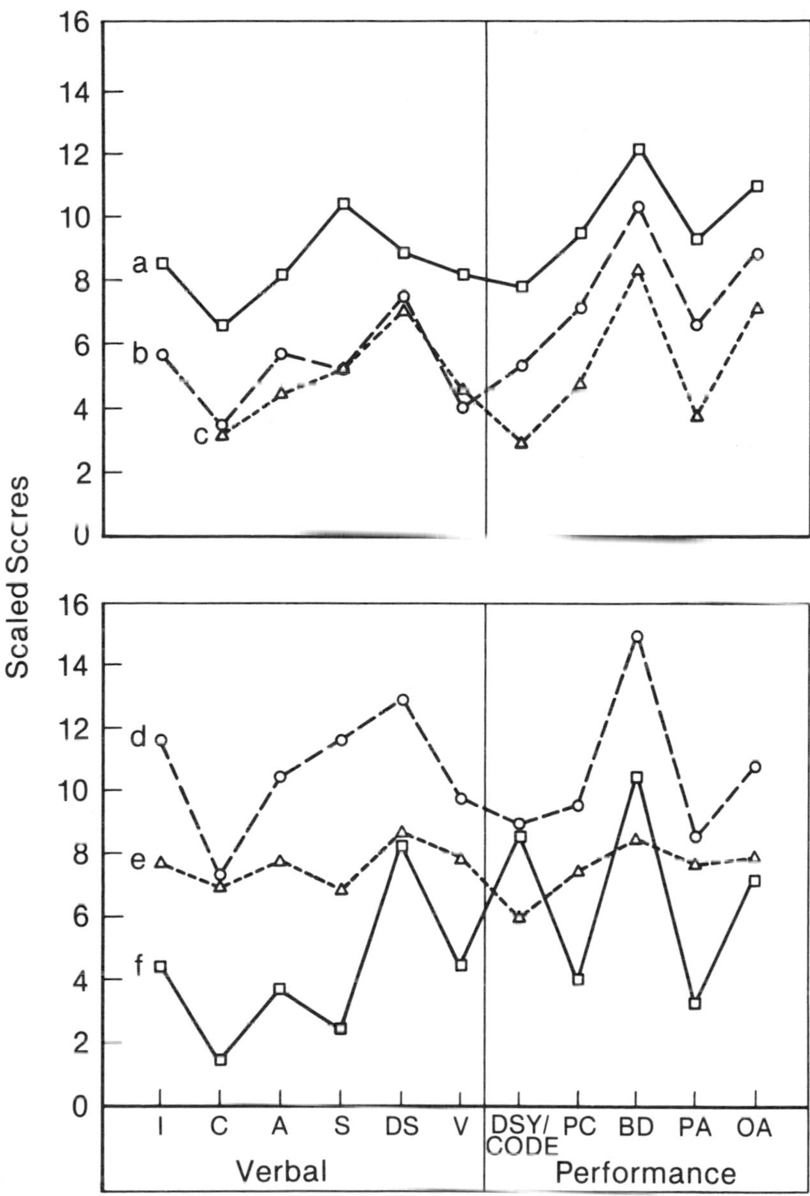

Fig. 3-1. Wechsler profiles across studies.
I = Information; C = Comprehension; A = Arithmetic; S = Similarities; DS = Digit Span; V = Vocabulary; DSY = Digit Symbol; Code = Coding; PC = Picture Completion; BD = Block Design; PA = Picture Arrangement; OA = Object Assembly.

[a] = Freeman *et al.* (1985), ages 6–12, $n = 21$. [b] = Lincoln *et al.* (1988), ages 8–29, $n = 33$. [c] = Lockyer & Rutter (1970), mean age = 15, $n = 63$. [d] = Rumsey & Hamburger (1988), ages 18–39, $n = 10$. [e] = Szatmari *et al.* (1989), ages 7–32, mean = 22, $n = 17$. [f] = Narita & Koga (1987), mean age = 10, $n = 45$.

WAIS, WAIS-R). When profiles from independent studies are plotted (see Figure 3-1), striking similarities are seen despite differences in the versions of this scale, the ages studied, and data analysis (Freeman, Lucas, Forness, & Ritvo, 1985; Lincoln, Courchesne, Kilman, Elmasian & Allen, 1988; Lockyer & Rutter, 1970; Narita & Koga, 1987; Rumsey & Hamburger, 1988; Szatmari, Tuff, Finlayson, & Bartolucci, 1990). These group data show depressed scores on Comprehension and Picture Arrangement and elevated scores on Block Design and Digit Span. Moreover, similarities are seen across American, English, and Japanese samples. This pattern differs from those associated with developmental language disorder, severe developmental dyslexia, schizophrenia in children, dysthymia, and oppositional disorder (Asarnow, Tanguay, Bott, & Freeman, 1987; Lincoln *et al.*, 1988; Rumsey & Hamburger, 1990), but is similar to that seen in Asperger syndrome, whose core feature is social impairment (Szatmari *et al.*, 1990) and which may be a variant of autism (Wolff & Barlow, 1980).

Test profiles vary with developmental level. Patients with Full Scale IQs under 85 show higher scores on performance than on verbal subtests, while patients with IQs above 85 show no overall lowering of verbal subtests (Szatmari *et al.*, 1990). The studies illustrated in Figure 3-1 are consistent with this finding.

The strengths and deficits on both verbal and performance subtests and lack of overall verbal-performance differences in the highest functioning patients suggest that differences between rote and abstract reasoning are more specifically characteristic of autism than are verbal–nonverbal discrepancies. This is supported by Lincoln *et al.*'s (1988) factor analytic study of 33 high-functioning patients, which suggested a dichotomy of poor comprehension of social and context-relevant information versus asocial/noncontextual information on the Wechsler.

Wechsler profiles also vary in the degree of unevenness found across studies. The sample studied by Szatmari *et al.* (1990) showed less unevenness despite similarity in shape. One might expect the degree of unevenness to correlate with deficits on neuropsychological test measures, though this relationship has not been studied.

Thus, there are characteristic uneven cognitive skills even in the highest-functioning autistic patients, with similarities and some differences among groups at different developmental levels. Verbal-performance discrepancies are more characteristic of patients with IQs under 85. More pronounced unevenness may be seen in classic Kanner's cases.

ATTENTION

Attention consists of several processes, dependent on the integrity of different neural systems. One model, derived from factor analyzed neuropsychological test data (Mirsky, 1987), proposes four elements: (1) the ability to *sustain* attention/concentration; (2) a *focus–execute* function, defined as the perceptual ability to scan stimulus material rapidly and to make a verbal or skilled motor response quickly; (3) an *encode* aspect having to do with registration, recall, and mental manipulation of numeric information; and (4) the ability to *shift* attention in a flexible and adaptive manner. The sustain element is thought to be subserved by the reticular formation of the brainstem, midbrain, and thalamus; the encode element by the hippocampus; the shift element by the prefrontal and possibly medial frontal cortex and anterior cingulate; and the focus–execute element by the inferior parietal, superior temporal, and striatal regions.

Clinically, autistic patients have been noted to show unusually narrow attention and difficulty in shifting attention. Autistic children may engage in overfocused, repetitive play for lengthy periods of time, underreacting to distractions in the environment. High-functioning adults show perseverative speech and underrespond to interviewer attempts to change the topic of conversation (Rumsey, Andreasen & Rapoport, 1986; Rumsey, Rapoport, & Sceery, 1985). These observations suggest good sustained attention, but deficient flexibility in shifting attention.

While there is little neuropsychological research on attention in high-level autism, a large literature on "stimulus overselectivity" in lower-functioning patients (reviewed in Lovaas, Koegel, & Schreibman, 1979) has demonstrated unusually narrow breadth of attention. This has, however, been related to IQ and chronological age, with patients having lower IQs and younger children being more overselective than those with higher IQs or older children (Gersten, 1983; Lovaas *et al.*, 1979).

Several studies of high-functioning patients have reported deficits on the Wisconsin Card Sorting Test (Prior & Hoffman, 1990; Rumsey, 1985; Steel, Gorman, & Flexman, 1984; Szatmari *et al.*, 1990), which loads on the shift element (Mirsky, 1987). In contrast, performance on the Digit Span, Arithmetic, and Digit Symbol subtests of the Wechsler scales—tests that load on the encode element—is reported intact in high-functioning autistic persons (Lincoln *et al.*, 1988; Lockyer & Rutter, 1970; Rumsey & Hamburger, 1988). Such patients also perform well on the Continuous Performance Test, a measure of sustained attention (R. F. Asarnow, personal communication). For the focus–execute dimension, the limited available data is mixed with one report of poor performance on the Trailmaking Test (Rumsey & Hamburger, 1988) and several of relatively intact Digit Symbol performance (Lincoln *et al.*, 1988; Lockyer & Rutter, 1970; Rumsey & Hamburger, 1988). Thus, the limited data suggest that the shift element and possibly the focus–execute element (subserved by the prefrontal and temporoparietal/striatal regions, respectively) are selectively impaired in autistic individuals, but additional research on attention is needed.

MEMORY AND LEARNING

Kanner (1943) was impressed by the good rote memories observed clinically in autistic patients. Delayed echolalia suggested memory as a frequent "splinter skill." Studies of lower-functioning samples (Frith, 1970; Hermelin & O'Connor, 1970;

Prior & Chen, 1976) have confirmed remarkably intact rote memory in autistic children relative to both retarded and normal controls, but difficulty with initial processing, rule extraction, and meaningful material. The latter deficits implicate higher-level cognitive deficiencies, rather than difficulty with the retention of information. Based on such findings, Damasio and Maurer (1978) hypothesize a potential for normal memory with a higher-order defect in the governance of perception, storage, and retrieval.

Yet analogies between autism and amnesic syndromes resulting from damage to limbic structures, including the hippocampus and medial diencephalic structures (dorsomedial nucleus, mammillary bodies, fornix), have been claimed (Boucher & Warrington, 1976; DeLong, 1976; Hauser, DeLong, & Rosman, 1975). Amnesiacs require numerous trials to learn new material and are highly sensitive to the effects of delay on recall, showing rapid forgetting. In autism, Boucher reported deficits in forced-choice recognition of pictures—but not on several tests of cued recall, nor on paired-associate learning of unrelated words (Boucher & Warrington, 1976)—and reduced primacy learning (i.e., recall of words early in a list) with no overall memory deficits relative to normal controls (Boucher, 1981).

Hauser *et al.* (1975) likened the autistic child's inability to learn and profit from experience to a congenital Korsakoff syndrome and to the Kluver–Bucy syndrome with its incapacity for adaptive social behavior and loss of recognition of the significance of others. DeLong (1976) further proposed that children with unilateral left-sided lesions might show deficiencies in verbal memory and other left hemisphere skills without compensatory transfer to the right hemisphere. Those with bilateral lesions would show global retardation with depression of both right and left hemisphere skills.

Three studies have examined memory and learning in high-level autism. Ameli, Courchesne, Lincoln, Kaufman, & Grillon (1988) examined visual recognition memory in 16 high-functioning autistic adolescents and adults and age-, sex- and Performance IQ-matched controls. Effects of stimulus meaningfulness were assessed by comparing memory for meaningful pictures versus meaningless nonsense shapes. Both an immediate and a one-minute delayed recall condition were employed to assess the effects of delay on memory.

Differences between patients and controls were seen primarily with regard to meaningless shapes, suggesting poorer encoding in autism. Unlike effects seen in amnesia, delay failed to differentially affect recall. Patient performance correlated moderately and significantly with both Performance IQ, on which group differences just missed significance ($p < .06$), and with performance on the Benton Visual Retention Test. Patients' Verbal IQs ranged from 54 to 111. Thus, verbal and/or nonverbal intelligence may have contributed to the selective deficits seen.

Rumsey and Hamburger (1988) examined 10 very high-functioning men with verbal and nonverbal memory tests. A Selective Reminding Test, consisting of 12 unrelated words to be learned over 12 trials, and portions of the Wechsler Memory Scale shown to be sensitive to memory deficits in amnesia (Butters *et al.*, 1988) were used. Paragraphs (logical-memory subtest) and designs from the Wechsler were used with immediate and 30-minute delayed recall conditions.

No group differences were seen on measures of long-term storage or consistent long-term retrieval on the Selective Reminding Test. A weak, marginally significant ($p = .0474$) difference was seen on the Wechsler Memory Scale when four scores (paragraphs versus designs × immediate versus delayed) were combined. Though no interactions reached significance, the largest group differences were seen on immediate recall of paragraphs, where difficulty with the initial processing of complex verbal paragraphs appeared to be the primary contributor to poor performance. Information produced on immediate recall was not lost or forgotten over the 30-minute delay, unlike results in amnesia (Butters *et al.*, 1988).

Finally, Zaucha, Asarnow, and Neuchterlein (unpublished data) compared autistic, schizophrenic, and normal men (with estimated IQs of 70 to 126) on word-list learning tasks designed to assess the effects of rehearsal on recall. Even with higher estimated IQs in the normal controls relative to both patient groups, the autistic group showed normal levels of recall across all conditions—unlike the schizophrenics, who showed impaired recall across conditions. Both autistic and schizophrenic patients rehearsed less than controls, but this decreased performance only in the schizophrenics. Thus, the repetition of an item seemed to benefit later recall more in the autistic group. Only the autistic group showed a significant correlation between the number of rehearsals and recall. The investigators' interpretation was that the autistic group was likely encoding words at a literal level, while the controls and schizophrenics were using semantic and associative features.

These studies of high-functioning patients suggest intact consolidation and retrieval of memories and argue against parallels between autism and temporal lobe amnesia. They do not, however, rule out the involvement of medial temporal lobe structures in autism, as the behavioral effects of developmental neuropathology may differ from those seen with large acquired lesions.

Qualitative differences in the initial processing and encoding of information may parallel findings in lower-functioning samples, suggesting continuity across developmental levels. Rote memory, unaltered by active encoding or deeper levels of processing, may be characteristic of autism. Some investigators (Lucci, Fein, Holevas, & Kaplan, 1988) have hypothesized that good rote or "high fidelity" memory seen in autistic savants may be due to hyperfunction of, or an overreliance on, the hippocampal functioning. This is discussed later in the section on exceptional abilities.

LANGUAGE, SEQUENTIAL PROCESSING, AND SENSORY–MOTOR FUNCTION: THE LEFT HEMISPHERE HYPOTHESIS

Several investigators (Blackstock, 1978; Dawson, 1983; Prior, 1979; Tanguay, 1976) have hypothesized left hemisphere dysfunction on the basis of language deficits in autism (which frequently result in low Verbal IQs relative to Performance

IQs) and deficits in sequential, analytic, and symbolic processing (which may be linked to left hemisphere dysfunction) (Lezak, 1983). Relative strengths in visuospatial abilities—as measured by Block Design, Object Assembly, and formboards—and relative talents in music have been interpreted as evidence of relatively intact right hemispheric functioning (Prior, 1979; Prior & Bradshaw, 1975).

However, heterogeneity in language skills and in patterns of preserved visuospatial versus deficient language skills is seen (Fein, Humes, Kaplan, Lucci, & Waterhouse, 1984). Language delays, particularly in phonology and syntax, may result from concomitant mental retardation (Bartak, Rutter, & Cox, 1977; Cantwell, Baker, & Rutter, 1978; Cohen, Caparulo, & Shaywitz, 1976; Tager-Flusberg, 1981; Waterhouse & Fein, 1982). Because good recovery of language in young children with maldeveloped left hemispheres suggests that the right hemisphere is able to take over considerable language function (Hecaen, 1976), continuing language impairment in autism suggests bilateral dysfunction.

In addition, task demands, rather than linguistic or spatial content, may determine performance. Thus, lower Verbal IQs may result from judgmental and organizational demands of verbal tasks, as contrasted with performance tasks, which frequently involve copying a model (Fein *et al.*, 1984). Social and contextual aspects of information processing appear to be more influential than verbal-performance distinctions in high-functioning subjects (Lincoln *et al.*, 1988).

Hoffmann and Prior (1982) tested a "left hemisphere hypothesis" in 10 high-functioning autistic children with Leiter ("nonverbal") IQs of 76 to 109. Relative to chronological and mental age-matched normal controls with average to superior IQs, the autistic children showed deficits on large number of putative left hemisphere tests, with intact performance on three of four right hemisphere tests. However, the "left hemisphere" tests (Categories, Progressive Figures, Seashore Rhythm, Trails B, WISC verbal subtests, Rhyming Test, Weigl Color Form Sorting Test) were complex, and performance on them is subject to disruption by other than left hemisphere lesions. Behaviors suggestive of frontal dysfunction (e.g., poor planning and lack of strategies) were also noted.

Szatmari *et al.* (1990) found relative verbal deficits to be characteristic of patients with Full Scale IQs between 70 and 85. However, neither his nor Rumsey and Hamburger's group with IQs above 85 showed substantial differences between language and visuospatial functioning. In contrast, deficits in abstract flexibility were characteristic. Additional language measures in Rumsey and Hamburger's (1988) study documented only mild language deficits in 10 very high-functioning men who showed more striking pragmatic disturbances and dysprosodies.

Two studies have compared simultaneous versus sequential processing, thought to reflect predominant right and left hemispheric functioning, respectively, in high-level autism. Both used the Kaufman Assessment Battery for Children (K-ABC; Kaufman, O'Neal, Avant, & Long, 1987), for which there is some limited evidence of differential hemispheric processing (Lewandowski & de Rienzo, 1985; Morris & Bigler, 1987).

Freeman *et al.* (1985) examined a very high-functioning sample of 21 autistic children (ages 6 to 12 years), all with Performance IQs above 70 and with a mean Full Scale IQ of 97. No significant differences between sequential and simultaneous processing scores were seen, despite significant Verbal–Performance IQ differences on the WISC (mean Verbal IQ = 90, Performance IQ = 105, $p < .01$) in this same group. Variability across subtests of the K-ABC was seen, with lowest scores on Riddles (which involves abstract reasoning) and highest scores on Reading Decoding.

In comparing 20 autistic (mean Verbal IQ = 57, Performance IQ = 85) and 20 language-disordered (mean Verbal IQ = 82, Performance IQ = 97) children, Allen, Lincoln, and Kaufman (1991) found that both groups performed better on tests of simultaneous than sequential processing, with no significant differences between groups. The autistic children had lower Full Scale IQs and more depressed Verbal IQs than the language-disordered children. The autistic sample was also lower functioning and more verbally impaired than that studied by Freeman. Thus, it may be that differences in simultaneous versus sequential processing on the K-ABC are seen only in the more verbally impaired autistic children, who tend to have Full Scale IQs under 85 or so.

To test the left hemisphere hypothesis independent of cognitive deficits, studies of sensory and motor functioning on the two sides of the body have been used. Dawson (1983) tested sensory-perceptual and motor functioning in autistic boys and men (Full Scale IQs 40–113). Overall the autistic group performed more poorly with the right hand, suggesting left-lateralized hemispheric dysfunction. However, the four patients with Full Scale IQs above 70, three of whom had Full Scale IQs above 90, failed to show lateralized dysfunction.

Szatmari's high-functioning sample (IQs >70) (Szatmari *et al.*, 1990) performed poorly with the dominant hand (presumably the right hand in most cases) and failed to show a dominant hand advantage on the Grooved Pegboard, but handedness was not reported. Differences between the two hands appeared to be reduced substantially (and thus more normal) in patients with IQs above 85, though data here was reported only for a combined group of autistic and Asperger's patients. Eight high-functioning subjects with a strong hand preference (five right, three left) studied by Rumsey and Hamburger (1988) showed a trend ($p < .06$) toward decreased speed and coordination on the Grooved Pegboard, as well as a trend ($p < .07$) toward worse performance with the nondominant hand, which varied across subjects. No evidence of consistently lateralized dysfunction was seen on sensory-perceptual measures, which were the same as those used by Dawson (1983).

Studies of language, simultaneous versus sequential processing, and sensory and motor functions then do not as a whole provide strong support for a left hemisphere hypothesis. More complex cognitive tasks, such as those used in Hoffman and Prior's (1982) study, involve elements dependent on the integrity of many different brain regions and circuits. Patients with IQs over 85 show intact language with more striking extralinguistic than linguistic disturbances, no differences between simultaneous and sequential processing, and no consistently lateralized sensory–motor dysfunction. Overall, patients with more language impairment and IQs under 85 have more findings compatible with greater left than right hemisphere involvement than do those with higher IQs.

PRAGMATIC DEFICITS AND DYSPROSODIES

Pragmatic skills (social uses of speech) are truly deviant, not merely delayed, and are more specifically impaired in autism than are linguistic skills (Tager-Flusberg, 1981). Delayed echolalia, repetitions of one's own utterances, thinking aloud/action accompaniments, metaphorical language, dysprosodies, paucity of spontaneous speech, overly literal speech, social inappropriateness, and perseverative speech are all specifically associated with autism (Cantwell & Baker, 1978; Prior, 1977; Simmons & Baltaxe, 1975; Tager-Flusberg, 1981).

High-functioning patients show nonreciprocal speech, literalness, irrelevant speech, poor social awareness, lack of empathy, and inflexibility (Dewey & Everard, 1974). They may talk excessively without following the flow, give-and-take, or focus of conversation. Literalness involves the failure to understand the shifting meaning of words in context and the intent of questions and requests, particularly indirect ones. Thus, when asked "Do you have a hobby?" the autistic adolescent might simply answer "yes." Peculiar uses of speech and language, a tendency to talk to oneself, perseverative questions or topics, poverty of speech, flat intonation, word or phrase repetition, and use of stereotyped scripts have been documented in high-functioning adults with good language (Rumsey *et al.*, 1986; Rumsey *et al.*, 1985).

Dysprosodies—or disturbances of the stresses, inflections, and rhythm of speech—may encompass both propositional (syntactic) and affective intonation (Baltaxe & Simmons, 1983) and may implicate right anterior cortical or subcortical, extrapyramidal neural circuits (Cancelliere & Kertesz, 1984; Kent & Rosenbek, 1982; Ross & Mesulam, 1979). Whether such disturbances are receptive as well as expressive is unknown.

Two recent studies have focused on intonation in high-level autism. Fine, Bartolucci, Ginsberg, and Szatmari (1991) studied 20 autistic persons (ages 7 through 32) using loosely structured interviews coded blindly for intonation contours and stress patterns. While the basic grammatical patterning of sentences and mapping of intonation onto these patterns were intact, the use of intonation patterns capable of carrying special or notable meanings, or meanings to be mapped onto specific contexts, was impaired. Much less deviance was seen in the use of intonation patterns that fit many different contexts. The investigators hypothesized that high-functioning autistic speakers either (a) fail to assess contexts correctly, (b) have difficulty mapping intonation patterns onto contexts, or (c) are unaware of the communication value of specific intonation patterns.

Macdonald *et al.* (1989) tested both receptive and expressive components of affective intonation in 10 high-functioning autistic men. Subjects were asked to identify emotions conveyed by intonation in semantically neutral sentences using a multiple-choice format and were recorded while reading short passages. Relative to controls, the autistic patients were impaired on receptive and expressive tasks except for one receptive task using filtered speech. Lay raters described the autistic voices as sad (monotonous) and as odd. The lack of differences when using filtered speech, a more difficult condition for controls, appeared consistent with other reports that autistic persons are less affected by manipulations that make stimuli less meaningful than are controls (Hobson, Ouston, & Lee, 1988; Langdell, 1978).

The extralinguistic deficits seen in high-level autism suggest analogies to communication deficits seen in patients with acquired right hemisphere lesions. Such patients may display fluent, but tangential and perseverative speech, fail to organize speech to convey main ideas, and make socially inappropriate comments. They may fail to comprehend indirect requests, figurative language, connotative meanings, sarcasm, and humor, to draw inferences, and to comprehend and use propositional and emotional prosody and facial expression (Weylman, Brownell, & Gardner, 1988). With elementary linguistic functions intact, they have difficulty processing complex linguistic material and using context to assess meaning (Wapner, Hamby, & Gardner, 1981). We are therefore examining high-functioning adolescents and adults with a battery of tests shown to be sensitive to communication deficits associated with acquired right hemisphere lesions. Preliminary results (Rumsey & Hanahan, 1990) suggest several similarities.

To summarize, pragmatic deficits and dysprosodies are more specifically associated with autism than are linguistic deficits. These features are just beginning to be studied in high-level autism and suggest the possibility of right hemisphere or subcortical, extrapyramidal involvement. Intonation may be impaired both receptively and expressively, and dysprosodies may stem in part from higher-level cognitive deficits.

FACIAL EXPRESSION

Communication deficits in autism involve nonverbal as well as verbal modalities. High-functioning adults with autism show less spontaneous facial expression and fewer expressive gestures than controls (Rumsey *et al.*, 1986).

The perception and expression of facial emotion are believed to be subserved by right hemisphere and extrapyramidal circuits (Borod, Koff, & Caron, 1983; Rinn, 1984; Ross & Mesulam, 1979), with expression subserved more by anterior regions (Kolb & Milner, 1981). Damasio and Maurer (1978) have clinically described abnormal asymmetries of spontaneous facial expression ("reverse facial paralysis"), thought to be subserved by extrapyramidal circuits, in autism, with normal symmetry seen in voluntary facial expression.

Receptive and expressive deficits in facial emotion have been reported in mental retardation (Gray, Fraser, & Leudar, 1983; Maurer & Newbrough, 1987).

Some studies of the perception of facial emotion have found few differences in level of performance between autistic and retarded children matched for verbal ability, though differences in features attended to or in strategies may be present (Hertzig, Snow, & Sherman, 1989; Weeks & Hobson, 1987).

Two studies have examined facial emotion in high-level autism using tests. Smalley and Asarnow (1990) found a group of nine high-functioning autistic males (mean age 20 years) to be impaired on a matching-and-labeling task using photographs of emotional faces, while unimpaired on other "right hemisphere" visuospatial tests. However, these perceptual deficits were not independent of language deficits, as some comparisons lost statistical significance when vocabulary scores were used as a covariate, raising the issue of the contribution of verbal task demands to these findings.

Macdonald *et al.* (1989) found deficits in both the recognition and elicited expression of facial emotion in 10 high-functioning autistic persons (mean age 27 years). Expressive deficits retained significance with adjustments for differences in verbal functioning, and perceptual deficits were reduced only slightly ($p < .06$) by such adjustments.

ACADEMIC SKILLS

Reading, spelling, and calculation skills, all believed to be primarily subserved by the left hemisphere, may be remarkably intact in autism or even precocious as evidenced by hyperlexia, seen in a significant subgroup of autistic children (Goldberg, 1987; Whitehouse & Harris, 1984). Rumsey and Hamburger's (1990) sample showed good skills in all three areas, and patients studied by Szatmari *et al.* (1990) had excellent reading skills relative both to their own IQs and to the skills of outpatient psychiatric controls.

High-functioning autistic men differed from severely dyslexic men in one study (Rumsey & Hamburger, 1990), in which the former seemed to have intact just what the dyslexics lacked—good phonological skills, as manifested in phonetic spelling, and good rote auditory memory. That this finding extends to lower-functioning autistic individuals is suggested by the work of Frith and Snowling (1983), who found complementary deficits in autistic and dyslexic children and adolescents matched for reading age. The dyslexic group showed specific difficulties with phonological processing, but superior comprehension and use of semantic context. Conversely, the autistic group showed poor comprehension and poor use of semantic context.

Considerable neuropsychological and some neuropathological evidence suggests left temporal cortical dysfunction in dyslexia (Galaburda, Sherman, Rosen, Aboitiz, & Geschwind, 1985; Satz & Morris, 1981). In contrast, neuropathological studies of three autistic brains have found no pathology in left temporal cortex, even in patients with little or no speech (Bauman & Kemper, 1985, 1987; Coleman, Romano, Lapham, & Simon, 1985).

HANDEDNESS AND ANOMALOUS DOMINANCE

Hand preference is usually assessed by the number of skilled unimanual actions normally performed with each hand. Though frequently studied as a dichotomous variable, handedness is continuously distributed as a J-shaped curve with a majority of individuals expressing strong right preference; approximately 10%, moderate through strong left preference; and very few in the center or indifferent range (Annett, 1972; Hardyck & Petrinovich, 1977).

The term *pathological left-handedness* has been used to account for an increase in the incidence of left-handedness in epilepsy and mental retardation, where it may be associated with language deficits (Lucas, Rosenstein, & Bigler, 1989; Satz, Soper, Orsini, Henry, & Zvi, 1985). This concept refers to the hypothesized switch of manual preference in natural right-handers, or dextrals, because of early cerebral insult. Because of different base rates for handedness in the general population—that is, a higher incidence of right-handedness—an equal distribution of unilateral (right- and left-sided) lesions will result in more pathological left-handers than right-handers (Satz, 1973). Thus, an increased incidence of left-handedness in a population may result from nonlateralized early brain insult.

Several studies have reported a low incidence of right-handedness in autism, with estimates ranging from 35% to 43% right-handedness, 10% to 35% left-handedness, and 30% to 47% mixed (Colby & Parkison, 1977; Gillberg, 1983; Soper *et al.*, 1986; Tsai, 1982). Soper and his colleagues reported that more than 90% of this mixed handedness subgroup showed ambiguous handedness, defined by inconsistent preference within items on repeated testing, rather than ambidexterity (inconsistency only between items) (Soper *et al.*, 1986). However, ambiguous handedness appears to be linked to mental retardation (Soper *et al.*, 1986; Soper, Satz, Orsini, Van Grop, & Green, 1987; Tsai, 1982). More thorough reviews of the literature on handedness in autism are found in Bryson (1990) and in Fein *et al.* (1984).

The incidence of nonright-handedness in high-level autism (IQs > 70) is unknown. The only neuropsychological study of high-level autism to report handedness (Rumsey & Hamburger, 1988) found strong right-handedness, determined using pantomimed responses to verbal commands from the Halstead-Reitan battery, in only 5 of 10 patients, using an 85% criterion; three patients were left-handed, and two were mixed. Gillberg's (1983) study of handedness in autism included five patients with IQs over 70, three of whom showed mixed handedness—defined broadly as less than complete (100%) consistency in preference—while two were right-handed. Though limited and potentially biased, these observations suggest that anomalous handedness may exist in high-functioning patients.

EXCEPTIONAL ABILITIES

Kanner (1943) noted "islets of higher functioning," most notably good rote memory and visuospatial skills (e.g., ability to complete formboards and puzzles), in autistic children. Normal or near-normal skills frequently stand out against a background of language deficits and abnormal social behavior, and thus represent relative, rather than absolute, strengths. In rare instances, most notably in savants, skills may be superior when compared with the population at large.

While data are limited and definitions subjective, prevalence rates for savant skills have been estimated to be 0.06% among institutionalized retardates (Hill, 1977) and 9.8% in autism, with music, memory, and art (skills thought to be mediated predominantly by the right hemisphere) being the most frequent domains of talent (Rimland, 1978). The studies just cited used different methods, both involving questionnaire data, and neither diagnosed subjects in person nor for the other disorder. A predominantly male sex ratio for exceptional abilities similar to that associated with autism was reported by Hill (1978). Furthermore, Rimland (1978) reported a higher incidence of special talents in autistic children with classical Kanner syndrome than in other autistic children.

The lack of objective diagnostic criteria, their direct application, and epidemiologically based data preclude firm conclusions on the association of autism and savant skills. Nonetheless, commonalities in neuropsychological strengths (memory and certain "right hemisphere skills") in the two syndromes are worthy of further study.

While high-functioning patients show uneven Wechsler profiles, their relative strengths are not necessarily superior to those seen in normal controls. Matching by Full Scale IQ insures that some subtest scores will be high if others are low. Nonetheless, relative strengths on Wechsler Block Design and Digit Span subtests suggest visuospatial organization and rote memory as domains worthy of further study.

Watkins and Asarnow (unpublished data) designed tasks to separate out the analytic ("taking apart") versus synthetic ("putting together") demands of the Wechsler Block Design subtest. These tasks used pictorial representations of blocks to be visually taken apart versus visually combined and two levels of complexity, with a multiple-choice format. High-functioning autistic children were more accurate than normal and schizophrenic controls matched by Wechsler Block Design scores on all tasks, but slower than schizophrenic boys on complex synthetic tasks. In a study of memory reviewed earlier, Zaucha, Asarnow, and Nuechterlein (unpublished data) reported an increased benefit of rehearsal in autistic patients relative to normal and schizophrenic controls.

A case study of a high-functioning 29-year-old autistic male (WAIS Full Scale IQ 91) with extraordinary calculation abilities was reported by Steel *et al.* (1984). Perinatal history included fetal distress and probable anoxia. No significant difference was seen between Verbal IQ (94) and Performance IQ (89). Subtest scores ranged from a low of 4 on Comprehension to highs of 13 on Block Design, 16 on Digit Span, and 17 on Arithmetic, an impressive spread of more than four standard deviations. Superior performance was noted on Raven's Coloured Progressive Matrices and on the Wechsler Memory Scale, although the patient was unable to synthesize verbal information contained in paragraphs of the latter. Poor performance was noted on the Wisconsin Card Sorting Test, where he perseverated, and on Porteus Mazes and Rey Figures. The results resemble those seen in Rumsey and Hamburger's (1988) high-functioning autistic sample.

Theories concerning the etiology of savant skills include intense practice and repetition, genetic factors, and abnormal neuronal circuitry. Intense practice may stem from narrow, circumscribed interests, frequently seen in autism. Genetically based talents have been proposed in the case of "prodigious savants," those with supernormal talent (Hermelin & O'Connor, 1986; O'Connor & Hermelin, 1987; Treffert, 1988).

Hyperfunction or overreliance on hippocampal functioning for memory formation and/or accompanying neurotransmitter imbalances has been proposed as well. This might be triggered by dysfunction of some complementary structure such as the amygdala, thought to be involved in providing emotional significance to memories (Lucci *et al.*, 1988). This might involve overstimulation of some cholinergic, glutaminergic, or other neurotransmitter system or hypersensitivity of neuronal membranes (Oscar-Berman, 1988). Unusual neurotransmitter activity may involve visual association cortex in the case of visual calculators and left temporal cortex in the case of auditory calculators or verbal mnemonists (Oscar-Berman, 1988). Attentional dysfunction, involving deficient orienting, overly efficient gating of external stimuli, and an overfocus on internal stimuli, has also been proposed (Rimland & Fein, 1988). This might involve the reticular activating system, thalamus, hypothalamus, fronto-parietal cortex, and the hippocampus, thought to have an inhibitory effect on brainstem arousal mechanisms (Rimland & Fein, 1988, p. 486). And finally, Waterhouse (1988) has hypothesized "cortical rededication," or the reorganization of sensory association or polymodal association cortex, such that the exclusive use of tissue for one purpose comes to preclude its use for other activity.

PROBLEM SOLVING

Several studies of high-functioning autistic patients have reported poor performance on tests of frontal lobe functioning (including the Wisconsin Card Sorting Test, Milner Maze, and Porteus Mazes), as well as on Trailmaking, the Category Test, Colour Form Sorting, and other verbal and nonverbal problem-solving measures (Hoffmann & Prior, 1982; Prior & Hoffmann, 1990; Rumsey, 1985; Rumsey & Hamburger, 1988; Steel *et al.*, 1984; Szatmari *et al.*, 1990). Rumsey and Hamburger (1988) used several subtests from the Binet (Verbal and Picture Absurdities, Problem Situations, Plan of Search) to draw out defects in reasoning and problem solving (Lezak, 1983, p. 494). In sharp contrast to their good performances on a wide range of other measures, including tests of language and visuoperceptual organization, these subjects showed dramatic deficits across a wide range of problem-solving tasks. They showed an increased percentage of perseverative errors and decreased conceptual responding on the Wisconsin Card Sorting Test, but no difficulties with set maintenance.

Qualitatively, patient responses did not reflect poor language comprehension, but rather failures to integrate information and to draw inferences. "Plan of Search," which requires the subject to map out the route he or she would follow to search for a purse lost in a field, revealed disorganized, nonplanful approaches. Deficits on Picture Absurdities, which require identification of illogical or practically impossible aspects of anomalous pictures, revealed failures to focus selectively on relevant details and/or failures to integrate the elements of pictures. Hoffman and Prior (1982) noted qualitative evidence of frontal impairments (e.g., lack of plans for problem solving, omission of preliminary investigation of task requirements, fragmentary impulsive actions, difficulty in learning from experience, inability to benefit from feedback, inflexibility and perseveration, and lack of hypothesis testing) in their high-functioning autistic sample.

Szatmari *et al.* (1990) found impairments on the Wisconsin Card Sorting Test in a group of 17 autistic patients, all with IQs above 70, when compared with outpatient psychiatric controls with higher IQs. However, a combined group of 8 autistic subjects with IQs above 85 and 14 Asperger's patients failed to differ from the outpatient psychiatric controls with similar IQs whose diagnoses included attention-deficit disorder, anxiety disorder, and/or conduct disorder. The highest-functioning subgroup of autistic patients was not reported separately, but the mean for the combined autistic–Asperger's group with IQs greater than 85 fell one standard deviation below published age norms. Furthermore, frontal lobe dysfunction has been hypothesized in attention-deficit disorder, and poor Wisconsin Card Sorting performance documented in it (Chelune, Ferguson, Koon, & Dickey, 1986; Mattes, 1980). This failure to find significant differences in the highest-functioning subgroup might therefore be due to the inclusion of the Asperger's patients, who performed better than the autistic patients, or to the use of controls with attention-deficit disorder. Another possibility for conflicting findings are sampling differences, as Szatmari *et al.*'s (1990) sample showed a less uneven Wechsler profile than several other samples reported in the literature. Nonetheless, significant deficits were seen even in higher-functioning autistic and Asperger's patients on Wechsler subtests thought to reflect higher-order verbal and nonverbal problem solving.

Schneider and Asarnow (1987) also failed to find significant differences between high-functioning autistic and normal children on a modified version of the Wisconsin Card Sorting Test, but excluded from their analysis 4 of 15 children who perseverated throughout the test. The autistic group's performance fell between that of the controls and the schizophrenic children, who were significantly impaired.

Patients with frontal lesions, especially those of the dorsolateral prefrontal cortex, demonstrate remarkable impairment on the Wisconsin Card Sorting Test, even with preserved IQ scores and linguistic and visuoperceptual skills (Pendleton & Heaton, 1982; Robinson, Heaton, Lehman & Stilson, 1980; Zangwill, 1966). Poor Wisconsin Card Sorting Test performance seen in the presence of high IQs and intact language and visuospatial skills in autism (Rumsey & Hamburger, 1988) is impressive and compatible with the hypothesis of frontosubcortical dysfunction.

Furthermore, Szatmari, Bartolucci, Bremner, Bond, and Rich (1989) reported significant correlations between Wisconsin Card Sorting Test performance and social outcomes in their follow-up study of high-functioning autistic persons (ages 17 to 34).

The above findings, along with motor deficits, have led Rumsey and Hamburger (1988) and Szatmari *et al.* (1990) to propose frontosubcortical dysfunction as a basis for autism. Because of its connections with subcortical structures, selective deficits in higher-level problem solving can result from neuropathology that is entirely subcortical. Impaired performance on the Wisconsin Card Sorting Test and the Milner Maze has been demonstrated in subcortical dementias such as Parkinson's disease (Delis, Direnfeld, Alexander, & Kaplan, 1982; Lees & Smith, 1983) and may occur even in mildly affected patients with intact memory functions (Lees & Smith, 1983).

Based on behavioral analogies to adults with acquired lesions, Damasio and Maurer (1978) have proposed that autism is due to dysfunction in bilateral neural structures that include mesolimbic cortex in the mesial frontal and temporal lobes, the neostriatum, and the anterior and medial nuclear groups of the thalamus. Other hypothesized subcortical sites of dysfunction in autism include the brainstem, thalamus, and neostriatum (Ornitz, 1983) and the cerebellum (Courchesne, Yeung-Courchesne, Press, Hesselink, & Jernigan, 1988).

Courchesne (1987) has hypothesized that in autism, as in epilepsy, abnormal neural activity interferes with otherwise normal neural systems. A dysfunctional reticulo-thalamic-cortical activating system might over time create a fluctuating disturbance that may result in anomalous connections and frequent excitation of limited cortical zones with selective inhibition of other patches of cortex. Such a fluctuating disturbance might interfere most with language, social knowledge, and problem solving, by virtue of their dependence on context and temporal processing.

COMPARISONS TO OTHER DISORDERS

The studies of high-level autism reviewed above indicate neuropsychological profiles that differ from those associated with schizophrenia (in children and in adults), developmental language disorders, and developmental dyslexia. Autistic children are more impaired in language and abstracting skills than are schizophrenic children, but show less distractibility, less reduced information-processing capacity, and differences in memory processing (Asarnow *et al.*, 1987; Schneider & Asarnow, 1987; Watkins & Asarnow, unpublished data; Zaucha *et al.*, unpublished data). Relative to persons with developmental language disorders, they show unique Wechsler profiles suggesting impairments in both verbal and nonverbal comprehension of social and contextual information (Lincoln *et al.*, 1988). Relative to severely dyslexic adults, they show superior rote memory and basic academic skills (reading, spelling, and math), but severely impaired verbal and nonverbal problem-solving abilities (Rumsey & Hamburger, 1990). High-functioning people with autism share verbal and nonverbal impairments, similar Wechsler profiles, and good reading skills with Asperger's patients. However, they failed to show a dominant hand advantage on motor testing in one study (unlike the Asperger's patients), perform worse on the Wisconsin Card Sorting Test (Szatmari *et al.*, 1990), and show greater impairments in the use of intonation to denote special meanings or specific contexts (Fine *et al.*, 1991).

CONCLUSION

The small number of studies, small sample sizes, limited success in controlling for intelligence, and sample heterogeneity make the following conclusions preliminary. Nonetheless, some answers to the questions posed at the beginning of this chapter are available. Cognitive deficits are seen in high-level autism, debunking the myth that this subgroup of autistic patients is intellectually normal.

Wechsler profiles, consistent across studies, suggest that relative verbal deficits in patients with IQs in the 70–85 range disappear as IQs reach an average range. The characteristic peaks and valleys that persist into the average range reflect difficulties with social and context-relevant information, whether verbal or nonverbal.

Attentional dysfunction may selectively involve the shifting of attention and possibly its breadth. Memory dysfunction appears to involve problems with the encoding of information rather than with consolidation and retention. Communication deficits specifically associated with high-level autism include pragmatic deficits and dysprosodies, some of which may stem from failures to appreciate context. While verbal task demands may have contributed to the findings, there is some evidence of impaired perception and expression of facial emotion. Basic reading, spelling, and calculation skills appear to be intact. Anomalous handedness is a possibility, but little data is available. Manual speed and coordination may be reduced even in the highest-functioning patients, though evidence concerning lateralized motor dysfunction is contradictory and perhaps complicated by anomalous hand dominance. While rote memory and visuospatial skills represent relative strengths, the existence of supernormal skills and possible relationships to savant skills have not been convincingly demonstrated. Deficits in higher-level problem solving, including deficits on several frontal lobe measures, have been reported.

Similarities to lower-functioning groups are suggested by Wechsler profiles and good rote memory but probable problems with encoding. Differences are seen predominantly in the degree of language impairment, and there is less evidence (cognitive and sensory–motor) of dysfunction lateralized to the left hemisphere in the highest functioning subgroup.

The neuropsychological profile seen in autism differs from that in several other developmental and childhood-onset neuropsychiatric disorders, as discussed above. The disorder with greatest similarity is Asperger syndrome, a disorder with prominent social impairment (though some differences are seen here as well). This is not surprising, as the diagnostic validity of Asperger's as a syndrome distinct from autism is controversial (Szatmari, Bartolucci, & Bremner, 1989; Wolff & Barlow, 1980).

Neuropsychological profiles associated with high-level autism suggest dissimilarities from temporal lobe amnesia and provide little evidence that neocortical dysfunction is limited to the left hemisphere. Paradoxically, both communication deficits associated with right hemisphere syndromes and strengths suggestive of intact right hemisphere functioning are seen. The findings reviewed above suggest shared characteristics with frontal syndromes and/or subcortical dementias, including possible deficits in the ability to shift attention, higher-level problem solving, and motor functioning in the absence of substantial linguistic impairment, agnosia, amnesia, or acalculia (Cummings & Benson, 1984).

Differences between acquired and developmental neuropathology and their effects on psychological functioning limit generalizations based on behavioral similarities. Hopefully, neuroimaging—particularly functional neuroimaging with positron emission tomography—will enable us to link neuropsychological profiles to physiological measures of brain function in autism and other developmental disorders.

REFERENCES

Altman, D. G. (1982). *Statistics and ethics in medical research.* London: British Medical Association.

Allen, M., Lincoln, A., & Kaufman, A. S. (1991). Sequential and simultaneous processing capabilities of high-functioning autistic children and language-impaired children. *Journal of Autism and Developmental Disorders, 21,* 483–502.

Ameli, R., Courchesne, E., Lincoln, A., Kaufman, A. S., & Grillon, C. (1988). Visual memory processes in high-functioning individuals with autism. *Journal of Autism and Developmental Disorders, 18,* 601–615.

Annett, M. (1972). The distribution of manual asymmetry. *British Journal of Psychology, 63,* 343–348.

Asarnow, R. F., Tanguay, P. E., Bott, L., & Freeman, B. J. (1987). Patterns of intellectual functioning in non-retarded autistic and schizophrenic children. *Journal of Child Psychology and Psychiatry, 28,* 273–280.

Baltaxe, C. A. M., & Simmons, J. Q. (1983). Communication deficits in the adolescent and adult autistic. *Journal of Speech & Hearing Disorders, 40,* 439–458.

Bartak, L., & Rutter, M. (1976). Differences between mentally retarded and normally intelligent autistic children. *Journal of Autism and Childhood Schizophrenia, 2,* 109–120.

Bartak, L., Rutter, M., & Cox, A. (1977). A comparative study of infantile autism & specific developmental language disorders: III. Discriminant function analysis. *Journal of Autism and Childhood Schizophrenia, 7,* 383–396.

Bauman, M., & Kemper, T. L. (1985). Histoanatomic observation of the brain in early infantile autism. *Neurology, 35,* 866–874.

Bauman, M. L., & Kemper, T. L. (1987). Limbic involvement in a second case of early infantile autism. *Neurology, 37*(Suppl. 1), 147.

Blackstock, E. G. (1978). Cerebral asymmetry and the development of early infantile autism. *Journal of Autism and Childhood Schizophrenia, 8,* 339–353.

Borod, J. C., Koff, E., & Caron, H. S. (1983). Right hemisphere specialization for the expression and appreciation of emotion: A focus on the face. In E. Perecman (Ed.), *Cognitive processes in the right hemisphere*. New York: Academic Press.

Boucher, J. (1981). Immediate free recall in early childhood autism: Another point of behavioural similarity with the anmestic syndrome. *British Journal of Psychology, 72,* 211–215.

Boucher, J., & Warrington, E. K. (1976). Memory deficits in early infantile autism: Some similarities to the amnestic syndrome. *British Journal of Psychology, 67,* 73–87.

Bryson, S. E. (1990). Autism and anomalous handedness. In S. Coren (Ed.), *Left-handedness: Behavioural implications and anomalies* (Advances in Psychology Series). New York: Elsevier Science Publishers B. V./North-Holland Book Series.

Butters, N., Salmon, D. P., Cullum, C. M., Cairns, P., Troster, A. I., & Jacobs, D. (1988). Differentiation of amnesic and demented patients with the Wechsler Memory Scale-Revised. The *Clinical Neuropsychologist, 2,* 133–148.

Cancelliere, A., & Kertesz, A. (1984). *Evidence for non-specific hemispheric involvement in emotional expression and comprehension*. Presented at the Body for the Advancement of Brain, Behaviour and Language Enterprises, Niagara Falls, Ontario.

Cantwell, D., & Baker, L. (1978). Imitations & echoes in autistic and dysphasic children. *Journal of American Academy of Child Psychiatry, 17,* 614–624.

Cantwell, D., Baker, L., & Rutter, M. (1978). A comparative study of infantile autism and specific developmental receptive language disorder. IV: Analysis of syntax and language function. *Journal of Child Psychology and Psychiatry, 19,* 351–362.

Chelune, G. J., Ferguson, W., Koon, R., & Dickey, T. O. (1986). Frontal lobe disinhibition in attention deficit disorder. *Child Psychiatry and Human Development, 16,* 221–234.

Cohen, D. J., Caparulo, B. K. & Shaywitz, B. A. (1976). Primary childhood aphasia and childhood autism. *Journal of the American Academy of Child Psychiatry, 15,* 604–645.

Colby, K. M., & Parkison, C. (1977). Handedness in autistic children. *Journal of Autism and Childhood Schizophrenia, 7,* 3–9.

Coleman, P. D., Romano, J., Lapham, L., & Simon, W. (1985). Cell counts in the cerebral cortex of an autistic patient. *Journal of Autism and Developmental Disorders, 15,* 245–255.

Courchesne, E. (1987). A neurophysiological view of autism. In E. Schopler & G. B. Mesibov (Eds.), *Neurobiological issues in autism* (pp. 285–324). New York: Plenum.

Courchesne, E., Yeung-Courchesne, R., Press, G. A., Hesselink, J. R., & Jernigan, T. L. (1988). Hypoplasia of cerebellar vermal lobules VI and VII in autism. *New England Journal of Medicine, 318,* 1349–1354.

Cummings, J. L., & Benson, D. F. (1984). Subcortical dementia: Review of an emerging concept. *Archives of Neurology, 41,* 874–879.

Damasio, A. R., & Maurer, R. G. (1978). A neurological model for childhood autism. *Archives of Neurology, 35,* 777–786.

Dawson, G. (1983). Lateralized brain dysfunction in autism: Evidence from the Halstead–Reitan neuropsychological battery. *Journal of Autism and Developmental Disorders, 13,* 269–286.

Delis, D., Direnfeld, L., Alexander, M. P., & Kaplan, E. (1982). Cognitive fluctuations associated with on–off phenomenon in Parkinson disease. *Neurology, 32,* 1049–1052.

DeLong, G. (1976). A neuropsychological interpretation of infantile autism. In M. Rutter & E. Schopler (Eds.), *Autism: A reappraisal of concepts and treatment* (pp. 207–218). New York: Plenum.

Dewey, M. A., & Everard, M. P. (1974). The near-normal autistic adolescent. *Journal of Autism and Developmental Disorders, 4,* 348–356.

Fein, D., Humes, M., Kaplan, E., Lucci, D., & Waterhouse, L. (1984). The question of left hemisphere dysfunction in infantile autism. *Psychological Bulletin, 95,* 258–281.

Fein, F., Pennington, B., Markowitz, P., Braverman, M., & Waterhouse, L. (1986). Toward a neuropsychological model of infantile autism: Are the social deficits primary? *Journal of the American Academy of Child Psychiatry, 25,* 198–212.

Fine, J., Bartolucci, G., Ginsberg, G., & Szatmari, P. (1991). The use of intonation to communicate in subjects with pervasive developmental disorders. *Journal of Child Psychology and Psychiatry, 32,* 771–782.

Freeman, B. J., Lucas, J. C., Forness, S. R., & Ritvo, E. R. (1985). Cognitive processing of high-functioning autistic children: Comparing the K-ABC and the WISC-R. *Journal of Psychoeducational Assessment, 4,* 357–362.

Frith, U. (1970). Studies in pattern detection in normal and autistic children. II. Reproduction and production of color sequences. *Journal of Experimental Child Psychology, 10,* 120–135.

Frith, U., & Snowling, M. (1983). Reading for meaning and reading for sound in autistic and dyslexic children. *British Journal of Developmental Psychology, 1,* 329–342.

Galaburda, A. M., Sherman, G. F., Rosen, G. D., Aboitiz, F., & Geschwind, N. (1985). Developmental dyslexia: Four consecutive patients with cortical anomalies. *Annals of Neurology, 18,* 222–233.

Gersten, R. (1983). Stimulus overselectivity in autistic, trainable mentally retarded, and non-handicapped children: Comparative research controlling chronological (rather than mental) age. *Journal of Abnormal Child Psychology, 11,* 61–76.

Gillberg, C. (1983). Autistic children's hand preferences: results from an epidemiological study of infantile autism. *Psychiatry Research, 10,* 21–30.

Goldberg, T. E. (1987). On hermetic reading abilities. *Journal of Autism and Developmental Disorders, 17,* 29–44.

Goldman-Rakic, P., & Rakic, P. (1984). Experimental modification of gyral patterns. In N. Geschwind & A. M. Galaburda (Eds.), *Cerebral dominance: The biological foundations.* Cambridge, MA: Harvard University Press.

Gray, J. M., Fraser, W. L., & Leudar, I. (1983). Recognition of emotion from facial expression in mental handicap. *British Journal of Psychiatry, 142,* 566–571.

Hardyk, C., & Petrinovich, L. F. (1977). Left-handedness. *Psychological Bulletin, 84,* 385–404.

Hauser, S. L., DeLong, G. R., & Rosman, N. P. (1975). Pneumographic findings in the infantile autism syndrome: A correlation with temporal lobe disease. *Brain, 98,* 677–688.

Hecaen, H. (1976). Acquired aphasia in children and the ontogenesis of hemispheric functional specialization. *Brain and Language, 3,* 114–134.

Hermelin, B., & O'Connor, N. (1970). *Psychological experiments with autistic children.* Oxford: Pergamon.

Hermelin, B., & O'Connor, N. (1986). Idiot savant calendrical calculators: Rules and regularities. *Psychological Medicine, 16,* 1–9.

Hertzig, M. E., Snow, M. E., & Sherman, M. (1989). Affect and cognition in autism. *Journal of the American Academy of Child and Adolescent Psychiatry, 28,* 195–199.

Hill, A. L. (1977). Idiot savants: Rate of incidence. *Perceptual and Motor Skills, 44,* 161–162.

Hill, A. L. (1978). Savants: Mentally retarded individuals with special skills. In N. R. Ellis (Ed.), *International review of research in mental retardation, vol. 9.* New York: Academic Press.

Hobson, R. P., Ouston, J., & Lee, A. (1988). What's in a face? The cause of autism. *British Journal of Psychology, 79,* 441–453.

Hoffmann, W. L., & Prior, M. R. (1982). Neuropsychological dimensions of autism in children: A test of the hemispheric dysfunction hypothesis. *Journal of Clinical Neuropsychology, 4,* 27–41.

Kanner, L. (1943). Autistic disturbances of affective contact. *Nervous Child, 2,* 217–250.

Kaufman, A. S., O'Neal, M. R., Avant, A. H., & Long, S. W. (1987). Introduction to the Kaufman Assessment Battery for Children (K-ABC) for pediatric neuroclinicians. *Journal of Child Neurology, 2,* 3–16.

Kent, R. D., & Rosenbek, J. C. (1982). Prosodic disturbance and neurologic lesion. *Brain and Language, 14,* 259–291.

Kolb, B. (1989). Brain development, plasticity, and behavior. *American Psychologist, 44,* 1203–1212.

Kolb, B., & Milner, B. (1981). Observations on spontaneous facial expression after focal cerebral excisions and after intracarotid injection of sodium amytal. *Neuropsychologia, 19,* 491–503.

Langdell, T. (1978). Recognition of faces: An approach to the study of autism. *Journal of Child Psychology and Psychiatry, 19,* 255–268.

Lees, A. J., & Smith, E. (1983). Cognitive disorders in the early stages of Parkinson's disease. *Brain, 106,* 257–270.

Lewandowski, L. J., & de Rienzo, P. J. (1985). WISC-R and K-ABC performances of hemiplegic children. *Journal of Psychoeducational Assessment, 3,* 215–221.

Lezak, M. D. (1983). *Neuropsychological assessment* (2nd ed.). New York: Oxford University Press.

Lincoln, A. J., Courchesne, E., Kilman, B. A., Elmasian, R., & Allen, M. (1988). A study of intellectual abilities in high-functioning people with autism. *Journal of Autism and Developmental Disorders, 18,* 505–524.

Lockyer, L., & Rutter, M. (1970). A five- to fifteen-year follow-up study of infantile psychosis: IV. Patterns of cognitive ability. *British Journal of Social and Clinical Psychology, 9,* 152–163.

Lovaas, O. I., Koegel, R. L., & Schreibman, L. (1979). Stimulus overselectivity in autism: A review of research. *Psychological Bulletin, 86,* 1236–1254.

Lucas, J. A., Rosenstein, L. D., & Bigler, E. D. (1989). Handedness and language among the mentally retarded: Implications for the model of pathological left-handedness and gender differences in hemispheric specialization. *Neuropsychologia, 27,* 713–723.

Lucci, D., Fein, D., Holevas, A., & Kaplan, E. (1988). Paul: A musically gifted autistic boy. In L. K. Obler & D. Fein (Eds.), *The exceptional brain: Neuropsychology of talent and special abilities* (pp. 310–324). New York: Guilford.

Macdonald, H., Rutter, M., Howlin, P., Rios, P., LeCouteur, A., Evered, C., & Folstein, S. (1989). Recognition and expression of emotional cues by autistic and normal adults. *Journal of Child Psychology and Psychiatry, 30,* 865–877.

Mattes, J. A. (1980). The role of frontal lobe dysfunction in childhood hyperkinesis. *Comprehensive Psychiatry, 21,* 358–369.

Maurer, H., & Newbrough, J. R. (1987). Facial expressions of mentally retarded and non-retarded children: I. Recognition by mentally retarded and non-retarded adults and II. Recognition by non-retarded adults with varying experience with mental retardation. *American Journal of Mental Deficiency, 91,* 505–515.

Mirsky, A. F. (1987). Behavioral and psychophysiological markers of disordered attention. *Environmental Health Perspectives, 74,* 191–199.

Morris, J. M., & Bigler, E. D. (1987). Hemispheric functioning and the Kaufman Assessment Battery for Children: Results in the neurologically impaired. *Developmental Neuropsychology, 3,* 67–79.

Narita, T., & Koga, Y. (1987). Neuropsychological assessment of childhood autism. *Advances in Biological Psychiatry, 16,* 156–170.

O'Connor, N., & Hermelin, B. (1987). Visual and graphic abilities of the idiot savant artist. *Psychological Medicine, 17,* 79–90.

Ornitz, E. (1983). The functional neuroanatomy of infantile autism. *International Journal of Neuroscience, 19,* 85–124.

Oscar-Berman, M. (1988). Superior memory: Perspective from the neuropsychology of memory disorders. In L. K. Obler & D. Fein (Eds.), *The exceptional brain: Neuropsychology of talent and special abilities* (pp. 212–217). New York: Guilford.

Pendleton, M. G., & Heaton, R. K. (1982). A comparison of the Wisconsin Card Sorting Test and the Category Test. *Journal of Clinical Psychology, 38,* 392–396.

Prior, M. (1977). Psycholinguistic disabilities of autistic and retarded children. *Journal of Mental Deficiency Research, 21,* 37–45.

Prior, M. (1979). Cognitive abilities and disabilities in infantile autism: A review. *Journal of Abnormal Child Psychology, 7,* 357–380.

Prior, M., & Bradshaw, J. L. (1975). Hemispheric functioning in autistic children. *Cortex, 15,* 73–81.

Prior, M. R., & Chen, C. S. (1976). Short-term and serial memory in autistic, retarded, and normal children. *Journal of Autism and Childhood Schizophrenia, 6,* 121–131.

Prior, M. R., & Hoffmann, W. (1990). Brief report: Neuropsychological testing of autistic children through an exploration with frontal lobe tests. *Journal of Autism and Developmental Disorders, 20,* 581–590.

Rimland, B. (1978). Savant capabilities of autistic children and their cognitive implications. In G. Serban (Ed.)., *Cognitive defects in the development of mental illness.* New York: Brunner-Mazel.

Rimland, B., & Fein, D. (1988). Special talents of autistic savants. In L. K. Obler & D. Fein (Eds.), *The exceptional brain: Neuropsychology of talent and special abilities* (pp. 474–492). New York: Guilford.

Rinn, W. E. (1984). The neuropsychology of facial expression: A review of the neurological and psychological mechanisms for producing facial expressions. *Psychological Bulletin, 95,* 52–77.

Robinson, A. L., Heaton, R. K., Lehman, R. A., & Stilson, D. W. (1980). The utility of the Wisconsin Card Sorting Test in detecting and localizing frontal lobe lesions. *Journal of Consulting and Clinical Psychology, 48,* 604–614.

Ross, E. D. & Mesulam, M. (1979). Dominant language functions of the right hemisphere? Prosody and emotional gesturing. *Archives of Neurology, 36,* 144–148.

Rumsey, J. (1985). Conceptual problem-solving in highly verbal, nonretarded autistic men. *Journal of Autism and Developmental Disorders, 15,* 23–36.

Rumsey, J. M., Andreasen, N. C., & Rapoport, J. L. (1986). Thought, language, communication, and affective flattening in autistic adults. *Archives of General Psychiatry, 43,* 771–777.

Rumsey, J. M., & Hamburger, S. D. (1988). Neuropsychological findings in high-functioning men with infantile autism, residual state. *Journal of Clinical and Experimental Neuropsychology, 10,* 201–221.

Rumsey, J. M., & Hamburger, S. D. (1990). Neuropsychological divergence of high-level autism and severe dyslexia. *Journal of Autism and Developmental Disorders, 20,* 155–168.

Rumsey, J. M., & Hanahan, A. P. (1990). Getting it "right": Performance of high-functioning autistic adults on a right-hemisphere battery. *Journal of Clinical and Experimental Neuropsychology, 12,* 81.

Rumsey, J., Rapoport, J. L., & Sceery, W. (1985). Autistic children as adults: Psychiatric, social, and behavioral outcomes. *Journal of the American Academy of Child Psychiatry, 24,* 465–473.

Rutter, M. (1983). Cognitive deficits in the pathogenesis of autism. *Journal of Child Psychology and Psychiatry, 24,* 513–531.

Rutter, M. (1987). The role of cognition in child development and disorder. *British Journal of Medical Psychology, 60,* 1–16.

Satz, P. (1973). Left-handedness and early brain insult: An explanation. *Neuropsychologia, 11,* 115–117.

Satz, P., & Morris, R. (1981). Learning disability subtypes: A review. In F. J. Pirozzola & M. C. Wittrock (Eds.), *Neuropsychological and cognitive processes in reading* (pp. 109–141). Orlando, FL: Academic Press.

Satz, P., Soper, H. V., Orsini, D. L., Henry, R. R., & Zvi, J. C. (1985). Handedness subtypes in autism: Some putative etiological markers. *Psychiatric Annals, 15,* 447–450.

Schneider, S. G., & Asarnow, R. F. (1987). A comparison of cognitive/neuropsychological impairments of nonretarded autistic and schizophrenic children. *Journal of Abnormal Child Psychology, 15,* 29–45.

Simmons, J., & Baltaxe, C. (1975). Language patterns of adolescent autistics. *Journal of Autism and Childhood Schizophrenia, 5,* 331–351.

Smalley, S. L., & Asarnow, R. F. (1990). Brief Report: Cognitive sub-clinical markers in autism. *Journal of Autism and Developmental Disorders, 20,* 271–278.

Soper, H. V., Satz, P., Orsini, D. L., Henry, R. R., Zvi, J., & Schulman, M. (1986). Handedness patterns in autism suggest subtypes. *Journal of Autism and Developmental Disorders, 16,* 155–167.

Soper, H. V., Satz, P., Orsini, D. L., Van Gorp, W. G., & Green, M. F. (1987). Handedness distribution in a residential population with severe or profound mental retardation. *American Journal of Mental Deficiency, 92,* 94–102.

Steel, J. G., Gorman, R., & Flexman, J. E. (1984). Neuropsychiatric testing in an autistic mathematical idiot-savant: Evidence for nonverbal abstract capacity. *Journal of the American Academy of Child Psychiatry, 23,* 704–707.

Szatmari, P., Bartolucci, G., & Bremner, R. (1989). Asperger's syndrome and autism: Comparisons on early history and outcome. *Developmental Medicine and Child Neurology, 31,* 709–720.

Szatmari, P., Bartolucci, G., Bremner, R., Bond, S., & Rich, S. (1989). A follow-up study of high-functioning autistic children. *Journal of Autism and Developmental Disorders, 19,* 213–225.

Szatmari, P., Tuff, L., Finlayson, M. A. J., & Bartolucci, G. (1990). Asperger's syndrome and autism: Neurocognitive aspects. *Journal of the American Academy of Child Psychiatry, 29,* 130–136.

Tager-Flusberg, H. B. (1981). On the nature of linguistic functioning in early infantile autism. *Journal of Autism and Developmental Disorders, 11,* 45–56.

Tanguay, P. E. (1976). Clinical and electrophysiological research. In E. Ritvo (Ed.), *Autism: Diagnosis, research, management* (pp. 75–84). New York: Spectrum.

Treffert, D. A. (1988). The idiot savant: A review of the syndrome. *American Journal of Psychiatry, 145,* 563–572.

Tsai, L. Y. (1982). Brief report: Handedness in autistic children and their families. *Journal of Autism and Developmental Disorders, 12,* 421–423.

Wapner, W., Hamby, S., & Gardner, H. (1981). The role of the right hemisphere in the apprehension of complex linguistic materials. *Brain and Language, 14,* 15–33.

Waterhouse, L. (1988). Speculations on the neuroanatomical substrate of special talents. In L. K. Obler & D. Fein (Eds.), *The exceptional brain: Neuropsychology of talent and special abilities* (pp. 493–512). New York: Guilford.

Waterhouse, L., & Fein, D. (1982). Language skills in developmentally disabled children. *Brain and Language, 15,* 307–333.

Watkins, J. M., & Asarnow, R. F. (unpublished data). *Information-processing strategies in schizophrenic and autistic children: I. Componential analysis.* Manuscript submitted for publication.

Weeks, S. J., & Hobson, R. P. (1987). The salience of facial expression for autistic children. *Journal of Child Psychology and Psychiatry, 28,* 137–151.

Weylman, S. T., Brownell, H. H., & Gardner, H. (1988). "It's what you mean, not what you say": Pragmatic language use in brain-damaged patients. In F. Plum (Ed.), *Language, communication and the brain.* New York: Raven.

Whitehouse, D., & Harris, J. C. (1984). Hyperlexia in infantile autism. *Journal of Autism and Developmental Disorders, 14,* 281–289.

Wolff, S., & Barlow, A. (1980). Schizoid personality in childhood: A comparative study of schizoid, autistic and normal children. *Annual Progress in Child Psychiatry & Child Development,* 396–417.

Zangwill, O. L. (1966). Psychological deficits associated with frontal lobe lesions. *International Journal of Neurology, 5,* 396–402.

Zaucha, K. M., Asarnow, R. F., & Nuechterlein, K. H. (unpublished data). *The role of rehearsal in the free recall performance of non-retarded adult autistic and schizophrenic patients.*

4

Neurological Localization in Autism

NANCY J. MINSHEW

INTRODUCTION

The location of the neuropathology responsible for the clinical syndrome of autism has been a hotly debated topic since the 1960s, when evidence for central nervous system involvement was first given serious consideration. Since that time, three fundamentally different localizations have been hypothesized for the primary neuropathology in autism: the brainstem–cerebellar circuitry, the limbic system, and the circuitry of the cerebral cortex. In the last decade, there have been major shifts in the data available to support each of these localizations and, consequently, in the theories themselves. Although there continues to be some degree of support for abnormalities at each of these levels within the neuraxis, the evolving body of scientific research appears to suggest primary involvement of forebrain structures in autism and, in particular, in the distributed neural network involved in complex information processing. However, examination of existing data also highlights the real paucity of data related to the neurobiologic issues and the need for research to target specific hypotheses on the location and mechanism of the primary pathophysiology in autism, to accumulate a substantial research data base on these issues, and to interpret these data across test modalities and across the spectrum of autism in order to ascertain the essential nature and location of the neurobiology.

High-functioning individuals with autism have played a central role in recent neurobiologic research, due to their greater capacity for testing and lower prevalence of associated disorders. Some methodologies are feasible regardless of level of function, but others are dependent on a high level of function, and hence many key questions can only be addressed by study of this subgroup. The research focus

NANCY J. MINSHEW • Western Psychiatric Institute and Clinic, University of Pittsburgh School of Medicine, Pittsburgh, Pennsylvania 15213.

High-Functioning Individuals with Autism, edited by Eric Schopler and Gary B. Mesibov. Plenum Press, New York, 1992.

on high-functioning autistic individuals is a recent strategy made possible by improvements in the clinical definition of this syndrome and the renewed appreciation of the continuity in this syndrome across the range of severity. Support for the continuity between low- and high-functioning individuals with autism is based on their common presentation in the preschool years, the case-to-case continuity in the clinical syndrome across the severity spectrum, the coexistence in multiplex families of high- and low-functioning offspring with autism, and the ability to develop qualitative descriptors of the core deficits that are equally applicable to low- and high-functioning individuals. Indeed, variation in severity is a characteristic of most biologic disorders, and experience has shown that variability in severity alone has not been a reliable indicator of etiologic diversity. Due to the clinical unity of this syndrome, the neurological localization proposed for the syndrome of autism is the same regardless of level of function. The most obvious evidence for the validity of this tenet is the presence of identical neuropathologic findings in high- and low-functioning autistic individuals.

Although variability in the biology proposed solely on the basis of severity has not been shown to be a valid strategy, it is important to consider whether it is likely from a neurologic standpoint that there is only one localization for this particular clinical syndrome, or many. Heterogeneity has often been emphasized in connection with autism, but this conclusion has been largely based on variability in clinical severity, the presence in a small minority of cases of a variety of associated disorders that are thought to be etiologic, and inadequate definition of the clinical syndrome. These factors have been significantly reduced as a result of the improved characterization of the clinical deficits that has occurred over the past decade. Reexamination of secondary cases of autism in light of these clinical advances has unfortunately not been systematically conducted, but in two disorders where this has been done—fragile-X syndrome and Rett syndrome—the clinical distinctions from autism have become increasingly apparent. Homogeneity in the pathophysiology of the majority of cases of autism is highly likely because of the specificity of structural–functional relationships in the central nervous system and the specificity and complexity of the clinical deficits defining this syndrome. Heterogeneity may still exist within the clinical syndrome of autism (and therefore in the pathophysiology) as a result of clinical phenocopies, particularly in lower-functioning autistic individuals in whom it is difficult to establish the specific qualitative nature of their deficits and abnormal behavior, and in high-functioning individuals in whom the nature of the deficits has not been sufficiently defined to distinguish autism from closely related disorders. Heterogeneity may also continue to exist in the form of multiple etiologic factors that have the capacity to trigger the same pathophysiology.

This chapter will review the theories and existing structural, functional, and neurologic data relevant to localization in autism, and to consider the likely role of various sites within the neuraxis in the pathophysiology of autism. Neuropsychological data also play a central role in assessing localization and will be taken into consideration in this analysis, but have been reviewed already in Chapter 3. The purpose of this chapter is to provide a clearer view of the existing data relevant to localization and pathophysiology, to bring into focus the various hypotheses, and to make apparent the data that are needed if the various hypotheses are to be definitively addressed by future research.

THE BRAINSTEM IN AUTISM

A brainstem origin for autism has been espoused in various forms since the 1960s. The original data supporting these theories, and the theories themselves, played a major role in shifting scientific opinion on the origin of autism from family environment to innate biologic abnormalities of the brain. However, the originally reported brainstem abnormalities have since been traced to the presence of associated neurologic disorders in the autistic subject groups and to methodologic problems. In addition, some of the early hypotheses regarding the neuropsychologic mechanism for the clinical deficits have also been contradicted by emerging data. The early pattern of abnormalities has now been supplanted by tentative reports of subtle oculovestibular abnormalities and cerebellar hypoplasia on MRI. In consideration of these developments in the data, the revised brainstem theories emphasize attentional abnormalities at the cortical level resulting from abnormal brainstem projections.

Brainstem Theories

A brainstem localization for the pathophysiology of autism was originally proposed in three theories—the sensory inconstancy theory, the "whisper of the bang" theory, and the neurological model of Damasio and Maurer (1978). The sensory inconstancy theory proposed that the fundamental deficit in autism was fluctuation in sensory input and sensory perception as a result of erratic sensory transmission through the brainstem (Ornitz & Ritvo, 1968). When subsequent research provided evidence of intact sensory transmission, this theory was revised to propose abnormalities originating in the brainstem attentional system as giving rise to selective deficits in attention at the cortical level (Ornitz, 1985, 1989). Both versions of this theory focus on the exaggerated response to some sensory stimuli and the hyporesponsiveness to other aspects of the environment.

The "whisper of the bang" theory proposed that abnormalities in ascending projections from the brainstem adversely influenced fetal forebrain development, and that brainstem abnormalities in the form of abnormal auditory evoked potentials and oculovestibular reflexes constituted the residual evidence of the early brainstem malformation (Tanguay & Edwards, 1982).

From a different perspective, Damasio and Maurer (1978) proposed a neurologic model of autism based on a detailed analysis of the clinical syndrome from a behavioral neurology viewpoint that suggested that the clinical deficits were related to dysfunction in medial frontal and medial temporal cortex. Since the forebrain structures clinically implicated in their model constituted the entire projection area of ascending mesencephalic dopaminergic neurons, Damasio and Maurer further postulated that forebrain dysfunction in primary cases of autism was the result of a neurotransmitter imbalance in dopaminergic mesencephalic projections.

Evidence of Intrinsic Brainstem Dysfunction

Initial studies of brainstem auditory evoked potentials (BAEPs) (Fein, Skoff, & Mirsky, 1981; Gillberg, Rosenhall, & Johansson, 1983; Ornitz, Mo, Olson, & Walter, 1980; Ornitz & Walter, 1975; Rosenblum *et al.,* 1980; Skoff, Mirsky, & Turner, 1980; Student & Sohmer, 1978, 1979; Tanguay, Edwards, Buchwald, Schwafel, & Allen, 1982; Taylor, Rosenblatt, & Linschoten, 1982), oculovestibular reflexes, and eye movements (Colbert, Koegler, & Markham, 1959; Ornitz, 1974, 1978; Piggott, Purcell, Cummings, & Caldwell, 1976; Pollack & Krieger, 1958; Ritvo *et al.,* 1969) in autistic subjects reported significant abnormal findings that have since been traced to the methodology used and the presence of associated neurologic disorders in the autistic subjects. These limitations were the product of the times and the evolving state of these technologies. The BAEP abnormalities reported by these studies have been determined to be the result of (a) the inclusion of a substantial proportion of autistic subjects with acquired brain damage and peripheral nerve deafness; (b) the failure to match control and autistic subjects on the basis of sex; (c) the use of invalid and unreliable measurements; (d) the failure to control for the effects of temperature; and (e) the failure to consider clinical normative values in the interpretation of the findings (Courchesne, Yeung-Courchesne, Hicks, & Lincoln, 1985; Rumsey, Grimes, Pikus, Duara, & Ismond, 1984). In addition, the magnitude of the reported abnormalities was small and included both shortened and prolonged latencies. Similarly, the reported oculovestibular abnormalities have been attributed to subject selection, failure to control for the effects of visual fixation, and the use of idiosyncratic response measures (Ornitz, 1985).

Recent studies of brainstem auditory evoked responses using current methodology and subject screening for associated disorders have reported normal latencies in autistic individuals regardless of level of function (Courchesne, Yeung-Courchesne, *et al.,* 1985; Grillon, Courchesne, & Akshoomoff, 1989; Rumsey *et al.,* 1984). Recent oculovestibular data has revealed only minor abnormalities (Minshew, Furman, Goldstein, & Payton, 1990; Ornitz, 1985) that are not ordinarily considered clinically significant. Recent auditory, visual, and somatosensory evoked-potential and neuropsychologic studies have provided documentation of consistent sensory transmission to the cortex as well as accurate and consistent sensory perception by autistic individuals (Courchesne, Kilman, Galambos, & Lincoln, 1984; Courchesne, Lincoln, Kilman, & Galambos, 1985; Grillon *et al.*, 1989; Minshew, Goldstein, & Payton, 1989; Rumsey & Hamburger, 1988).

Evidence of Structural Abnormalities

Research radiologic evaluations of posterior fossa structures have been uncommon until recently, due to the limitations imposed on computerized axial tomography (CT) by the surrounding bone. Magnetic resonance imaging (MRI) does not have this constraint, and hence has made available the technology for assessing the radiologic anatomy of the posterior fossa. One CT study did report an increase in the width of the upper and middle portions of the fourth ventricle and some cerebellar atrophy on CT scans of autistic children (Bauman, LeMay, Bauman, & Rosenberger, 1985). MRI studies of the posterior fossa in autism have yielded inconsistent reports of alterations in the size of the brainstem and the fourth ventricle. In a series of studies, Gaffney and colleagues (Gaffney, Kuperman, & Tsai, 1989; Gaffney, Kuperman, Tsai, & Minchin, 1988; Gaffney, Kuperman, Tsai, Minchin, & Hassanein, 1987; Gaffney, Tsai, Kuperman, & Minchin, 1987) reported: (a) an increase in the size of the fourth ventricle, a decrease in the size of the pons, and no change in the size of the cerebellum on planimetric measurements from *midsagittal* MRI in autistic subjects; (b) an increase in the size of the fourth ventricle with a decrease in the size of the cerebellum on *coronal* scans; and (c) no change in any posterior fossa structures on *axial* scans. Ritvo and Garber (1988) and Garber *et al.* (1989), on the other hand, found no changes in the size of the fourth ventricle or cerebellum on midsagittal MRI in autistic subjects compared to normal controls. Hashimoto, Tayama, Mori, Fujino, Miyazaki, and Kuroda (1989), studying autistic subjects with uncomplicated mental retardation and controls, found a smaller brainstem in the mentally retarded group compared to both the autistic and control groups, but no significant change in the size of the brainstem in the autistic group.

These MRI studies highlight some of the methodologic problems with this evolving technology that need to be addressed in order to achieve valid and meaningful radiologic findings. First, planimetric or area measurements made from two-dimensional images of three-dimensional, irregularly shaped structures are of limited validity. In addition, many of the structures of interest are quite small, increasing the impact of resolution limits. Two-dimensional analysis methods will eventually be replaced in research studies by volume-imaging methods that collect three-dimensional data sets using 1 mm isotropic (cubic) voxels. The ability to view a structure in any plane from the same data set will improve visualization, and the 1 mm voxel will reduce the edge effect over current methods. Volumetric measurements can be made in two orthogonal planes to provide an index of the validity of the measurements.

A second significant limitation of imaging studies to date relates to the methods used for selection of controls and the lack of population norms. There are three parameters—age, sex, and IQ (Full Scale, Verbal and/or Performance, depending on the structural–functional correlations under consideration)—that have a potent effect on CNS function and, therefore, have the most likelihood of impacting on structural measurements independent of disease status. It is therefore necessary to take each of these factors into account when selecting controls for autistic subjects and during data analysis. The most problematic of these matching variables is IQ, when IQ falls in the mentally retarded range. The mentally retarded population is a very diverse and heterogenous population with usually undefined deficits and etiologies, the impact of which on MRI measurements are unknown. There are no simple solutions to this issue, but an average-IQ comparison group should probably be considered in addition to a mentally retarded group. In autistic subjects, the disparity between Verbal and Performance IQ is also a factor that should be addressed in the context of the structural–functional issues of the study. However, the larger issue in relation to controls at present is the lack of clinical normative values for the measurements being generated. The range of values in the normal population, the effect of age, sex, and IQ on these values, and the clinical correlations with abnormal values are all significant unknowns. Two studies that have provided some normative data (Schaefer *et al.*, 1990; Schaefer, Thompson, Bodensteinet, Gingold, Wilson, & Wilson, 1991) on a few midline structures have also found significant variability in the size of these structures within the normal population.

The resolution of these methodologic problems is essential to imaging research. However, their resolution will not remove the inherent limitation of gross structural measurements as an index of the integrity of CNS structures. Many subcellular structural, metabolic, and dynamic abnormalities will not be reflected in measurable differences in the overall size of a brain structure.

The neuropathologic anatomy of the brainstem has been investigated by Bauman and Kemper (1985, 1986), who noted essentially the absence of abnormality in the brainstem, including in the inferior olivary nuclei that have connections with abnormal cerebellar structures.

Neurological Localization and the Brainstem

At present, then, there is no compelling evidence for functional or structural abnormalities of the brainstem in autism. Furthermore, there is no clinical or neurologic evidence to support a direct or indirect role of the brainstem in the pathogenesis of autism. The brainstem is a compact structure of densely packed motor and sensory tracts and cranial nerve nuclei. The central area contains structures involved in respiration, heart rate, and arousal. Brainstem dysfunction classically results in clinical syndromes characterized by a combination of signs referable to sensory and motor tracts and cranial nerve nuclei; involvement of medullary structures is associated with basic alterations in vital functions and level of consciousness. These signs are absent in autism. Furthermore, neither acquired disease of the brainstem (stroke, trauma, or tumor) nor congenital dysplasia of the brainstem (Arnold-Chiari malformation) is known to cause the types of clinical deficits seen in autism. Hence, there is no existing evidence that a structurally abnormal brainstem or the projections from such an abnormal brainstem give rise to clinical findings of the type associated with autism. Similarly, there is no support for a neurotransmitter imbalance in mesencephalic dopaminergic neurons as a cause for autisticlike signs and symptoms, since individuals with Parkinson's disease and individuals with pharmacologic alterations in the CNS dopamine system do not develop the signs or symptoms of autism. In addition, there has been no consistent evidence of CSF alterations in dopamine metabolism in autism, nor does pharmacologic manipulation of the dopamine system in autistic individuals result in improvement of the core signs and symptoms of autism.

Summary

In conclusion, there does not appear to be evidence at present of any significant structural or functional abnormalities of the brainstem in autism, nor is there precedence in the neurology literature to support a connection between the brainstem or its development and autism. Minor abnormalities may exist in sophisticated measures of oculovestibular and oculomotor function, but these abnormalities are subtle and do not fall in the clinically significant range; certainly their magnitude relative to the severity of this clinical syndrome would not support an etiologic relationship. Finally, there is clear documentation of the integrity and constancy of sensory transmission to the cortex and of elementary sensory perception, making it unlikely that autism is the consequence of sensory inconstancy. Further investigation of sensory perceptual and attentional abilities in autism is needed to address hypothesized deficits in these functions.

THE CEREBELLUM IN AUTISM

A cerebellar origin for autism has been recently proposed, based on the initial reports of MRI abnormalities. However, these radiologic findings are dependent on a control group that was selected from radiologic files and have not yet been replicated. As with the brainstem, there is little neurologic or clinical evidence to support a primary role for the cerebellum in autism.

Cerebellar Theories

A cerebellar theory of the pathogenesis of autism was recently proposed based on the observation of hypoplasia of vermal lobules VI and VII on sagittal MRI (Courchesne, Hesselink, Jernigan, & Yeung-Courchesne, 1987; Courchesne, Yeung-Courchesne, Press, Hesselink, & Jernigan, 1988). This theory initially hypothesized intrinsic dysfunction of the cerebellum as the direct cause of the clinical syndrome of autism, emphasizing the role of the cerebellum in learning paradigms and speech modulation. This theory was subsequently modified to reflect better both the MRI findings and their prior cognitive evoked-potential findings and now hypothesizes that abnormal cerebellar projections result in an abnormality in cortical mechanisms for selective attention (Courchesne, Lincoln, *et al.*, 1985; Courchesne, Lincoln, Yeung-Courchesne, Elmasian, & Grillon, 1989).

Evidence of Structural Abnormalities

Recent neuropathologic and neuroimaging studies have provided evidence of structural abnormalities in the cerebellar hemispheres and in the vermis, respectively. Bauman and Kemper (1985, 1986, 1990) have reported bilateral and symmetric atrophy of the lateral and inferior regions of the cerebellar hemispheres (neocerebellar cortex) characterized by marked loss of Purkinje cells and a moderate loss of granule cells in seven autopsy cases. In five cases, these findings were confined to the neocerebellar cortex, but in one case there was more widespread involvement of the hemispheres, and in one case the vermis was also affected. In addition, the cerebellar roof nuclei (which are connected to neocerebellar cortex) contained reduced numbers of neurons, and the remaining neurons appeared small and pale. Areas of the inferior olivary nucleus in the brainstem with connections to the abnormal cerebellar cortex failed to show retrograde cell loss. The loss of Purkinje cells with preservation of the olivary neurons suggests that this pathological process in the cerebellum probably occurred prior to the establishment of the close relationship between the olivary neurons and the Purkinje cells at 30 weeks of gestation. The primary neuropathologic abnormality in the cerebellum in autism appears to be in the inferior and lateral region of the hemisphere or neocerebellar cortex, and the findings in the roof nuclei and the olivary nuclei appear to be secondary to this abnormality. Further examination of the histologic features of this cerebellar circuitry in autism suggests that it represents the persistence of a fetal pattern of circuitry due to the failure to develop more mature circuitry, and this fetal circuitry appears to be subject to premature deterioration in adolescence or early adulthood (Raymond, Bauman, & Kemper, 1989). This cerebellar abnormality does not appear to be related to clinical severity, and in fact, the highest-functioning case had the most extensive involvement of the cerebellar hemispheres.

Courchesne and colleagues (Courchesne, Hesselink, *et al.*, 1987; Courchesne *et al.*, 1988) have reported hypoplasia of cerebellar vermal lobules VI and VII and of the paramedian regions of the cerebellar hemispheres (Murakami, Courchesne, Press, Yeung-Courchesne, & Hesselink, 1989) on MRI of 18 high-functioning young adult autistic individuals as compared to controls drawn from radiologic files. These abnormalities were not related to the clinical severity of the autism. Other investigators studying a younger autistic population (6–22 years) have not found MRI differences in vermal size (Gaffney *et al.*, 1988; Garber *et al.*, 1989; Ritvo & Garber, 1988). A decrease in the size of the cerebellum was reported in the coronal plane (Gaffney, Tsai, *et al.*, 1987), but not in the sagittal or axial planes (Gaffney, Kuperman, *et al.*, 1987, 1988, 1989). One CT study (Bauman *et al.*,

1985) also reported cerebellar atrophy. Further studies are clearly needed to resolve these discrepancies and to determine the distribution, prevalence, and time course of cerebellar MRI abnormalities.

At present, it appears that the structural abnormalities described by neuropathologic and imaging methods may be separate phenomena, since there is little overlap in the distribution of the abnormalities reported by these two methods. The neuropathologic studies have reported abnormalities of the inferior and lateral portions of the cerebellar hemispheres (pars lateralis), whereas the MRI abnormalities have involved the posterior region of the vermis and the pars intermedia of the hemisphere. The neuroanatomic observations suggest that the abnormal cerebellar circuits represent persistence of fetal circuitry, and hence will be intact in early life but subject to deterioration later on. In contrast, Courchesne and colleagues propose that the cerebellar abnormalities will be maximal in early life and attenuated in later life, paralleling the severity of the clinical course in autism. The fundamental differences between these theories provide an excellent opportunity for hypothesis testing through studies of cerebellar size and function in relation to chronological age.

Evidence of Cerebellar Dysfunction

Data on cerebellar function in autistic individuals have been very limited thus far. In a recent study of oculovestibular function in autistic children, Ornitz (1985) reported a statistically significant abnormality in only one parameter, the time constant for vestibulocular reflex phase values. This parameter is dependent on the function of the inferior vermis and the oculovestibular pathways in the brainstem. Although there was a statistically significant difference between the autistic and control groups, only two autistic subjects had values that were outside two standard deviations of the normative data.

Minshew *et al.* have recently completed an assessment of oculomotor function (pursuit, saccades, and optokinetic reflexes), oculovestibular function, posturography, motor dexterity, and grip strength in 20 high-functioning autistic individuals between 6 and 40 years of age and in 20 age-, IQ-, sex-, and race-matched controls (Minshew, Furman, Goldstein, & Payton, 1990). No statistically significant differences between the autistic and control groups were present on any parameter when the two groups were compared. When the subjects were divided into those under and over 12 years of age, minor but statistically significant differences were found between autistics and controls over the age of 12 years on two posturography parameters, one oculovestibular parameter, and both motor parameters, but not between groups under the age of 12 years. The data from this study suggest that the overall function of the cerebellum and oculovestibular system in autism is intact, but that there may be subtle abnormalities in diffusely represented pathways between the posterior fossa and the cerebral cortex that may be age related.

Neurological Localization and the Cerebellum

At present, there is neuropathologic evidence of minor structural abnormalities in the neocerebellar cortex of the cerebellar hemispheres that appear to reflect the failure of a more mature pattern of circuitry to develop. In addition, there appears to be a tendency for deterioration to occur in this immature circuitry during adolescence or early adulthood. To date, these findings have not correlated with clinical severity, and the time course for the deterioration is similarly inconsistent with a primary role for these abnormalities in the genesis of the clinical syndrome of autism. Radiologic abnormalities of the cerebellum have been inconsistent, and the major study by Courchesne *et al.* (1988) and Murakami, Courchesne, Press, Yeung-Courchesne, & Hesselink (1989) is based on a single sample of autistic subjects and on controls selected from radiologic files. Hence, these findings await confirmation. That these abnormalities were not present in the study of a younger population runs counter to a cerebellar basis for this clinical syndrome, as the syndrome is most severe early in life. Functional studies of the cerebellar–brainstem circuitry have been largely remarkable for the absence of significant abnormalities, except for very minor abnormalities in parameters dependent on diffusely represented pathways.

From a clinical perspective, there are subtle signs referable to the motor system during the first two years of life that could be the result of cerebellar dysfunction. The early mild clumsiness of gait (when the subjects first begin to walk) and the subtle hypotonia are consistent with, but not exclusive to, a cerebellar localization. These signs could also be the result of "cerebral hypotonia." The deep tendon reflexes in autism are variable, making it difficult to distinguish a cerebral versus cerebellar origin. However, these signs are a subtle and variable part of the clinical syndrome and are not part of the diagnostic criteria for autism.

Studies of the role of the cerebellum in learning have suggested that the cerebellum may play a role in classical conditioned reflex responses, visuospatial learning, and the modulation of affective behavior through connections with the limbic system (Heath, Dempsey, Fontana, & Myers, 1978; LaLonde & Botez, 1986; Leaton & Supple, 1986a, b; Leiner, Leiner, & Dow, 1986; McCormick & Thompson, 1984; Ornitz & Walter, 1975; Thompson, 1983, 1986). The relationship between these findings and the abstraction, language, symbolic play, and social deficits that characterize autism would appear to be remote. There is no data to implicate the cerebellum in the particular types of cognitive and linguistic deficits that characterize autism. Second, congenital absence of the cerebellum is not associated with autism, nor is autism associated with the removal of cerebellar vermal tumors during early childhood.

Summary

In conclusion, the neuropathologic and functional abnormalities of the cerebellum reported to date are minor and do not appear to be clinically significant or to be directly related to the clinical manifestations of autism. The radiologic abnormalities are inconsistent but appear at this time to be more prominent in later life, as do the neuropathologic and functional abnormalities. Although more data clearly are needed to verify these trends, the existing data and the neurologic evidence do not appear to support a significant role for the cerebellum in autism at this time. Rather, the cerebellar abnormalities are more consistent with a marker of a more generalized aberration in neuronal development and could reflect the functional or developmental overlap between the forebrain and the cerebellum.

THE LIMBIC SYSTEM IN AUTISM

The limbic system has been proposed to play a primary role in the pathogenesis of autism, initially in terms of a congenital amnesic theory but more recently in terms of its role in transferring information between sensory cortex and association cortex. Neuropsychologic and language studies have documented the integrity of basic memory processes and have defined specific deficits in social, language, and cognitive areas that cannot be explained at a limbic level. Neuropathologic studies have described histologic abnormalities of the hippocampus and functionally related subcortical structures that are characterized by an underdevelopment of the dendritic tree. These data, together with the pattern of histoanatomic abnormalities observed in the limbic system and related subcortical structures, appear to be most consistent with involvement of the neural network involved in complex information processing (of which the limbic system is a significant component).

Limbic Theories

A limbic localization for the pathogenesis of autism has been proposed for the past 15 years. The original limbic theory, proposing that autism was the result of a congenital amnesic syndrome, was largely based on observations of hippocampal atrophy on pneumoencephalography (Aakrog, 1968). This theory proposed that autism was the result of the congenital absence of the capacity to learn, which resulted in the failure to acquire social, language, and cognitive skills. This theory was substantially strengthened by the report of autisticlike behavior in monkeys following bilateral neonatal medial temporal ablation. Although there was no clinical documentation of an amnesic syndrome in autism, there were reports of memory deficits in autistic children based primarily on the failure of their memories to benefit from cues (Boucher, 1981; Boucher & Warrington, 1976). When later pneumoencephalographic (PEG) studies found predominately unilateral left hippocampal atrophy in autistic individuals, the amnesic theory was modified to postulate primary left temporal lobe dysfunction impeding the acquisition of language as the primary pathophysiologic mechanism in autism (DeLong, 1978). The recent report of bilaterally symmetric neuropathologic abnormalities of the hippocampus and related structures has renewed consideration of the role of memory deficits and the limbic system in the pathogenesis of autism (Bauman & Kemper, 1985).

A nonamnesic limbic theory of the pathogenesis of autism also has been proposed. Damasio and Maurer (1978) emphasized the role of mesolimbic cortex in the transfer of information from primary sensory cortex to association cortex and subcortical structures and in the affective labeling of information during the process of learning. The central relationship of the limbic system to cortical, subcortical, and brainstem structures also was emphasized by Bauman and Kemper (1985) in their description of histoanatomic abnormalities of the limbic system in autism.

Evidence of Structural Abnormalities

The earliest evidence for structural abnormalities of the hippocampus in autism was provided by PEG studies between the 1950s and 1970s, which reported a significant incidence of lateral ventricular enlargement that appeared, in at least some cases, to be related to atrophy of the underlying hippocampal contour (Aakrog, 1968; Hauser, DeLong, & Rosman, 1975; Melchior, Dyggve, & Gylstorff, 1961). However, the more recent neuroimaging studies involving CT and MRI have not found evidence of hippocampal atrophy (Damasio, Maurer, Damasio, & Chui, 1980; Hier, LeMay, & Rosenberger, 1979). In one CT study in which autistic subjects were classified as primary or secondary cases of autism, Damasio *et al.* (1980) observed that structural abnormalities of the brain were confined to those autistic individuals with acquired brain damage. In retrospect, the hippocampal atrophy found in the early PEG studies is likely related to the prevalence of acquired brain damage in the autistic subjects, a factor that has been found to be responsible for a number of the neurobiologic abnormalities reported prior to the 1980s.

Evidence of histologic abnormalities involving the limbic system and related subcortical structures in two autopsy cases of autism was recently reported by Bauman and Kemper (1985). In the forebrain, histoanatomic abnormalities were found in all areas of the hippocampus and subiculum, in the mammillary body, and in selective areas of the septum and the amygdaloid complex (see Figure 4-1). The cytoarchitecture in these areas was characterized by reduced neuronal cell size and increased cell packing density. The neurons appeared immature and their dendritic development truncated. These abnormalities involved hippocampus and functionally related subcortical areas that together project to association cortex and to brainstem reticular structures. Although these observations represent a significant contribution to autism research, the neuropathologic studies are limited by the small number of cases examined so far and the absence of neurochemical studies that might provide more insight on the status of dendritic connections and neurotransmitters.

Attempts to image the hippocampus have been frustrated by the difficulty in visualizing this small structure in sufficient anatomic detail to allow valid measurements of its volume. A recent change in the positioning of the head with respect to

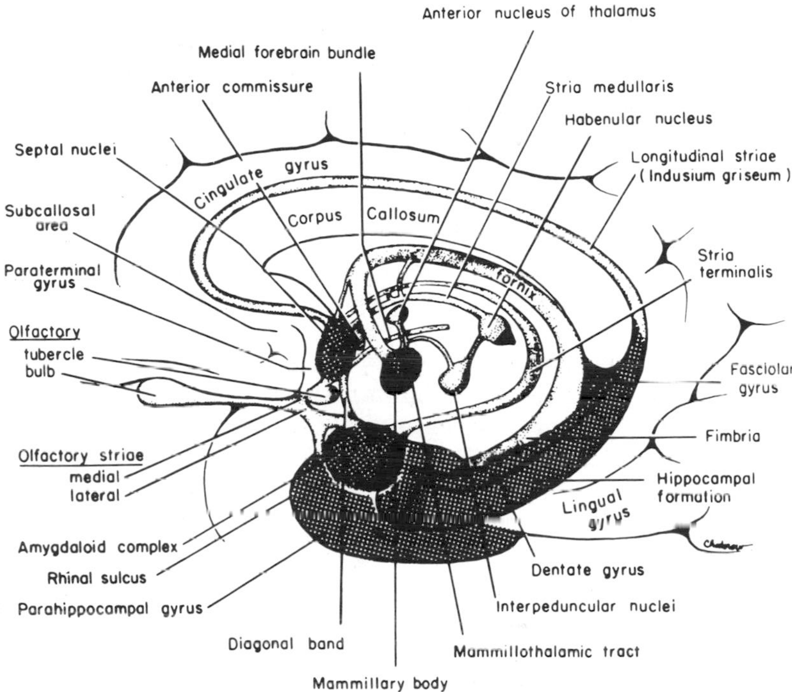

Fig. 4-1. Schematic drawing of the medial view of the right hemisphere shows areas of the limbic system (shaded areas) that have been found to be abnormal in autism. (Adapted from Carpenter, MB: *Core Text of Neuroanatomy*. Baltimore, Williams and Wilkins, 1972. Used with permission.)

the imaging plane has significantly improved hippocampal image quality and will likely lead to volume measurements of this structure in the near future (Press, Amaral, & Squire, 1989).

Evidence of Functional Abnormalities

Perhaps the most commonly cited data in support of limbic dysfunction and an amnesic etiology in autism are the reports of autisticlike behavior in monkeys resulting from congenital medial temporal lobe ablation (Bachevalier, 1990; Mishkin, 1978). Although this lesion model produces significant deficits in social behavior in monkeys, there are substantial reservations regarding its applicability to autism, largely related to the difficulty in determining if the behavioral abnormalities seen in the monkeys represent the same clinical phenomenon seen in humans with autism. Even in low-functioning children, the diagnosis of autism is often difficult, due to the inability to determine if their abnormal behavior has the deviant qualities specific to autism. In addition, autism is defined by a constellation of specific and complex impairments, and the presence of only one or two of the manifestations is not sufficient to differentiate this syndrome from other disorders in humans—and hence not in monkeys, either. However, the most direct evidence on the relevance of this lesioned-monkey model to autism is the case study reported by Maurer (1989) and the neuropsychologic studies of memory in autism. Maurer (1989) has described in detail the deficits in a child with congenital bilateral infarction of medial temporal structures and an amnesic syndrome. Although this child has severe behavior problems as a consequence of the amnesic syndrome, her fundamental social and nonverbal communication skills are intact, and her severe behavior problems have responded to training of habit memory and appropriate structuring of the environment. Nonetheless, this case study and the lesioned-monkey model do suggest that bilateral hippocampal destruction in humans could produce a clinical phenocopy of autism that would be relatively difficult to distinguish from autism in low-functioning patients. As the neuropsychological characteristics of autism are better defined, such acquired cases are likely to be recognized and differentiated from autism.

Neuropsychologic studies of memory in testable autistic individuals have provided evidence for the integrity of basic memory functions and the absence of an amnesiac disorder in autistic individuals (Ameli, Courchesne, Lincoln, Kaufman, & Grillon, 1989; Lockyer & Rutter, 1970; Minshew, Goldstein, & Payton, 1989; Rumsey & Hamburger, 1988; Rutter, 1988). These studies, as well as earlier work, are reviewed in detail in Chapter 3. Clinical observations also substantiate the fundamental integrity of memory in autistic individuals. Many of the classical clinical manifestations of autism are indicative of the integrity of basic memory functions (e.g., their focus on minute details; the remarkable factual repertoire of verbal autistic individuals; and the dramatic reaction of lower-functioning autistic individuals to very minor changes in their environment, with calming when the change is restored to its original state).

Neurological Localization

There is clear neuroanatomic evidence for involvement of the hippocampus and related subcortical structures in the pathophysiology of autism. However, neither the clinical syndrome nor the neuropsychologic studies of memory in autism have supported an amnesic disorder, making an amnesic theory untenable in autism. Furthermore, a limbic localization is not sufficient to explain the type and complexity of deficits seen in autism.

One version of the nonamnesic limbic theory has proposed that a primary deficit exists in the association of emotional "valence," or value, with information. This theory proposes that autistic individuals do not respond to people because the limbic system does not attach the appropriate emotional value to human contact. This theory presupposes that the clinical deficits in autism are all socially based, which is clearly not the case. The cumulated evidence on this clinical syndrome documents concurrent deficits in cognitive, language, and social skills (Rutter, 1988); there is no evidence that any one of these deficits has primacy either in time or in severity (Minshew & Payton, 1988a, b; Minshew & Rattan, 1991). Secondly, such a theory also presumes that the comprehension of information is intact, since failure to react in a normal way to stimuli cannot be attributed to a failure to associate emotional value with stimuli if the individual's ability to understand the information is significantly impaired. Neuropsychologic studies have clearly documented deficits in cognitive and language function that seriously impair the autistic individual's understanding of incoming information.

The more prevalent theory regarding the role of the limbic system in autism is based on the role of the limbic system in the transfer of information between primary sensory cortex and association cortex (Bauman & Kemper, 1985; Damasio & Maurer, 1978). However, regardless of the mechanism proposed, a primary limbic localization is insufficient to explain the clinical syndrome of autism. Deficits have been documented in a number of higher cortical functions fundamental to this clinical syndrome that cannot be explained by dysfunction at the limbic level. Deficits in the comprehension as well as the use of pragmatic, prosodic, and nonverbal language are particularly difficult to localize to limbic and subcortical structure, as are the specific types of deficits in abstraction, problem solving, judgment, symbolic play, and social skills seen in autism.

An alternative interpretation of the histologic findings and the role of the limbic system in autism is suggested by the nature of the histologic abnormalities. The fundamental histoanatomic abnormality reported in the forebrain is the increase in neuronal cell packing density and the underdeveloped appearance of the neurons. Since the number of neurons appears to be normal, the increase in cell packing density is most likely due to a reduction in the neuropil or the neuronal connections to and from the neurons in these structures. This interpretation of the histologic abnormalities is supported by the recent report of truncation of the dendritic tree of these neurons on Golgi preparations, suggesting a curtailment in the development of neural connectivity. These findings suggest that the neuropathologic changes in the limbic system may be a part of or a reflection of a more generalized defect in the connectivity of the neural network involved in complex information processing.

Summary

There is clear documentation of histologic abnormalities of the limbic system and related subcortical structures. However, neuropsychologic studies have not documented deficits in the classical functions associated with the limbic system, and in addition, the deficits present cannot be accounted for by dysfunction at this level. Rather, it appears the histologic abnormalities observed may be part of a more generalized defect in the connectivity of the neural network involved in complex information processing.

THE CEREBRAL CORTEX IN AUTISM

The cerebral cortex has been primarily implicated in the pathogenesis of autism in the neurologic model of Damasio and Maurer (1978) and on the basis of recent neurophysiologic and neuropsychologic data. Structural abnormalities have not yet been identified in cerebral cortex, although a recent nuclear magnetic resonance (NMR) spectroscopy study has reported metabolic abnormalities in the dorsal prefrontal cortex in autism that correlate well with cognitive and language dysfunction. Neuropsychologic, psychologic, and language studies have provided further definition of the deficits associated with autism and suggest fundamental problems with complex information processing but integrity of information acquisition mechanisms. The pattern of these deficits and the absence of focal neurologic deficits associated with localized dysfunction in association cortex suggest primary involvement in autism of a distributed neural network for complex information processing.

Cortical Theories

The cerebral cortex, other than the limbic system, has been secondarily implicated in a number of the theories already discussed, but has only infrequently been proposed as a primary site of the neurobiology in autism. The first major reference to the cerebral cortex in autism was Damasio and Maurer's (1978) proposal of a mesofrontal and mesotemporal localization for many of the social, language, and behavioral abnormalities in autism. This model also proposed involvement of the basal ganglia to explain certain of the other behavioral and motor manifestations. This formulation was based on a clinical analysis of the signs and symptoms of autism, and on analogies drawn to the neurologic localization literature.

In the ensuing decade, neurobiologic findings suggesting intrinsic abnormalities of the cortex have resulted in three cortically based theories. The first of these theories proposed a deficit in auditory processing by parietal cortex based on the initial observation of attenuation or absence of auditory P300s in autism (Novick, Kurtzberg, & Vaughan, 1979; Novick, Vaughan, Kurtzberg, & Simson, 1980). The second theory proposed a primary clinical and biological deficit in cortical selective-attention mechanisms, citing the neurophysiological abnormalities involving frontal and parietal cortex elicited by selective-attention paradigms (Ciesielski, Courchesne, & Elmasian, 1990; Courchesne, Elmasian, & Yeung-Courchesne, 1987; Courchesne *et al.*, 1989; Grillon *et al.*, 1989). A third theory—based on the evoked-potential abnormalities involving parietal and frontal cortices, the aphasic pattern of language development in autism, and the predominate involvement of higher cortical functions in autism—postulated generalized dysfunction of association cortex and the network of intra- and interhemispheric connections involved in complex information processing (Minshew, Goldstein, & Payton,

1989; Minshew & Payton, 1988; Minshew, Payton, & Sclabassi, 1986). This theory was recently restated to propose primary involvement of a distributed neural network for complex information processing, because of the absence of focal deficits involving association cortex (such as those that characterize the syndrome of developmental learning disabilities of the right hemisphere) and the predominance of deficits involving the recognition of complex patterns in information as opposed to the retention of facts.

Evidence of Functional Abnormalities

The first neurobiologic evidence of intrinsic dysfunction of the cerebral cortex was the bilaterally symmetric attenuation or absence of auditory P300 potentials in autistic individuals, despite their ability to attend to and correctly identify the odd stimuli (Novick *et al.*, 1979). This P300 abnormality was subsequently confirmed and further defined by several other laboratories (Courchesne *et al.*, 1984; Courchesne, Lincoln, Kilman, & Galambos, 1985). Abnormalities in a second cognitive potential—the frontally distributed negative component Nc—were first reported by Courchesne, Hesselink, *et al.* (1987), who observed the absence of auditory and visual Nc in autistic individuals, despite their ability to attend to and correctly classify the stimuli. These findings have been replicated in a second autistic population by Ciesielski *et al.* (1990). The P300 and Nc abnormalities have been observed with both auditory and visual paradigms, but the predominant effect appears to be in the auditory modality.

Other evidence of functional abnormalities involving the cortex has been reported, but must be considered preliminary based on inconsistencies in the data and the small number of subjects studied so far. One PET study of 12 young adult autistic men reported an increase in 2-fluoro-2-deoxy-D-glucose (FDG) uptake, and in turn in the metabolic rate for glucose in frontal, parietal, temporal, and occipital cortex, and hippocampus, thalamus, and basal ganglia (Rumsey *et al.*, 1985). Although statistically significant, there was a large degree of overlap in the data between the autistic and control groups. Further analysis of the data from 15 autistic men revealed fewer interhemispheric correlations between homologous regions in the frontal and parietal lobes, and decreased intrahemispheric correlations between the frontal and parietal lobes and the striatum and thalamus (Horwitz, Rumsey, Grady, & Rapoport, 1987). These findings are particularly interesting because of the overlap with the neuropathologic observations showing involvement of many of the same functionally related structures.

Similar trends were noted in a second FDG PET study of 16 autistic children, but were not statistically significant (De Volder, Bol, Michel, Cogneau, & Goffinet, 1987). A third PET study of six autistic adults failed to show any differences in cerebral blood flow, oxygen consumption, or glucose metabolism (Herold, Frackowiak, LeCouteur, Rutter, & Howlin, 1988). All of these studies were performed under resting conditions, which may account for the discrepancies between the findings. Cortical activation techniques are needed to complete this evaluation and may resolve the discrepancies between these studies. PET studies of receptor binding unfortunately have not been reported in autism but, together with the analogous neuropathologic studies, are particularly important to the evaluation of neuronal function and histology in autism.

One study has reported the results of *in vivo* phosphorus-31 (^{31}P) NMR spectroscopy in 11 high-functioning autistic adolescents and adults and 11 closely matched normal controls. Phosphorus-31 NMR spectroscopy can be used to investigate *in vivo* high-energy phosphate metabolism and membrane phospholipid metabolism in the brain by determining the levels of phosphocreatine (PCr), adenosine di- and triphosphates (ADP, ATP), inorganic orthophosphate, the labile high-energy molecules, and the levels of the phosphomonoesters and phosphodiesters (the building blocks and breakdown products of membrane phospholipids). This study reported statistically significant decreases in the PCr and ATP levels and a borderline-significant ($p < 0.07$) increase in the level of phosphodiesters in the dorsal prefrontal cortex of the autistic subject group under resting conditions, suggesting an increase in high-energy phosphate utilization and a possible alteration in brain phospholipid metabolism (Minshew, Pettegrew, *et al.*, 1989). These alterations in the labile energy molecules are consistent with the increase in 2-FDG uptake reported by the PET study of Rumsey *et al.* (1985) and are the opposite of the metabolic hypofrontality that has been observed with ^{31}P NMR spectroscopy in first-break schizophrenic individuals (Pettegrew, Keshavan, & Panchalingam, 1989). When these metabolic findings were compared with performance of the subjects on the Wisconsin Card Sorting Test, the California Verbal Learning Test, the Token Test, and the Test of Language Competence, a number of correlations were present in the autistic group that were not present in the control group. In essence, as cognitive performance declined in the autistic group, the levels of the labile energy molecules and the phosphodiesters rose in the brain, indicating declining energy utilization and an increasing disturbance in membrane phospholipid metabolism.

Neuropsychological, psychological, and language studies have provided further documentation and definition of the cognitive, language, and social deficits in autism (Rutter, 1988), which have significant implications for neural localization. Neuropsychological studies have defined a fundamental cognitive deficit in autism that has been characterized generally, if somewhat inadequately, as a deficit in abstraction. Hence, autistic individuals have been reported to perform poorly on subtests of the Wechsler Intelligence Scales that require verbal abstraction or comprehension, sequencing, and coding, but perform well on subtests dependent on short-term rote memory and visuospatial abilities (Hoffman & Prior, 1982; Lincoln, Courchesne, Kilman, Elmasian, & Allen, 1988; Lockyer & Rutter, 1970; Rumsey & Hamburger, 1988; Rutter, 1988). Autistic individuals have also been shown to make relatively little use of meaning in their memory and thought processes. In addition, they have greater difficulty with the analysis of complex temporal sequences, in contrast to spatial sequences (Courchesne *et al.*, 1989; Fyffe & Prior, 1978; Hermelin, 1976; Hermelin & O'Connor, 1970; Kanner, 1943; Rumsey & Hamburger, 1988; Rutter, 1988; Wing, 1976). Recent neuropsychologic studies have reported deficits on the Wisconsin Card Sorting Test, the Goldsetin–Scheerer Object Sorting Test, and the Trailmaking Test of the Halstead–Reitan Neuropsychology Test Battery (Minshew, Goldstein, & Rattan, 1989; Rumsey & Hamburger, 1988) that suggest problems with inferential or conceptual processing. Studies of memory have provided documentation of the integrity of rote memory functions, the absence of an amnesic syndrome, and the presence of deficits in complex memory processes dependent on an encoding strategy that would facilitate retrieval (Courchesne *et al.*, 1989; Minshew, Goldstein, & Rattan, 1989).

In a clinical extension of the cognitive deficits, Baron-Cohen, Leslie, and Frith (1985, 1986) have reported that autistic individuals are unable to make basic predictions regarding the beliefs or viewpoints that others will have about an event, a cognitive ability that normally develops by 4 years of age. Similarly, Minshew and colleagues have proposed that the cognitive deficit may underlie many of the behavioral abnormalities in the restricted-range-of-interests-and-activities symptom category (Minshew & Payton, 1988a). That is, the failure to understand the symbolic meaning of toys could underlie the lack of interest in toys and the abnormal nature of toy play; the inability to predict the consequences of change could underlie the difficulty in coping with change; the interest in the elementary sensory aspects of objects and in few topics and the focus on details could be the result of the absence of more advanced cognitive analytic capabilities. Language studies have documented deficits in the comprehension of pragmatic, semantic and syntactical language and in the understanding of the conceptual and contextual meanings of sentences and passages, despite comprehension of the meaning of the individual words (Dawson, 1983; Frith & Snowling, 1983; Fyffe & Prior, 1978; Hermelin, 1976; Hermelin & O'Connor, 1970; Lockyer & Rutter, 1970; Minshew, Goldstein, & Payton, 1989; Rumsey, 1985; Rutter, 1988). Deficits also have been recently documented in the comprehension and expression of affective prosody (MacDonald *et al.*, 1989). Finally, recent neuropsychologic and neurophysiologic studies have provided evidence of intact attention and sensory perception (Courchesne *et al.*, 1984; Courchesne, Lincoln, *et al.*, 1985; Grillon *et al.*, 1989; Minshew, Goldstein, & Rattan, 1989; Rumsey & Hamburger, 1988).

In summary, neuropsychologic, psychologic, and language studies have documented deficits in higher cortical functions, primarily involving the detection of complex patterns (e.g., complex information processing). These studies have also provided preliminary evidence of the basic integrity of information acquisition processes (e.g., memory, sensory perception, and attention). Finally, this body of data has provided evidence that the deficits in cognition, language, and social behavior are concurrent. The evidence has not supported any one deficit as being primary either in time or in severity; developmental progress in each of the areas is generally proportionate and linked, suggesting a common neural basis for these deficits (Minshew & Payton, 1988b; Minshew & Rattan, 1991).

Evidence of Structural Abnormalities

Evidence of anatomic abnormalities of the cortex outside of the hippocampus and cingulate gyrus have not yet been reported. The pertinent imaging measurements—sulcal volume as an indirect measurement of cortical volume, and cortical volume measured directly—are either under way or pending new developments in MRI technology. More sophisticated histologic studies including cell counts and neurochemistry also are pending, as are PET studies of receptor content and distribution and further ^{31}P NMR spectroscopy studies.

Neurological Localization

At the present time, there is clinical, language, and neuropsychological evidence of concurrent widespread deficits in complex information processing and neurophysiologic evidence of abnormalities in multimodal (heteromodal) association cortices, but an absence of the focal deficits that may be seen with localized dysfunction of association cortex. The deficits are bilaterally symmetric and do not support a hemispheric theory but suggest more widespread deficits in information processing. This pattern of deficits may be consistent with dysfunction in the distributed neural network for complex information processing.

Current mathematical models of brain information processing propose that the more complex aspects of information analysis are accomplished by distributed neural networks; one such model proposes a parallel circuitry design and parallel distributed processing. A parallel circuit design provides for the concurrent and integrated analysis of information by multiple subcircuits, a design that is maximally suited for the detection of complex patterns. A serial circuit design is, on the other hand, best suited to number crunching but is poor at detecting complex patterns (Mesulam, 1985). The current clinical, neuropsychological, and neurophysiologic evidence in autism suggests that there may be a fundamental deficit in the development of the distributed neural network necessary for complex information processing. In high-functioning autistic individuals, the data suggest that information processing may be operating primarily in a serial mode without the benefit of the parallel distributed processing network. In low-functioning autistic individuals, the more severe deficits of social, language, and cognitive function suggest that there may be an absence of both serial and parallel information processing circuitry, including the fundamental connections with association cortex.

Summary

A review of the neurobiologic literature in autism relevant to neurologic localization highlights histologic abnormalities in the hippocampus and functionally related subcortical structures that are indicative of underdevelopment of the neuronal dendritic tree, neurophysiologic abnormalities of parietal and frontal cortex, and a pattern of deficits in higher cortical functions consistent with a generalized problem in the detection of complex patterns in information. Studies also have provided evidence of the integrity of the basic mechanisms involved in information acquisition. Evidence for abnormalities at lower levels in the central nervous system is insufficient at this time and in the context of the neurologic literature to support an etiologically significant role for these structures in autism. Based on the available evidence, it appears that autism may be the consequence of a developmental failure in the distributed neural network involved in complex information processing, and that the histologic abnormalities observed in the forebrain may reflect their role in this system. The available data also documents the need for further research to address each of the hypotheses for the pathogenesis of autism, as the data are very limited in many areas.

REFERENCES

Aakrog, T. (1968). Organic factors in infantile psychoses and borderline psychoses. *Danish Medical Bulletin, 15,* 283–288.

Ameli, R., Courchesne, E., Lincoln, A., Kaufman, A. S., & Grillon, C. (1988). Visual memory process in high-functioning individuals with autism. *Journal of Autism and Developmental Disorders, 18*(4), 601–615.

Bachevalier, J. (1990). Memory loss and socio-emotional disturbances following neonatal damage of the limbic system in monkeys: An animal model for childhood autism. In *Advances in Psychiatry, Vol. 1: Schizophrenia.* New York: Raven.

Baron-Cohen, S., Leslie, A. M., & Frith, U. (1985). Does the autistic child have a "theory of mind"? *Cognition, 21,* 37–46.

Baron-Cohen, S., Leslie, A. M., & Frith, U. (1986). Mechanical, behavioral and intentional understanding of picture stories in autistic children. *British Journal of Developmental Psychology, 4,* 113–125.

Bauman, M. L., & Kemper, T. L. (1985). Histoanatomic observations of the brain in early infantile autism. *Neurology, 35,* 866–874.

Bauman, M. L., & Kemper, T. L. (1986). Developmental cerebellar abnormalities: A consistent finding in early infantile autism. *Neurology, 36,* 190.

Bauman, M. L., & Kemper, T. L. (1989). Abnormal cerebellar circuitry in autism? *Neurology, 39*(1), 186.

Bauman, M. L., & Kemper, T. L. (1990). Limbic and cerebellar abnormalities are also present in an autistic child of normal intelligence. *Neurology, 40*(1), 359.

Bauman, M. L., LeMay, M., Bauman, R. A., & Rosenberger, P. B. (1985). Computerized tomographic (CT) observations of the posterior fossa in early infantile autism. *Neurology, 35*(1), 247.

Boucher, J. (1981). Immediate free recall in early childhood autism: Another part of behavioral similarity with the amnestic syndrome. *British Journal of Psychiatry, 72,* 211–215.

Boucher, J., & Warrington, E. K. (1976). Memory deficits in early infantile autism: Some similarities to the amnesic syndrome. *British Journal of Psychiatry, 67,* 73–87.

Ciesielski, K. T., Courchesne, E., & Elmasian, R. (1990). Effects of focused selective attention tasks on event-related potentials in autistic and normal individuals. *Electroencephalography and Clinical Neurophysiology, 75,* 207–220.

Colbert, E. G., Koegler, R. R., & Markham, C. H. (1959). Vestibular dysfunctions in childhood schizophrenia. *Archives of General Psychiatry, 1,* 600–617.

Courchesne, E., Elmasian, R. O., & Yeung-Courchesne, R. (1987). Electrophysiological correlates of cognitive processing: P3b and Nc, basic, clinical and developmental research. In A. M. Halliday, S. R. Butler, & R. Paul (Eds.), *A textbook of clinical neurophysiology*. Sussex, England: John Wiley & Sons.

Courchesne, E., Hesselink, J. R., Jernigan, T. L., & Yeung-Courchesne, R. (1987). Abnormal neuroanatomy in a non-retarded person with autism. *Archives of Neurology, 44,* 335–341.

Courchesne, E., Kilman, B. A., Galambos, R., & Lincoln, A. J. (1984). Autism: Processing of novel auditory information assessed by event-related brain potentials. *Electroencephalography and Clinical Neurophysiology, 59*(3), 238–248.

Courchesne, E., Lincoln, A. J., Kilman, B. A., & Galambos, R. (1985). Event-related brain potential correlates of the processing of novel visual and auditory information in autism. *Journal of Autism and Developmental Disorders, 15*(1), 55–76.

Courchesne, E., Lincoln, A. J., Yeung-Courchesne, R., Elmasian, R., & Grillon, C. (1989). Pathophysiologic findings in non-retarded autism and receptive developmental language disorders. *Journal of Autism and Developmental Disorders, 19,* 1–17.

Courchesne, E., Yeung-Courchesne, R., Hicks, G., & Lincoln, A. J. (1985). Functioning of the brain stem auditory pathway in non-retarded autistic individuals. *Electroencephalography and Clinical Neurophysiology, 51,* 491–501.

Courchesne, E., Yeung-Courchesne, R., Press, G. A., Hesselink, J. R., & Jernigan, T. L. (1988). Hypoplasia in cerebellar vermal lobules VI and VII in autism. *New England Journal of Medicine, 318,* 1349–1354.

Damasio, A. R., & Maurer, R. G. (1978). A neurological model for childhood autism. *Archives of Neurology, 35,* 777–786.

Damasio, H., Maurer, R. G., Damasio, A. R., & Chui, H. C. (1980). Computerized tomographic scan findings in patients with autistic behavior. *Archives of Neurology, 37,* 504–510.

Dawson, G. (1983). Lateralized brain function in autism: Evidence from the Halstead–Reitan Neuropsychological Battery. *Journal of Autism and Developmental Disorders, 13,* 369–386.

DeLong, G. R. (1978). A neuropsychological interpretation of infantile autism. In M. Rutter & E. Schopler (Eds.), *Autism*. New York: Plenum.

De Volder, A., Bol, A., Michel, C., Cogneau, M., & Goffinet, A. M. (1987). Brain glucose metabolism in children with the autistic syndrome: Positron tomography analysis. *Brain Development, 9,* 581–587.

Fein, D., Skoff, B., & Mirsky, A. F. (1981). Clinical correlates of brainstem dysfunction in autistic children. *Journal of Autism and Developmental Disorders, 11,* 303–315.

Frith, U., & Snowling, M. (1983). Reading for meaning and reading for sound in autistic and dyslexic children. *British Journal of Developmental Psychology, 1,* 329–343.

Fyffe, C., & Prior, M. R. (1978). Evidence of language recoding in autistic children: A re-examination. *British Journal of Psychiatry, 69,* 393–403.

Gaffney, G. R., Kuperman, S., & Tsai, L. Y. (1989). Forebrain structure in infantile autism. *Journal of the American Academy of Child and Adolescent Psychiatry, 28*(4), 534–537.

Gaffney, G. R., Kuperman, S., Tsai, L. Y., & Minchin, S. (1988). Morphological evidence for brainstem involvement in infantile autism. *Biological Psychiatry, 24,* 578–586.

Gaffney, G. R., Kuperman, S., Tsai, L. Y., Minchin, S., & Hassanein, K. M. (1987). Midsagittal magnetic resonance imaging of autism. *British Journal of Psychiatry, 151,* 831–833.

Gaffney, G. R., Tsai, L. Y., Kuperman, S., & Minchin, S. (1987). Cerebellar structure in autism. *American Journal of Disorders of Childhood, 141,* 1330–1332.

Garber, H. J., Ritvo, E. R., Chiu, L. C., Griswold, V. J., Kashanian, A., Freeman, B. J., & Oldendorf, W. H. (1989). A magnetic resonance imaging study of autism: Normal fourth ventricle size and absence of pathology. *American Journal of Psychiatry, 146,* 532–534.

Gillberg, C., Rosenhall, U., & Johansson, E. (1983). Auditory brainstem responses in childhood psychosis. *Journal of Autism and Developmental Disorders, 13,* 181–195.

Grillon, C., Courchesne, E., & Akshoomoff, N. (1989). Brainstem and middle latency auditory evoked potentials in autism and developmental language disorder. *Journal of Autism and Developmental Disorders, 19*(2), 255–269.

Hashimoto, T., Tayama, M., Mori, K., Fujino, K., Miyazaki, M., & Kuroda, Y. (1989). Magnetic resonance imaging in autism: Preliminary report. *Neuropediatrics, 20,* 142–146.

Hauser, S. L., DeLong, G. R., & Rosman, N. P. (1975). Pneumographic finding in the infantile autism syndrome: A correlation with temporal lobe disease. *Brain, 98,* 667–688.

Heath, R. G., Dempsey, C. W., Fontana, C. J., & Myers, W. A. (1978). Cerebellar stimulation: Effects on septal region, hippocampus, and amygdala of cats and rats. *Biological Psychiatry, 113,* 501–529.

Hermelin, B. (1976). Coding and the sense modalities. In L. Wing (Ed.), *Early childhood autism: Clinical, educational and social aspects* (2nd ed.). Oxford: Pergamon.

Hermelin, B., & O'Connor, N. (1970). *Psychological experiments with autistic children.* Oxford: Pergamon.

Herold, S., Frackowiak, R. S. J., LeCouteur, A., Rutter, M., & Howlin, P. (1988). Cerebral blood flow and metabolism of oxygen and glucose in young autistic adults. *Psychological Medicine, 18,* 823–831.

Hier, D. B., LeMay, M., & Rosenberger, P. B. (1979). Autism and unfavorable left–right asymmetries of the brain. *Journal of Autism and Developmental Disorders, 9,* 153–159.

Hoffman, W. L., & Prior, M. R. (1982). Neuropsychological dimensions of autism in children: A test of the hemispheric dysfunction hypothesis. *Journal of Clinical Neuropsychology, 4,* 27–41.

Horwitz, B., Rumsey, J. M., Grady, C., & Rapoport, S. I. (1987). Interregional correlations of glucose utilization among brain regions in autistic adults. *Annals of Neurology, 22,* 118.

Kanner, L. (1943). Autistic disturbance of affective contact. *Nervous Child, 2,* 217–250.

LaLonde, R., & Botez, M. I. (1986). The role of the cerebellum in visuospatial learning: Experimental studies. *Neurology, 36*(1), 263.

Leaton, R. N., & Supple, W. F. (1986a). Cerebellar vermis: Essential for long-term habituation of the acoustic startle response. *Science, 232,* 513–515.

Leaton, R. N., & Supple, W. F. (1986b). Long-term habituation of acoustic startle following lesions of the cerebellar vermis or cerebellar hemisphere. *Abstracts of the Society for Neuroscience, 12,* 978.

Leiner, H. C., Leiner, A. L., & Dow, R. S. (1986). Does the cerebellum contribute to mental skills? *Behavioral Neuroscience, 100,* 443–454.

Lincoln, A. J., Courchesne, E., Kilman, B. A., Elmasian, R., & Allen, M. (1988). A study of intellectual abilities in high-functioning people with autism. *Journal of Autism and Developmental Disorders, 18*(4), 505–524.

Lockyer, L., & Rutter, M. (1970). A five-year follow-up study of infantile psychosis: IV. Patterns of cognitive ability. *British Journal of Social and Clinical Psychology, 9,* 152–163.

MacDonald, H., Rutter, M., Howlin, P., Rios, P., LeCouteur, A., Evered, C., & Folstein, S. (1989). Recognition and expression of emotional cues by autistic and normal adults. *Journal of Child Psychology and Psychiatry, 30,* 865–877.

Maurer, R. G. (1989, February). *A case of congenital amnesic syndrome: A counter-example to theories of limbic system dysfunction as a case of autism.* Presented at the International Neuropsychological Society meeting.

McCormick, D. A., & Thompson, R. F. (1984). Cerebellum: Essential involvement in the classically conditioned eyelid response. *Science, 223,* 296–299.

Melchior, J. C., Dyggve, H. V., & Gylstorff, H. (1961). Pneumoencephalographic examination of 207 mentally retarded patients. *Danish Medical Bulletin, 12,* 38–42.

Mesulam, M. (1985). Patterns in behavioral neuroanatomy: Association areas, the limbic system, and hemispheric specialization. *Principles of Behavioral Neurology,* 1–70.

Minshew, N. J., Furman, J. M., Goldstein, G., & Payton, J. B. (1990). The cerebellum in autism: A central role or an epiphenomenon? *Neurology, 40*(1), 173.

Minshew, N. J., Goldstein, G., & Payton, J. B. (1989). Abstraction and memory deficits in non-retarded autistics: A fundamental deficit? *Neurology, 39*(1), 136.

Minshew, N. J., & Payton, J. B. (1988a). New perspectives in autism, part I: The clinical spectrum of autism. *Current Problems in Pediatrics, 18,* 563–610.

Minshew, N. J., & Payton, J. B. (1988b). New perspectives in autism, part 2: The differential diagnosis and neurobiology of autism. *Current Problems in Pediatrics, 19,* 615–694.

Minshew, N. J., Payton, J. B., & Sclabassi, R. J. (1986). Cortical neurophysiologic abnormalities in autism. *Neurology, 36*(1), 194–195.

Minshew, N. J., Pettegrew, J. W., Panchalingam, K., Payton, J. B., Kaplan, D., & Wolf, G. (1989). *Metabolic alterations in the dorsal prefrontal cortex of normal IQ autistics*. Presented at the Society of Magntic Resonance in Medicine meeting.

Minshew, N. J., & Rattan, A. I. (1991). The clinical syndrome of autism. In I. Rapin & S. Segalowitz (Eds.), *Handbook of Neuropsychology*. Amsterdam: Elsevier.

Mishkin, M. (1978). Memory in monkeys severely impaired by combined but not by separate removal of amygdala and hippocampus. *Nature, 273,* 297–298.

Murakami, J. W., Courchesne, E., Press, G. A., Yeung-Courchesne, R., & Hesselink, J. R. (1989). Reduced cerebellar hemisphere size and its relationship to vermal hypoplasia in autism. *Archives of Neurology, 46,* 689–694.

Novick, B., Kurtzberg, D., & Vaughan, H. G. (1979). An electrophysiological indication of defective information storage in childhood autism. *Psychiatry Research, 1,* 101–108.

Novick, B., Vaughan, H. G., Kurtzberg, D., & Simson, R. (1980). An electrophysiologic indication of auditory processing deficits in autism. *Psychiatry Research, 3,* 107–114.

Ornitz, E. M. (1974). The modulation of sensory input and motor output in autistic children. *Journal of Autism and Childhood Schizophrenia, 4,* 197–215.

Ornitz, E. M. (1978). Neurophysiologic studies. In M. Rutter & E. Schopler (Eds.), *Autism: A reappraisal of concepts and treatment*. New York: Plenum.

Ornitz, E. M. (1985). Neurophysiology of infantile autism. *Journal of the American Academy of Child Psychiatry, 24*(3), 251–262.

Ornitz, E. M. (1989). Autism at the interface between sensory and information processing. In G. Dawson (Ed.), *Autism: Nature, diagnosis and treatment*. New York: Guilford.

Ornitz, E. M., Mo, A., Olson, S. T., & Walter, D. O. (1980). Influence of click sound pressure direction on brainstem responses in children. *Audiology, 19,* 245–254.

Ornitz, E. M., & Ritvo, E. R. (1968). Perceptual inconstancy in early infantile autism. *Archives of General Psychiatry, 18,* 76–98.

Ornitz, E. M., & Walter, D. O. (1975). The effect of sound pressure waveform on human brainstem auditory evoked responses. *Brain Research, 92,* 490–498.

Pettegrew, J. W., Keshavan, M., & Panchalingam, K. (1989). ^{31}P NMR studies in schizophrenia. *Biological Psychiatry, 25*(1), 15.

Piggott, L., Purcell, G., Cummings, G., & Caldwell, D. (1976). Vestibular dysfunction in emotionally disturbed children. *Biological Psychiatry, 11,* 719–729.

Pollack, M., & Krieger, H. P. (1958). Oculomotor and postural patterns in schizophrenic children. *Archives of Neurology and Psychiatry, 79,* 720–726.

Press, G. A., Amaral, D. G., & Squire, L. R. (1989). Hippocampal abnormalities in amnesic patients revealed by high-resolution magnetic resonance imaging. *Nature, 341*(6237), 54–57.

Raymond, G., Bauman, M., & Kemper, T. (1989). The hippocampus in autism: Golgi analysis. *Annals of Neurology, 26*(3), 483–484.

Ritvo, E. R., & Garber, H. J. (1988). Cerebellar hypoplasia and autism. *New England Journal of Medicine, 319*(17), 1152–1154.

Ritvo, E. R., Ornitz, E. M., Eviatar, A., Markham, C. H., Brown, M. B., & Mason, A. (1969). Decreased postrotatory nystagmus in early infantile autism. *Neurology, 19,* 653–658.

Rosenblum, S. M., Arick, J. R., Krug, D. A., Stubbs, E. G., Young, N. B., & Pelson, R. O. (1980). Auditory brainstem evoked responses in autistic children. *Journal of Autism and Developmental Disorders, 10,* 215–225.

Rumsey, J. M. (1985). Conceptual problem-solving in highly verbal nonretarded autistic men. *Journal of Autism and Developmental Disorders, 15,* 23–36.

Rumsey, J. M., Duara, R., Grady, C., Rapoport, J. L., Margolin, R. A., Rapoport, S. I., & Cutler, N. R. (1985). Brain metabolism in autism. *Archives of General Psychiatry, 42,* 448–455.

Rumsey, J. M., Grimes, A. M., Pikus, A. M., Duara, R., & Ismond, D. (1984). Auditory brainstem responses in pervasive developmental disorders. *Biological Psychiatry, 19,* 1403–1417.

Rumsey, J. M., & Hamburger, S. D. (1988). Neuropsychological findings in high-functioning men with infantile autism, residual state. *Journal of Clinical and Experimental Neuropsychology, 10,* 201–221.

Rutter, M. (1988). Biological bases of autism: Implications for intervention. In F. J. Menolascino & J. A. Stark (Eds.), *Preventive and curative intervention in mental retardation.* New York: Paul H. Brooks.

Schaefer, G. B., Thompson, J. N., Bodensteiner, J. B., Gingold, M., Wilson, M., & Wilson, D. (1991). Age related changes in the relative growth of the posterior fossa. *Journal of Child Neurology, 6,* 15.

Schaefer, G. B., Thompson, J. N., Bodensteiner, J. B., Hamza, M., Tucker, R., Marks, W. A., Gay, C. T., and Wilson, D. (1990). Quantitative morphometric analysis of brain growth utilizing quantitative analysis of magnetic resonance imaging. *Journal of Child Neurology, 5,* 127.

Skoff, B. F., Mirsky, A. F., & Turner, D. (1980). Prolonged brainstem transmission time in autism. *Psychiatry Research, 2,* 157–166.

Student, M., & Sohmer, H. (1978). Evidence from auditory nerve and brainstem evoked responses for an organic brain lesion in children with autistic traits. *Journal of Autism and Child Schizophrenia, 8,* 13–20.

Student, M., & Sohmer, H. (1979). Erratum. *Journal of Autism and Developmental Disorders, 9*(3), 309.

Tanguay, P. E., & Edwards, M. R. (1982). Electrophysiological studies of autism: The whisper of the bang. *Journal of Autism and Developmental Disorders, 12,* 177–184.

Tanguay, P. E., Edwards, R. M., Buchwald, J., Schwafel, J., & Allen, V. (1982). Auditory brain stem evoked responses in autistic children. *Archives of General Psychiatry, 38,* 174–180.

Taylor, M. J., Rosenblatt, B., & Linschoten, L. (1982). Auditory brainstem response abnormalities in autistic children. *Journal of Canadian Science and Neurology, 9,* 429–434.

Thompson, R. F. (1983). Neuronal substrates of simple associative learning: Classical conditioning. *Trends in Neuroscience, 6,* 270–275.

Thompson, R. F. (1986). The neurobiology of learning and memory. *Science, 223,* 941–947.

Wing, L. (1976). Diagnosis, clinical descriptions, and prognosis. In L. Wing (Ed.), *Early childhood autism: Clinical, educational, and social aspects* (2nd ed.). Oxford: Pergamon.

5

A Parent's View of More Able People with Autism

SUSAN MORENO

INTRODUCTION

I want you to try to see through my eyes for just a little while, so that I can help you understand the experience of parenting a more able autistic child. I will attempt to describe some of the feelings and situations that my husband, Marco, and I experienced both separately and together during the last 17 years, and to delineate some of the basic issues that are part and parcel of raising a more able person with autism. I will try to combine these experiences with those communicated to me by other parents around the country.

In this chapter I give my personal viewpoint about the major issues common to parents of more able autistic people. Then I give advice to nonparents on what to do and what not to do to be supportive of these parents. In the last section, I share what I consider to be the good things in my life that are a direct result of parenting my daughter, Beth, who is a more able person with autism.

Beth is currently a junior in high school who maintains a B average, plays the violin in her high school orchestra, and sings in her high school a cappella choir. She hopes to attend college after high school.

The material at the beginning of the chapter is so serious that it may weigh heavily upon parents of younger people with autism. For those parents, I anticipate that the last part of the chapter will cheer them substantially. A further cheerful note is that I have been dealing with these issues for 17 years, and I regard myself as definitely living a very happy and productive life.

The suggestions to people who are not parents are given in the spirit of cooperation and mutual respect that I share with my extended family, friends,

---

SUSAN MORENO • MAAP, P.O. Box 524, Crown Point, Indiana 46307.

High-Functioning Individuals with Autism, edited by Eric Schopler and Gary B. Mesibov. Plenum Press, New York, 1992.

teachers, and other professionals I have dealt with on behalf of my daughter. I would ask nonparents to please bear with all of the "do not" suggestions and accept them for their positive intent—that of making life a little easier for parents of these rare and wonderful people.

ISSUES IN THE PARENTING PROCESS

The experience of parenting a more able person with autism involves coping with may issues. Some of these issues are dealt with only once or twice in a lifetime. Many occur on a frequent basis. The difficulty or facility of dealing with these issues varies greatly from parent to parent, depending on the individual's personality, available emotional and financial support, availability of appropriate schooling and other services for the person with autism, and the level of difficulties of the autistic loved one.

The first issue that I vividly remember dealing with was that of *getting a diagnosis* on our daughter. We went through the typical experience of wondering if there was something wrong with our child, but being reassured by family and physicians that she was fine. This, of course, led us to the lovely conclusion that if there was nothing wrong with our child, then we must be the worst parents ever put on earth. After all, she didn't want to be cuddled, wouldn't look at us, screamed inconsolably for hours on end, and slept only about 2 hours in every 24.

When our daughter was 2, we moved to Los Angeles and encountered a pediatrician who said, "You seem like intelligent, caring parents. Therefore, although I don't see anything wrong with this child, your concerns should be addressed by thorough testing." He referred us to a diagnostic clinic in the area, where Beth received an excellent, multidisciplinary workup. We were so very lucky to find a pediatrician who listened to us and respected us as parents!

During this workup, we began to deal with the next issue—*how to cope with the medical and psychological bureaucracy*. It is, at best, a nightmare. In her book about raising her autistic daughter, Clara Park tells of attending clinics where her observations were disregarded, and another where they did not want even to meet her daughter during the initial diagnostic visit (Park, 1982). My husband and I were made to feel incompetent, unimportant, and a nuisance by many of the medical personnel who tested our daughter. Our suggestions about the best ways to get her cooperation and not upset her were ignored. Luckily, this was not true of the psychology staff that worked with us. Finally, we began to see ourselves as consumers and to speak up for her rights and comforts.

Next, we faced the issue of *receiving the diagnosis and the shock and mourning that followed*. The staff of the clinic that gave us Beth's diagnosis did so in a compassionate and supportive way. However, I remember that my shock was so great that my ears were ringing and my nose stung as if I had been hit in the head. An odd dialogue continuously raced through my brain: "Don't cry. Don't scream. Don't let these strangers see you crack. Remember to be polite—they are only trying to help." I think my shock was so great because I was one of those parents who had received some information about autism before the diagnosis. I knew that it was a serious, lifelong disability. Dr. Kenneth Moses (1987) claims that parents of disabled children go through a mourning process when they learn of their child's disability. It is as if the child they have dreamed about suddenly is missing, replaced by a child with a very different future. I definitely feel that this was the case for Marco and me. Our hearts broke; we felt angry, guilty, and afraid. This unique mourning is not an experience that goes in exact stages and then goes away. It stays with parents on and off and in varying degrees for the rest of their lives. Time and living may resolve it somewhat, but it still resurfaces when least expected.

We were fortunate that the staff at the diagnostic clinic in Los Angeles told us immediately that this autism was not our fault and that they felt we were good parents. They also offered us immediate help and information. This type of positive experience is still quite rare for the parents who write to me. Many of them are treated as failures who have produced damaged goods. Others are treated well, but do not get much direction on how to go about helping their child. We were given short, understandable books and articles to read about behavior management and autism. I emphasize the word *short* because giving parents whose time and energy are already taxed to their limits huge, technical books to read just further frustrates them. It is ludicrous to tell parents to read a 350-page book that is going to show them how to help their child when each day these parents face time-management problems greater than those of corporate executives.

The early years of parenting a more able person with autism are troubled times. A source of strength for people in time of trouble is *extended family and friends. This support system often fails* for parents of more able autistic people and becomes another issue.

One of my most painful memories is of hearing extended family members say, "There is nothing wrong with Beth; you are just imagining all of this." That was like being "gaslighted," as the old term goes. If only those family members would have said, "We love you. We trust you. We're sorry that you are so worried about her. We don't understand all of your concerns, but we care." The "you're just imagining this" dialogue made me think that on top of the fact that my daughter was acting crazy, I was crazy too. In fairness to my family, I think that they were denying what they could not yet handle.

Since we were suddenly serious most of the time and weren't always ready for fun and games, many of our more superficial friends dropped us socially. This was a hard thing to go through at the time, but I now look back on it as a refining process that showed us how precious our real friends were.

The issue of *where to go to get the best help* for a more able autistic child is one that begins with the parents' first awareness of symptoms. Basically, this problem never ends. The first step, in my opinion, is internal. Parents need to find and read as much pertinent information as possible. For parents of more able autistic children this is especially difficult, since there are still very few books that specifically address this population.

Parents then need to *learn about behavior management and begin to use it in their daily family life.* This often involves physically rearranging the home and changing their responses to behaviors that they may have been reacting to in a certain way for many years. In addition, the child's siblings have to learn to cope with the parents' need to deal with the autistic person's behaviors the instant they occur, which often makes siblings feel like second priorities. When this is added to the guilt and anger that siblings may feel about their autistic brother or sister, it can be devastating. Many Autism Society of America chapters have support groups for siblings to help them cope with all of this. In some marriages, one spouse or the other does not recognize the need for or merit of this behavior management and also feels neglected or unimportant. These adjustments are difficult, but not insurmountable. In addition, when families start to see some positive results from using behavior techniques, they usually become more cooperative and begin to work more like a team.

A good, simple book to help a family in this process is called *Families,* by Gerald Patterson (1971). Another good book is *Progress Without Punishment* (Donnellan, LaVigna, Negri-Shoultz, & Fassbender, 1988), which emphasizes positive approaches to managing behavior. I feel that the negative aspects of behavior management used with an autistic person will come back to haunt a family. With time, the autistic child may begin to think that whoever is bigger and stronger wins. This is certainly not a helpful lesson for someone to learn who may grow to be "bigger and stronger" and who has a high risk of becoming aggressive during adolescence. Teaching our more able autistic loved ones kindness through redirection and reinforcement of the behavior that others desire is certainly more palatable to both parents and caring professionals. These positive techniques sometimes take a little longer for the autistic person to respond to, but they do work and are the best way to go.

Next, parents must start to deal with the issue of *selecting the best school, teacher, and classroom* for their autistic child. This is difficult to discuss, because it is such an individual thing. Parents often call me and ask what we specifically did for our daughter. It is their hope that if they duplicate our efforts as much as possible, their child will progress as well as ours. However, what was right for our daughter as an individual and what was available for us to choose from may not be the same as the needs and options that some other parents may face.

Our daughter began her school experience in a multilabel special education classroom within a regular public school. I personally prefer placements that keep autistic children around nonhandicapped children as much as possible while still meeting their special needs. This sounds simple, but is tantamount to finding the Holy Grail. The individual child has to be considered very closely, objectively, and sensitively. What it all comes down to is that there are no absolute rights or wrongs when selecting these programs. Parents need to use their own parental instincts in combination with good professional advice. I hope that more professionals will realize that there is merit in parental instinct and judgment—after all, parents are the ones who live with these kids day and night.

I also hope that parents will find professionals they trust and then *listen* to them and respect their advice. Only when parents and professionals cooperate, respect one another, and work as a team are the child's very best interests served. When the parents and professionals fight and bicker, trying to prove who is more powerful, the innocent victim is the child.

In the meantime, both at home and at school, there is the constant issue of *teaching social skills*. In my opinion, there is nothing harder to teach, yet more important, than social skills. The context of social skills changes constantly and has an incalculable number of variables. People engaged in social interaction through conversation receive physical cues, auditory cues, visual cues, and sometimes kinesthetic, olfactory, and proprioceptive cues as well. They must read, interpret, and respond appropriately to these cues. In doing so, they must go back and reference a vast social and intellectual repertoire. Finally, each person engaged in conversation must have some sense of what the other participants are experiencing. This is sometimes called empathy. In discussing his conversational efforts during his high school years, a more able young man with autism said

> When I was in high school, I would hear other people say things which were accepted well. Then I would make the same type of remark, but often there was an exchange of glances. . . . Now when I interact in a group and am accepted in a normal way, I feel as though it is some kind of rare victory. . . . Sometimes I latch on to the wrong words as most important and shut out the ones the other person thought were important. It is not a question of hearing the words, but of knowing what is important in the situation and what the other person assumes I already know. (Dewey, 1980)

This is an extremely difficult field and an area of great need for our autistic loved ones. Yet few programs offer social skills training that is appropriate for more able autistic people, because social skills training for people with other disabilities (when it exists) does not emphasize empathy and social repertoire. If both parents and professionals were to begin this training with an autistic person by age 3, they still would never finish teaching all the needed skills. Therefore, as parents we end up doing a lot of this training at home, using techniques such as rehearsal and role-playing.

I also think that some social skills training can be done only by nonhandicapped peers. For example, I consider learning appropriate choices in dress to be a social skill which is best taught by peers. One day early in her high school career, Beth appeared before me ready for school wearing a huge T-shirt that hung below midcalf. The T-shirt had childlike writing on it saying, "See Dick surf." In addition, her outfit included black stretch pants, extra-bulky bobby socks and dirty high-top shoes. I tried in vain to talk Beth out of wearing the outfit, but our dialogue was merely upsetting her before she began what was always for her a challenging day. Therefore, I conceded. All day I worried about her being ridiculed by classmates who already found many of her behaviors to be odd and who would now find her mode of dress to be equally odd. My worst fears were confirmed when immediately after school a sophomore, who was one of Beth's peer mentors and a close friend of the family, called. "I wanted to talk to you about Beth's outfit today," she said. "I know," I replied. "I tried to talk her out of it before school. Did a lot of kids make fun of her?" "No!" she said. "I just wanted to know where you bought that great T-shirt!"

Every day parents deal with the issue of *what to tell family, friends, and peers* to help them better understand and support more able people with autism. When talking to young children about an autistic person, be very careful. Sometimes they latch on to a name they will use as a weapon for teasing later on. Again, this is a judgment call. I still wonder if it would have been better to explain our daughter's condition to the other children in her school when she began "regular" class. We waited to tell her class as a whole about her until she was in junior high. Before then, we did very basic explanations to a few individual peers. This was mainly because we kept hoping that she would "blend in" with her peers. In retrospect, I feel we made a serious error.

The next issue parents deal with is *learning how to deal realistically with hope*. An article comes out in the paper about a new medication or treatment philosophy, and parents may hope that they have found a "cure." Balancing reading as much new information as possible and not counting on finding a cure is difficult. According to Bennett Leventhal (1989) and many other leading experts in the field of research on autism, the syndrome of autism as we currently understand it is not curable. Parents must decide if this or that new idea should be tried with their child, and they must realize that they will be trying a new therapy—not a cure. I try new ideas if they are morally, intellectually, and financially reasonable to me, but I do not put all my hope on them because such extreme hope is likely to be dashed. That is a real tough lesson to learn.

Time management is often a horrendous problem. To manage a home, a spouse, a job, siblings, and an autistic child is a 30-hour-per-day job. Teachers should beware of expecting a lot of lesson plans to be followed at home. There are many daily activities—activities of daily living, as they are technically called—that go on in the home, and these are skills best taught in the home environment. This is where parents can be great teachers of their own children. These activities of daily living include personal hygiene, making a bed, cleaning a room, setting the table, doing laundry, and a million more things.

My daughter is 17 years old and she does her own laundry, washes and styles her own hair, applies makeup appropriately (according to her peers), can cook a complete meal, and cares for our cats. All those things are important skills that can be taught at home. People with autism are not going to be able to live with minimal supervision as adults if they cannot do these types of things for themselves. There are many abstract cognitive skills that they learn from these activities as well.

The issue of *whether or not to medicate* the more able person with autism may come up at any time. The need to use psychotropic, sedative, or stimulant medications may arise from poor attention span, hyperactivity, depression, or aggression. The hyperactivity and attention-span problems occur more often in younger people with autism. The depression and aggression are more often problems of adolescence and adulthood. The pros and cons of this issue could be debated at great length.

Parents who suspect that medication may be appropriate for their autistic loved one should consult with a trusted physician. However, ultimately this decision rests with the parents. Because the potential side effects of these medications are indeed serious, parents must weigh the potential benefits of a particular medication against its potential negative consequences.

Planning for the ultimate living environment of the more able person with autism is an immense issue for parents. Unfortunately, most parents are so busy dealing with many other challenging issues that they often put this planning off until much too late. Most parents begin to deal with this issue when their child is a teenager; some even wait until their autistic loved one is an adult. In fairness to those who have waited, many had no idea of how far their child could or would develop until well into, or even beyond, the child's adolescence. Planning done while their child was young might have turned out to be inappropriate later on.

Many of our very high-functioning people with autism even consider living in a group-home situation to be too restrictive for them. Some of the autistic adults who have contacted me through my newsletter are capable of managing their own bank accounts, cooking, housecleaning, doing laundry, obtaining and keeping a job, and using public transportation or even driving. These skills make living in their own apartments or homes a viable option for them. However, parents must still secure job coaches, supportive mentors, and other personnel to help them when things go wrong. Usually the parent ends up doing these things for the autistic person, but parents are not immortal. Therefore, the problem remains of who will do these things for the autistic person when the parents are gone. Many parents think that the siblings will handle these responsibilities. But what if the sibling moves to another part of the country, becomes disabled, or dies? Or perhaps the sibling's job or spouse may prohibit him or her from caring for the autistic loved one.

Let me end the discussion of this particular issue with a piece of advice to parents: Always count on your autistic child's siblings to care *about* your child. Never count on your autistic child's siblings to care *for* your child.

Along with planning for where the autistic person will live as an adult comes *legal and financial planning*. Again, parents should consult with appropriate lawyers, insurance representatives, and other qualified and trusted professionals to deal competently with this issue.

I have mentioned that some autistic teenagers and adults do drive. The issue of *whether or not to encourage more able people with autism to obtain a driver's license* is very controversial. Some people with autism also have seizure disorders; this would prohibit their driving. However, others who do not have seizures may "space out" from time to time. Such episodes when they are not focused on their immediate environment could prove disastrous in a driving situation. In addition, most people with autism have difficulty controlling their tempers and knowing what to do in case of an emergency (e.g., an accident). These difficulties also could cause serious problems in driving. However, not being able to drive can limit the mobility and independence of the person with autism.

Many times, as people with autism improve in their awareness of the world around them, they become lonely and depressed. They become aware of how different they are from others. *Helping the autistic person cope with this loneliness and depression* is one of the most difficult issues a parent must face. This problem often occurs during adolescence, when the child is also coping with puberty and new schooling situations. This is a critical time for the parents to seek help and support from mentors, professionals, peer tutors, and peer companions (whether paid or volunteer).

As a rule, when more able autistic people improve in their social and environmental awareness, they gradually lose some or all of their exceptional skills, such as photographic memory and mental mathematical calculation. This can result in loss of peer support and in less enthusiasm or interest from some professionals.

A young man with autism sent me a poem he had written that I think most profoundly expresses the feeling of rejection that autistic people frequently experience. He uses the pen name of Jim Sinclair. Here is his poem:

I built a bridge
out of nowhere, across nothingness
and wondered if there would be something on the other side.

I built a bridge
out of fog, across darkness
and hoped that there would be light on the other side.

I built a bridge
out of despair, across oblivion
and knew that there would be hope on the other side.

I built a bridge out of helplessness, across chaos
and trusted that there would be strength on the other side.

I built a bridge
out of hell, across terror

and it was a good bridge, a strong bridge,
a beautiful bridge.
It was a bridge I built myself,
with only my hands for tools, my obstinacy for supports
my faith for spans, and my blood for rivets.

I built a bridge, and crossed it,
but there was no one there to meet me on the other side.

As parents, we continually deal with the many challenges of caring for our autistic children. As we and our children get older, we get tired and sometimes feel very worn out. For some parents, this happens earlier and is a bigger problem than for others. Regardless, throughout the parenting experience, parents must learn to deal with *fatigue*. Parents must find some time, however small, to rejuvenate and relax. For some parents this may mean an hour or so a day to themselves. For others this may mean one night a week to go out with friends. This may also mean a week's vacation. Time, availability of respite personnel, and finances will determine how well their needs are met.

During adolescence, it may become clear that the autistic person has areas of scholastic ability that could be pursued at a college level. Those autistic people who are mainstreamed into regular high school hear their classmates discussing which college they will attend and how much fun it will be. Many of these autistic people then want to do the same thing. A few of the most able people with autism do go to college, but usually their social skills deficits or their lack of independence skills cause parents to rule out college as a possibility. *Parents must weigh their autistic child's chances for success in college and then try to find a place that will accommodate their child's special needs.*

The most pervasive issue in *all* stages of parenting a more able person with autism is *learning to take reasonable and intelligent risks.* In order for more able people with autism to reach their highest potential, they must be exposed to everyday situations and responsibilities that will challenge—and sometimes exceed—their capabilities.

For example, in order to have a job, an autistic person must be able to get from home to the workplace. This may involve riding a bike, taking a bus, or even driving through the community. Realistically, not everyone whom they encounter during this commute will know that this person is handicapped. Therefore if the autistic person becomes upset, gets lost, or misses a bus, serious consequences could arise. In training an autistic person to make a commute, the time must eventually come when it is tried alone. This is a definite but necessary risk. Training about what to do in different situations will help prepare the autistic person for the trial run, but something unpredicted may still happen.

If the parent does not allow the autistic person to take these types of intelligent risks, an opportunity for developing important independence skills will be lost. When taking these risks results in psychological or physical pain for the autistic person, parents feel guilty, frustrated, defeated, depressed, or any combination of these feelings. Often extended family, friends, or professionals may judge the situation to indicate that the parent is cruel or incompetent. Regardless, parents must press on and continue to allow their child the dignity of reasonable and intelligent risks.

ADVICE FOR OTHERS WHO CARE

Caring friends, extended family, and professionals often want to know what they should and should not do to be as helpful and supportive as possible to parents of more able people with autism. Some of the advice that I offer here pertains to parenting any handicapped person. The rest is very uniquely specific to parenting a more able person with autism.

1. Do not say, "I know just how you feel." No matter how close you are to the parents, no matter how many parents of handicapped people you may have worked with, you still do not know how we feel. You can empathize with us, but you are not experiencing this process in our place.

2. Do try to include our autistic loved ones in your social gatherings or outings whenever appropriate. Some of my most painful memories of raising my daughter concern her being excluded from birthday and other parties of her classmates, family friends, and neighbors.

3. Do not say, "You must be a very wonderful person for God to have chosen you to have this child." We parents of handicapped children are no stronger, braver, or purer than anyone else. I personally would lose my faith in God if I thought that God chose me or my child to bear this burden. Basically, this well-meaning statement says to us parents that you think this situation hurts and taxes us less than it would you.

4. Do offer us a chance for respite whenever you feel you can. Even a break of an hour can be a great help. When we were living in California and our daughter was 2, a kind neighbor whom I barely knew called me one day when our daughter was about one and a half hours into what turned out to be a three-hour tantrum. I thought she was probably calling to complain about the noise. Instead she offered to come over and be with my daughter while I went to her house and took a swim in her pool. She explained that her teenage son had once had emotional problems that included tantrums, so she felt she could handle the noise and commotion. I did not take her up on her offer, but knowing that I could if necessary gave me the strength and courage to continue.

5. Do not offer unsolicited advice. We parents are often given unwanted and even stupid advice by people who think that they are experts on how to raise our children because their children are normal and ours are not. Our society imposes on parents of handicapped people the terrible prejudice that they have produced damaged goods and are thus inferior people and parents.

6. Do say that you care and ask how you may be of help.

7. Do not say, "But all teenagers/toddlers/young men/girls/etc. do that or have a problem with that." While it is true that what our more able autistic loved ones think, feel, or have difficulties with are common to others, it is the *degree* and *extent* of the difficulty and the impact that it has on their lives and ours that is so very different.

8. If a parent seems unduly upset or discouraged over a particular problem, remember that the problem you see is not the only one the parent is dealing with. The reality is that it is but one of a continual stream of problems.

9. When our autistic loved one is in an activity outside the home (e.g., scouting, church youth group, YMCA activity), do not assume we want to be there with them. This could be an excellent opportunity for the parent to have a break from the autistic person. I often felt that there was a sort of unspoken blackmail conveying the idea that if I wanted my handicapped child in an activity, then I must buy her way in by helping with the activity. I would not have minded if this happened with just one or two of her activities. However, this seemed to be the case in almost every activity.

10. Do not try to cheer a parent by saying, "You don't know for sure that [the autistic loved one] won't ever be able to . . . ." We all have hopes for our children, but we work hardest to habilitate and plan for them when we are *realistic* about their probable future limitations.

11. It is all right to say, "I wish I could say something to make it better, but I don't know what that might be. I hope that the future will be good to you and your child."

12. Regressed behavior in autistic loved ones often causes regressed behavior in parents. When a person with autism is experiencing a regression, parents experience a complete upheaval in their lives. People who have been friendly and supportive often stay away or completely sever their relationships with both the autistic person and the family. Professionals often question what the parents might be doing differently at home to "cause" the regression. This is at best accusatory, and at worst insulting and counterproductive.

During the regression of their autistic child, parents become fatigued, depressed, worried to the point of panic, and more emotional than usual. This tends to shorten our patience and our tempers. Unfortunately this is the time when we need to exercise the greatest strength, patience, and logic toward our autistic child and all with whom he or she comes in contact. All friends, loved ones, and professionals should try to be extra-supportive and patient during this difficult time. Times of regression are part and parcel of being autistic. Seldom, if ever, can the "cause" of the regression be traced to anything that the parent is doing.

13. Parenting any person with autism, regardless of functioning level, is a very challenging experience. Do not assume that because parents have a higher-functioning person with autism, they have fewer or smaller problems. Many parents have told me of incidents in which parents of lower-functioning people with autism have made them feel guilty about expressing their problems.

THE GOOD NEWS

This chapter contains a lot of information that could be depressing to those attempting to raise and nurture a more able person with autism. I want to end this with what I view as the good things in my life that have happened because of my daughter.

I waited five years before my daughter ever looked at me. That moment, in April of 1977, was absolutely miraculous. It was at bedtime, during her nightly bedtime story, right at the part when I would say, "and Beth went to sleep knowing that her Mommy and Daddy loved her." Then I said, "Oh, Beth, I wish that just once you'd tell me you loved me!" Suddenly, she opened her eyes, looked right into mine, and said, "love Mama." It was the most intensely joyous and miraculous experience that I have ever known in my life. For the first time in her young life, I knew that "someone was home." Only those who have lived with or worked closely with autistic people know exactly what I mean by that. I will never, ever take it for granted when she looks at me, and she does it a lot now.

I will never take for granted my daughter washing her hands. It took me six years to teach her that. Now I think that hand washing is the most amazing and wonderful thing. I am also raising another child, Mandy, who is 11. Through her, because of my experience with Beth, I have been able to see the miracle of normal human development.

I never take peace and quiet for granted. I never take smiles and hugs for granted. I never take laughter for granted. What I am trying to say is that I have learned an exquisite joy in very, very small things.

I have learned about human spirit from living with my daughter and seeing her try to help herself, just as much as we have tried to help her. I have learned a lot more about human dignity. And for all of the cruelty that Beth and our family have experienced, I have learned about human kindness from all of the wonderful people who have befriended Beth and who have been kind to us when we needed it most—people who suddenly and unexpectedly have come to our rescue when she was upset or who have included her in their social plans and outings. And I have learned about caring and commitment from the wonderful teachers who have given so much time and energy to Beth and to us.

I have learned that a few good friends are much more valuable than a long list of superficial friends. My friends have stood by me through the best and worst moments. What I appreciate most is their ability to know when I just need to have a good time instead of talking about deep issues. I have been blessed with bright and caring professional mentors who have made themselves accessible whenever I have needed encouragement, information, or advice.

My husband, Marco, has taught me that although the divorce statistics among parents of handicapped children are horrendous, this experience can instead make a marriage stronger than ever.

Those are good things in my life. If I could do it all over again, of course I would have my daughter be born normal, because she has been through such torture. But if my choice were to not have my daughter at all or to have her as she is, I would still choose to have my daughter and to live with autism.

REFERENCES

Dewey, M. (1980, September). *The socially aware autistic adult and child.* Talk given at Warwick, England.

Donnellan, A. M., LaVigna, G. W., Negri-Shoultz, N., & Fassbender, L. L. (Eds.). (1988). *Progress without punishment.* New York: Plenum.

Leventhal, B. (1991, July). *The biochemistry of autism.* Paper presented at the Annual Meeting of the Autism Society of America, Indianapolis.

Moses, K. (1987, Spring). The impact of childhood disability. *Ways Magazine,* 6–10.

Park, C. C. (1982). *The Siege* (3rd ed.). Boston: Little, Brown.

Patterson, G. R. (1971). *Families.* Champaign, IL: Research Press.

6

An Inside View of Autism

TEMPLE GRANDIN

INTRODUCTION

I am a 44-year old autistic woman who has a successful international career designing livestock equipment. I completed my Ph.D. in Animal Science at the University of Illinois in Urbana and I am now an Assistant Professor of Animal Science at Colorado State University. Early intervention at age 2½ helped me overcome my handicap.

Two of the subjects covered in this chapter are the frustration of not being able to speak and sensory problems. My senses were oversensitive to loud noise and touch. Loud noise hurt my ears and I withdrew from touch to avoid overwhelming sensation. I built a squeezing machine which helped me to calm my nerves and to tolerate touching. At puberty, horrible anxiety "nerve" attacks started and they became worse with age. Antidepressant medication relieved the anxiety. In the last section of the chapter directing my fixations into constructive activities and a career will be discussed along with the importance of a mentor. My skill and deficit areas are covered in detail. All my thinking is visual, like videos played in my imagination. Even abstract concepts such as getting along with other people are visualized through the use of door imagery.

LACK OF SPEECH

Not being able to speak was utter frustration. If adults spoke directly to me I could understand everything they said, but I could not get my words out. It was like

TEMPLE GRANDIN • Department of Animal Science, Colorado State University, Fort Collins, Colorado 80523.

High-Functioning Individuals with Autism, edited by Eric Schopler and Gary B. Mesibov. Plenum Press, New York, 1992.

a big stutter. If I was placed in a slight stress situation, words would sometimes overcome the barrier and come out. My speech therapist knew how to intrude into my world. She would hold me by my chin and made me look in her eyes and say *ball*. At age 3, *ball* came out "bah," said with great stress. If the therapist pushed too hard I threw a tantrum, and if she did not intrude far enough no progress was made. My mother and teachers wondered why I screamed. Screaming was the only way I could communicate. Often I would logically think to myself, "I am going to scream now because I want to tell somebody I don't want to do something."

It is interesting that my speech resembled the stressed speech in young children who have had tumors removed from the cerebellum. Rekate, Grubb, Aram, Hahn, and Ratcheson (1985) found that cancer surgeries that lesioned the vermis, deep nuclei, and both hemispheres of the cerebellum caused temporary speech loss in normal children. Vowel sounds were the first to return, and receptive speech was normal. Courchesne, Yeung-Courchesne, Press, Hesselink, and Jernigan (1988) reported that 14 out of 18 high- to moderate-functioning autistics had undersized cerebellar vermal lobules VI and VII. Bauman and Kemper (1985) and Ritvoe *et al.* (1986) also discovered that brains from autistics had lower than normal Purkinje cell counts in the cerebellum. In my own case an MRI scan revealed cerebellar abnormalities. I am unable to tandem walk (the standard "walk the line" test done by the police for drunken drivers). I end up toppling sideways, but my reactions are normal for other simple motor tests of cerebellar dysfunction.

Vestibular stimulation can sometimes stimulate speech in autistic children. Slowly swinging a child on a swing can sometimes help initiate speech (Ray, King, & Grandin, 1988). Certain types of smooth, coordinated movements are difficult for me, even though I appear normal to the casual observer. For example, when I operate hydraulic equipment that has a series of levers, I can operate one lever at a time perfectly. Coordinating the movement of two or three levers at once is impossible. This may also explain why I did not readily learn a musical instrument, even though I have innate musical talent for pitch and melody. The only musical instrument I mastered is whistling with my mouth.

RHYTHM AND MUSIC

Throughout elementary school my speech was still not completely normal. Often it took me longer than other children to start getting my words out. Singing, however, was easy. I have perfect pitch and I can effortlessly hum back the tune of a song I have heard only once or twice.

I still have many problems with rhythm. I can clap out a rhythm by myself, but I am unable to synchronize my rhythm with somebody else's rhythm. At a concert I am unable to clap in time with the music with the rest of the people. A lack of rhythm during autistic piano playing is noted by Park and Youderian (1974). Rhythm problems may be related to some autistic speech problems. Normal babies move in synchronization with adult speech (Condon & Sander, 1974). Autistics fail to do this. Condon (1985) also found that autistics and, to a lesser extent, dyslexics and stutterers have a defective orienting response. One ear hears a sound sooner than the other. The asynchrony between ears is sometimes over one second. This may help explain certain speech problems.

People still accuse me of interrupting. Due to a faulty rhythm sense, it is difficult to determine when I should break into a conversation. Following the rhythmic ebb and rise of a conversation is difficult.

AUDITORY PROBLEMS

My hearing is like having a hearing aid with the volume control stuck on "super loud." It is like an open microphone that picks up everything. I have two choices: turn the mike on and get deluged with sound, or shut it off. Mother reported that sometimes I acted like I was deaf. Hearing tests indicated that my hearing was normal. I can't modulate incoming auditory stimulation. Many autistics have problems with modulating sensory input (Ornitz, 1985). They either overreact or underreact. Ornitz (1985) suggests that some cognitive deficits could be caused by distorted sensory input. Autistics also have profound abnormalities in the neurological mechanisms that control the capacity to shift attention between different stimuli (Courchesne, 1989).

I am unable to talk on the phone in a noisy office or airport. Everybody else can use the phones in a noisy environment, but I can't. If I try to screen out the background noise, I also screen out the phone. A friend of mine, a high-functioning autistic, was unable to hear a conversation in a relatively quiet hotel lobby. She has the same problem I have, except worse.

Autistics must be protected from noises that bother them. Sudden loud noises hurt my ears like a dentist's drill hitting a nerve. A gifted, autistic man from Portugal wrote, "I jumped out of my skin when animals made noises" (White & White, 1987). An autistic child will cover his ears because certain sounds hurt. It is like an excessive startle reaction. A sudden noise (even a relatively faint one) will often make my heart race. Cerebellar abnormalities may play a role in increased sound sensitivity. Research on rats indicates that the vermis of the cerebellum modulates sensory input (Crispino & Bullock, 1984). Stimulation of the cerebellum with an electrode will make a cat hypersensitive to sound and touch (Chambers, 1947).

I still dislike places with confusing noise, such as shopping malls. High-pitched continuous noises such as bathroom vent fans or hair dryers are annoying. I can shut down my hearing and withdraw from most noise, but certain frequencies cannot be shut out. It is impossible for an autistic child to concentrate in a classroom if he is bombarded with noises that blast through his brain like a jet engine. High, shrill noises were the worst. A low rumble has no effect, but an exploding firecracker hurts my ears. As a child, my governess used to punish me by popping a paper bag. The sudden, loud noise was torture.

Even now, I still have problems with tuning out. I will be listening to a favorite song on the radio, and then realize I missed half of it. My hearing just shuts off. In college, I had to constantly keep taking notes to prevent tuning out. The young man from Portugal also wrote that carrying on a conversation was very difficult. The other person's voice faded in and out like a distant radio station (White & White, 1987).

TACTILE PROBLEMS

I often misbehaved in church, because the petticoats itched and scratched. Sunday clothes felt different than everyday clothes. Most people adapt to the feeling of different types of clothing in a few minutes. Even now, I avoid wearing new types of underwear. It takes me three to four days to fully adapt to new ones.

As a child in church, skirts and stockings drove me crazy. My legs hurt during the cold winter when I wore a skirt. The problem was the change from pants all week to a skirt on Sunday. If I had worn skirts all the time, I would not have been able to tolerate pants. Today I buy clothes that feel similar. My parents had no idea why I behaved so badly. A few simple changes in clothes would have improved my behavior.

Some tactile sensitivities can be desensitized. Encouraging a child to rub the skin with different cloth textures often helps. The nerve endings on my skin were supersensitive. Stimuli that were insignificant to most people were like Chinese water torture. Ayres (1979) lists many good suggestions on methods to desensitize the tactile system.

APPROACH–AVOID

In my book *Emergence: Labeled Autistic* (Grandin & Scariano, 1986), I describe craving pressure stimulation. It was an approach–avoid situation. I wanted to feel the good feeling of being hugged, but when people hugged me the stimuli washed over me like a tidal wave. When I was 5 years old, I used to daydream about a mechanical device I could get into that would apply comforting pressure. Being able to control the device was very important. I had to be able to stop the stimulation when it became too intense. When people hugged me, I stiffened and pulled away to avoid the all-engulfing tidal wave of stimulation. The stiffening up and flinching was like a wild animal pulling away. As a child, I used to like to get under the sofa cushions and have my sister sit on them. At various autism conferences, I have had 30 or 40 parents tell me that their autistic child seeks deep pressure stimuli. Research by Schopler (1965) indicated that autistic children prefer (proximal) sensory stimulation such as touching, tasting, and smelling to distal sensory stimulation such as hearing or seeing.

SQUEEZE MACHINE

At age 18 I built a squeezing machine. This device is completely lined with foam rubber, and the user has complete control over the duration and amount of pressure applied. A complete description of the machine is in Grandin (1983, 1984), and Grandin and Scariano (1986). The machine provides comforting pressure to large areas of the body.

It took me a long time to learn to accept the feeling of being held and not try to pull away from it. Reports in the literature indicate that autistics lack empathy (Bemporad, 1979; Volkmar & Cohen, 1985). I feel that the lack of empathy may be partially due to a lack of comforting tactual input.

One day about 12 years ago, a Siamese cat's reaction to me changed after I had used the squeeze machine. This cat used to run from me, but after using the machine, I learned to pet the cat more gently and he decided to stay with me. I had to be comforted myself before I could give comfort to the cat (Grandin, 1984).

I have found from my own experiences with the squeeze machine that I almost never feel aggressive after using it. In order to learn to relate to people better, I first had to learn how to receive comfort from the soothing pressure of the squeeze machine. Twelve years ago I wrote, "I realize that unless I can accept the squeeze

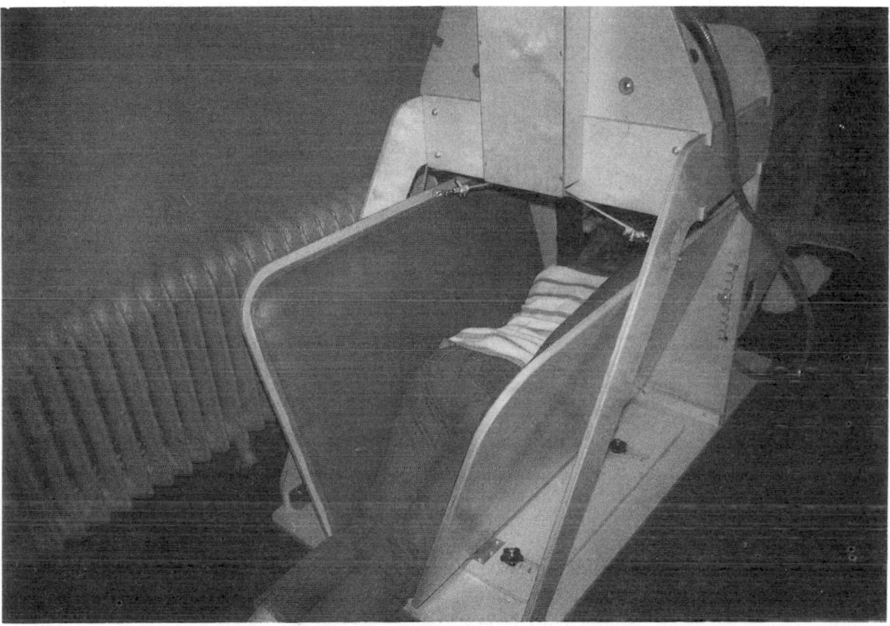

Fig. 6-1. Rear of squeeze machine. Pressure is applied to both sides of the person's body by padded sides.

machine I will never be able to bestow love on another human being" (Grandin, 1984). During my work with livestock, I find that touching the animals increases my empathy for them. Touching and stroking the cattle makes me feel gentle towards them. The squeeze machine also had a calming effect on my nervous system.

Squeeze machines have been in use in clinics working with autistic and hyperactive children (Figures 6-1 and 6-2). Lorna King, an occupational therapist in Phoenix, Arizona, reports that it has a calming effect on hyperactive behavior. Therapists have found that deep pressure stimulation has a calming effect (Ayres, 1979). Both animal and human studies have shown that pressure stimulation reduces nervous system arousal (Kumazawa, 1963; Melzack, Konrad, & Dubrobsky, 1969;

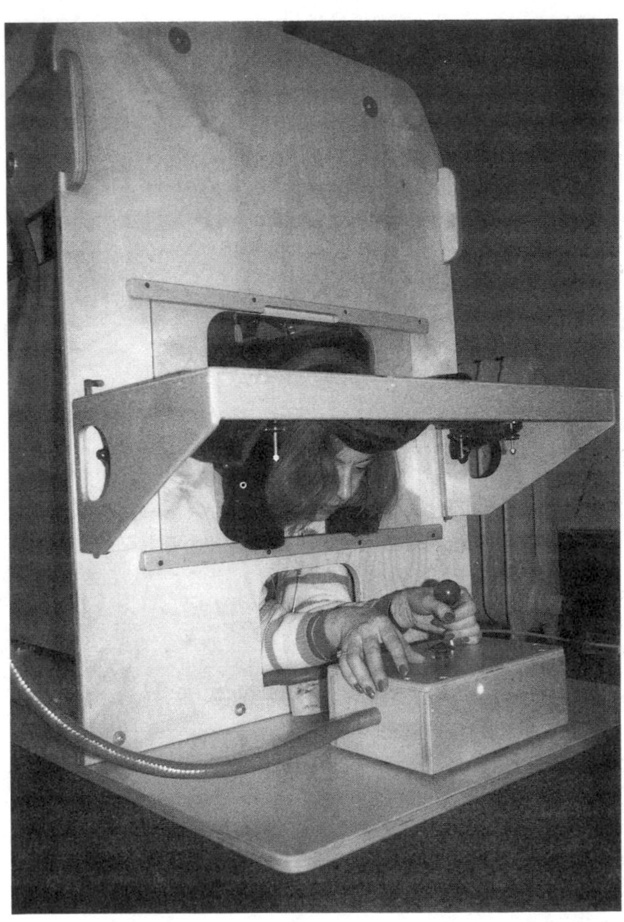

Fig. 6-2. Front view of the squeeze machine. The person using the machine has complete control over it.

Takagi & Kobagasi, 1956). Pressure on the sides of the body will induce relaxation in pigs (Grandin, Dodman, & Shuster, 1989).

ANXIETY AT PUBERTY

As a child I was hyperactive, but I did not feel "nervous" until I reached puberty. At puberty, my behavior took a bad turn for the worse. Gillberg and Schaumann (1981) describe behavior deterioration at puberty in many autistics. Shortly after my first menstrual period, the anxiety attacks started. The feeling was like a constant feeling of stage fright all the time. When people ask me what it is like I say, "Just imagine how you felt when you did something really anxiety provoking, such as your first public speaking engagement. Now just imagine if you felt that way most of the time for no reason." I had a pounding heart, sweaty palms, and restless movements.

The "nerves" were almost like hypersensitivity rather than anxiety. It was like my brain was running at 200 miles an hour, instead of 60 miles an hour. Librium and Valium provided no relief. The "nerves" followed a daily cycle and were worse in the late afternoon and early evening. They subsided late at night and early in the morning. The constant nervousness would go in cycles, with a tendency to be worse in the spring and fall. The "nerves" also subsided during menstruation.

Sometimes the "nerves" would manifest themselves in other forms. For weeks I had horrible bouts of colitis. When the colitis attacks were active, the feeling of "stage-fright" nerves went away.

I was desperate for relief. At a carnival I discovered that riding on the Rotor ride provided temporary relief. Intense pressure and vestibular stimulation calmed my nerves. Bhatara, Clark, Arnold, Gunsett, and Smeltzer (1981) have found that spinning in a chair twice each week reduces hyperactivity in young children.

While visiting my aunt's ranch, I observed that cattle being handled in a squeeze chute sometimes relaxed after the pressure was applied. A few days later I tried the cattle squeeze chute, and it provided relief for several hours. The squeeze machine was modeled after a squeeze chute used on cattle. It had two functions: (1) to help relax my "nerves" and (2) to provide the comforting feeling of being held. Prior to building the squeeze machine, the only other way I could get relief was strenuous exercise or manual labor. Research with autistics and mentally retarded clients has shown that vigorous exercise can decrease stereotypies and disruptive behavior (McGimsey & Favell, 1988; Walters & Walters, 1980). There are two other ways to fight the nerves: fixate on an intense activity, or withdraw and try to minimize outside stimulation. Fixating on one thing had a calming effect. When I was livestock editor for the *Arizona Farmer Ranchman,* I used to write three articles in one night. While I was typing furiously I felt calmer. I was the most nervous when I had nothing to do.

With age, the nerves got worse. Eight years ago, I had a stressful eye operation that triggered the worst bout of "nerves" in my life. I started waking up in the middle of the night with my heart pounding and obsessive thoughts about going blind.

MEDICATION

In the next section, I am going to describe my experiences with medication. There are many autism subtypes, and a medication that works for me may be useless for another case. Parents of autistic children should obtain medical advice from professionals who are knowledgeable of the latest medical research.

I read in the medical library that antidepressant drugs such as Tofranil (imipramine) were effective for treating patients with endogenous anxiety and panic (Sheehan, Beh, Ballenger, & Jacobsen, 1980). The symptoms described in this paper sounded like my symptoms, so I decided to try Tofranil. Fifty mg of Tofranil at bedtime worked like magic. Within a week, the feelings of nervousness started to go away. After being on Tofranil for four years I switched to 50 mg Norpramin (desipramine), which has fewer side effects. These pills have changed my life. Colitis and other stress-related health problems were cured.

Dr. Paul Hardy in Boston has found that Tofranil and Prozac (fluoxetine) are both effective for treating certain high-functioning autistic adolescents and adults. Both Dr. Hardy and Dr. John Ratey (personal communication, 1989) have learned that very small doses of these drugs must be used. These doses are usually much lower than the dose prescribed for depression. Too high a dose can cause agitation, aggression, or excitement, and too low a dose will have no effect. My "nerve" attacks would go in cycles, and I have had relapses while on the drug. It took will power to stick with the 50 mg dose and let the relapse subside on its own. Taking the medicine is like adjusting the idle screw on a car's carburetor. Before taking the drug, the engine was racing all the time. Now it runs at normal speed. I no longer fixate, and I am no longer "driven." Prozac and Anafranil (clomipramine) have been very effective in autistics who have obsessive–compulsive symptoms or obsessive thoughts which race through their heads. The effective doses for Prozac have ranged from two 20 mg capsules per week to 40 mg per day. Too high a dose will cause agitation and excitement. If an autistic person becomes agitated the dose should be lowered. Other promising drugs for aggressive autistic adolescents and adults are beta blockers. Beta blockers greatly reduce aggressive behavior (Ratey *et al.*, 1987).

SLOW IMPROVEMENT

During the eight years I have been taking antidepressants, there has been a steady improvement in my speech, sociability, and posture. The change was so gradual that I did not notice it. Even though I felt relief from the "nerves" immediately, it takes time to unlearn old behavior patterns.

Within the last year, I had an opportunity to visit an old friend who had known me before I started taking antidepressants. My friend, Billie Hart, told me I was a completely different person. She said I used to walk and sit in a hunched-over position and now my posture is straight. Eye contact had improved, and I no longer shifted around in my chair. I was also surprised to learn that I no longer seemed to be out of breath all the time, and I had stopped constantly swallowing.

Various people I have met at autism meetings have seen steady improvement in my speech and mannerisms throughout the eight-year period I have taken the medicines. My old friend, Lorna King, also noticed many changes. "Your speech used to seem pressured, coming in almost explosive bursts. Your old tendency to perseverate is gone" (Grandin & Scariano, 1986).

I had an odd lack of awareness of my oddities of speech and mannerisms until I looked at videotapes. I think videotapes could be used to help many high-functioning autistics with speech and social skills.

FAMILY HISTORY

There is much that can be learned from family history. During my travels to autism conferences, I have found many families with affective disorder in the family history. The relationship between autism and affective disorder has also been reported in the literature (Gillberg & Schaumann, 1981). Family histories of high-functioning autistics often contain giftedness, anxiety or panic disorder, depression, food allergies, and learning disorders. In many of the families I have interviewed the disorders were never formally diagnosed, but careful questioning revealed them.

My own family history contains nervousness and anxiety on both sides. My grandmother has mild depression, and Tofranil has also worked wonders for her. She is also very sensitive to loud noise. She told me that when she was a little girl, the sound of coal going down the chute was torture. My sister is bothered by confusing noise from several sources. On my father's side there is explosive temper, perseveration on one topic, extreme nervousness, and food allergies. Both sides of my family contain artists. There are also signs of immune system abnormalities in myself and my siblings. I had shingles in my thirties, and my brother had them at age 4. My sister had serious ear infections similar to the ear infections in many young autistics. My dad, brother, and myself all have eczema.

SENSORY DEPRIVATION SYMPTOMS

Animals placed in an environment that severely restricts sensory input develop many autistic symptoms such as stereotyped behavior, hyperactivity, and self-mutilation (Grandin, 1984). Why would an autistic and a lion in a barren concrete zoo cage have some of the same symptoms? From my own experience I would like to suggest a possible answer. Since incoming auditory and tactile stimulation often overwhelmed me, I may have created a self-imposed sensory restriction by withdrawing from input that was too intense. Mother told me that when I was a baby I stiffened and pulled away. By pulling away, I did not receive the comforting tactile input that is required for normal development. Animal studies show that sensory restriction in puppies and baby rats has a very detrimental effect on brain development. Puppies raised in a barren kennel become hyperexcitable, and their EEGs (brain waves) still contain signs of overarousal six months after removal from the kennel (Melzack & Burns, 1965). Autistic children also have a desynchronized EEG, which indicates high arousal (Hutt, Hutt, Lee, & Ounstead, 1965). Trimming the whiskers on baby rats causes the parts of the brain that receive input from the whiskers to become oversensitive (Simons & Land, 1987). The abnormality is relatively permanent; the brain areas are still abnormal after the whiskers grow back. Some autistics also have overactive brain metabolism (Rumsey *et al.*, 1985).

I often wonder, if I had received more tactile stimulation as a child would I have been less "hyper" as an adult? Handling baby rats produces less emotional adults who are more willing to explore a maze (Denenbert, Morton, Kline, & Grota, 1962; Ehrlich, 1959). Tactile stimulation is extremely important for babies and aids their development (Casler, 1965). Therapists have found that children who withdraw from comforting tactile stimulation can learn to enjoy it if their skin is carefully desensitized. Rubbing the skin with different cloth textures often helps. Deep pressure stimulation also reduces the urge to pull away.

I was born with sensory problems (due to cerebellar abnormalities), but perhaps secondary neurological damage is caused by withdrawal from touching. Autopsies of five autistic brains indicated that cerebellar abnormalities occur during fetal development, and many areas of the limbic systems were immature and abnormal (Bauman, 1989). The limbic system does not fully mature until two years after birth. Maybe withdrawal from touching made some behavior problems worse. In my book, I describe stupid "bathroom" fixations that got me into a lot of trouble. An interesting paper by McCray (1978) shows a link between a lack of tactual stimulation and excessive masturbation. Masturbation stopped when the children received more affection and hugging. Perhaps the "bathroom" fixation would never have occurred if I could have enjoyed affection and hugging.

Lately there has been a lot of publicity about holding therapy, where an autistic child is forcibly held and hugged until he stops resisting. If this had been done to me I would have found it highly aversive and stressful. Several parents of autistic children have told me that a gentler form of holding therapy is effective and it improved eye contact, language, and sociability. Powers and Thorworth (1985) report a similar result. Perhaps it would be beneficial if autistic babies were gently stroked when they pulled away. My reaction was like a wild animal. At first touching was aversive, and then it became pleasant. In my opinion, tactual defensiveness should be broken down slowly, like taming an animal. If a baby could be desensitized and learn to enjoy comforting tactile input, possibly future behavior problems could be reduced.

DIRECT FIXATIONS

Today I have a successful career designing livestock equipment because my high school science teacher, Mr. Carlock, used my fixation on cattle chutes to motivate me to study psychology and science. He also taught me how to use the scientific indexes. This knowledge enabled me to find out about Tofranil. While the school psychologist wanted to take my squeeze machine away, Mr. Carlock encouraged me to read scientific journals so I could learn why the machine had a relaxing effect. When I moved out to Arizona to go to graduate school, I went out to the feedlots to study the reactions of the cattle in squeeze chutes. This was the beginning of my career.

Today I travel all over the world designing stockyards and chutes for major meat-packing firms. I am a recognized leader in my field and have written over 100 technical and scientific papers on livestock handling (Grandin, 1987). If the psychologists had been successful in taking away my squeeze machine, maybe I would be sitting somewhere rotting in front of a TV instead of writing this chapter.

Some of the most successful high-functioning autistics have directed childhood fixations into careers (Bemporad, 1979; Grandin & Scariano, 1968; Kanner, 1971). When Kanner (1971) followed up his original 11 cases, there were two major successes. The most successful person turned a childhood fixation on numbers into a bank teller's job. The farmer who reared him found goals for his number fixation; he told him he could count the corn rows if he plowed the field.

Many of my fixations initially had a sensory basis. In the fourth grade, I was attracted to election posters because I liked the feeling of wearing the posters like a sandwich man. Occupational therapists have found that a weighted vest will often reduce hyperactivity.

Even though the poster fixation started out with a sensory basis, I became interested in the election. My teachers should have taken advantage of my poster fixation to stimulate an interest in social studies. Calculating electoral college points would have motivated me to study math. Reading could have been motivated by having me read newspaper articles about the people on the posters. If a child is interested in vacuum cleaners, then use a vacuum-cleaner instruction book as a text.

Another one of my fixations was automatic glass sliding doors. Initially I was attracted to the doors because I liked the sensation of watching them move back and forth. Then gradually the doors took on other meanings, which I will talk about in the next section. In a high-functioning adolescent, an interest in sliding doors could be used to stimulate science interests. If my teacher had challenged me to learn how the electronic box that opened the door worked, I would have dived head first into electronics. Fixations can be tremendous motivators. Teachers need to use fixations to motivate instead of trying to stamp them out. A narrow, fixated interest needs to be broadened into constructive activities. The principle can also be used with lower-functioning children; Simons and Sabine (1987) list many good examples.

Fixations need to be differentiated from stereotypies, such as hand flapping or rocking. A fixation is an interest in something external, such as airplanes, radio, or sliding doors. Engaging in stereotypic behavior for long periods of time may be damaging to the nervous system. In one experiment, pigs in a barren pen that engaged in large amounts of stereotyped rooting on each other had abnormal dendritic growth in the somatosensory cortex (Grandin, 1989).

VISUALIZATION

All my thinking is visual. When I think about abstract concepts such as getting along with people I use visual images such as the sliding glass door. Relationships must be approached carefully otherwise the sliding door could be shattered. Visualization to describe abstract concepts is also described by Park and Youderian (1974). As a young child I had visualizations to help me understand the Lord's Prayer. The "power and the glory" were high-tension electric towers and a blazing rainbow sun. The word *trespass* was visualized as a "No Trespassing" sign on the neighbor's tree. Some parts of the prayer were simply incomprehensible. The only nonvisual thoughts I have are of music. Today I no longer use sliding doors to understand personal relationships, but I still have to relate a particular relationship with something I have read—for example, the fight between Jane and Joe was like the U.S. and Canada squabbling over the trade agreement. Almost all my memories relate to visual images of specific events. If somebody says the word *cat,* my images are of individual cats I have known or read about. I do not think about a generalized cat.

My career as a designer of livestock facilities maximizes my talent areas and minimizes my deficits. I still have problems handling long strings of verbal information. If directions from a gas station contain more than three steps, I have to write them down. Statistics are extremely difficult because I am unable to hold one piece of information in my mind while I do the next step. Algebra is almost impossible, because I can't make a visual image and I mix up steps in the sequence. To learn statistics I had to sit down with a tutor and write down the directions for doing each test. Every time I do a *t*-test or a chi-square, I have to use the notes. I have no problem understanding the principles of statistics, because I can see the normal or skewed distributions in my head. The problem is I cannot remember the sequence for doing the calculations. I can put a regression line on a graph full of dots visually. The first time I tried it, I was off only a few degrees. I also have many dyslexic traits, such as reversing numbers and mixing up similar-sounding words such as *over* and *other*. Right and left are also mixed up.

Visual thinking is an asset for an equipment designer. I am able to "see" how all the parts of a project will fit together and see potential problems. It never ceases to amaze me how architects and engineers can make so many stupid mistakes in buildings. The disastrous accident where the catwalks at the Hyatt Regency fell and killed 100 people was caused by visualization errors. All the calculations were correct, but the architect's original design was impossible to build. Further visualization errors made during construction resulted in doubling the load on poorly designed fasteners. Academic requirements probably keep many visual thinkers out of these professions. Designing a piece of equipment with a sequential mind may be just as difficult for an engineer as statistics equations are for me. The sequential thinker can't see the whole. I have observed many incidents in industry where a brilliant maintenance man with a high school education designs a piece of equipment after all the Ph.D. engineers have failed. He may be an unrecognized visual thinker. There may be two basic kinds of thinking, visual and sequential. Farah (1989) concluded that "thinking in images is distinct from thinking in language." I have also had the opportunity to interview brilliant people who have very little visual thought. One professor told me that facts just come out of his mind instantly. To retrieve facts, I have to read them off a visualized page of a book or "play a video" of some previous event.

There is however, one area of visualization I am poor in. I often fail to recognize faces until I have known a person for a long time. This sometimes causes social problems, because I sometimes don't respond to an acquaintance because I fail to recognize them. Einstein was a visual thinker who failed his high school language requirement and relied on visual methods of study (Holton, 1971–1972). The theory of relativity was based on visual imagery of moving boxcars and riding on light beams. At an autism meeting I had the opportunity to visit some of Einstein's relatives. His family history has a high incidence of autism, dyslexia, food allergies, giftedness, and musical talent. Einstein himself had many autistic traits. An astute reader can find them in Einstein and Einstein (1987) and Lepscky (1982).

In my own family history, my grandfather on my mother's side was coinventor of the automatic pilot for airplanes, and on my father's side my great-grandfather was a maverick who started the largest corporate wheat farm in the world. My two sisters and one brother are all visual thinkers. One sister is dyslexic and is brilliant in the art of decorating houses. My brother can build anything but had problems with calculus when he tried to major in engineering. He is now a very successful banker and did well in all other subjects in college. My youngest sister is a sculptress and did well in school. My mother and grandparents on the mother's side were all good at higher math, and many people on my mother's side were well-known for intellect.

Drawing elaborate drawings of steel and concrete livestock stockyards is easy (Figure 6-3). I am able to visualize a motion picture of the finished facility in my imagination. However, drawing realistic human faces is very difficult. Figure 6-4 illustrates a buffalo-handling facility I designed. Since it was a government low-bid contract, every piece of steel had to be visualized and drawn on 26 sheets of detailed drawings. I am very proud of this job because I was able to accurately visualize everything prior to construction except for one little ladder. When I was a child, my parents and teachers encouraged my artistic talent. It is important to nurture talents.

Discussions with other high-functioning autistics have revealed visual methods of thinking on tasks that are often considered nonvisual. A brilliant autistic comput-

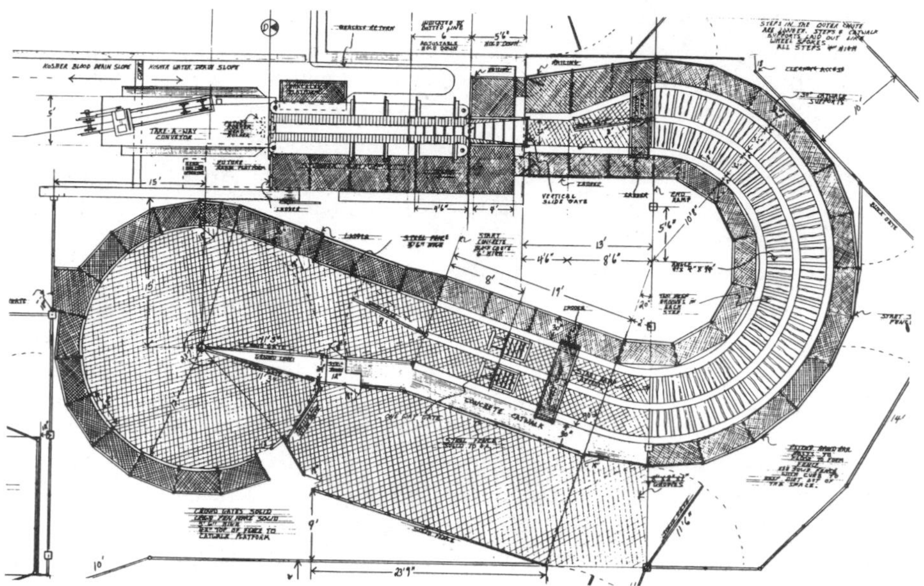

Fig. 6-3. Detailed drawing of a chute system the author designed for a large meat packing plant. The curves take advantage of natural circling behavior.

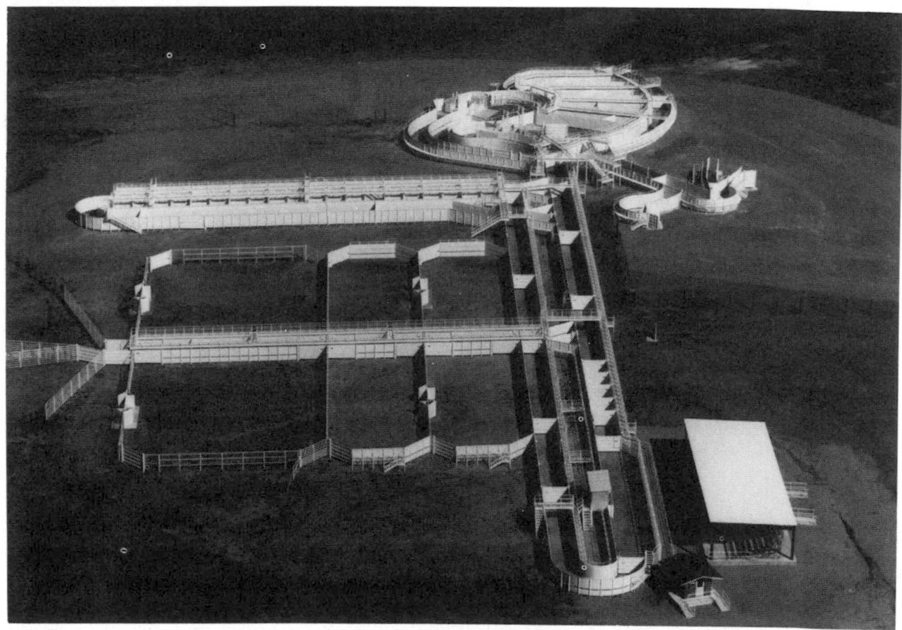

Fig. 6-4. Buffalo handling facility designed by the author for the U.S. Fish and Wildlife Service.

er programmer told me that he visualized the program tree in his mind and then just filled in the code on each branch. A gifted autistic composer told me that he made "sound pictures."

I was good at building things, but when I first started working with drawings it took time to learn how the lines on a drawing related to the picture in my imagination. When I built a house for my aunt and uncle, I had difficulty learning the relationship between symbolic markings on the drawings and the actual construction. The house was built before I learned drafting. Now I can instantly translate a drawing into a mental image of a finished structure. While agonizing over the house plans, I was able to pull up pictures out of my memory of a house addition that was built when I was eight. Mental images from my childhood memory helped me install windows, light switches, and plumbing. I replayed the "videos" in my imagination.

SAVANT SKILLS

Studies have shown that when autistic savants become less fixated and more social they lose their savant skills such as card counting, calendar calculation, or art skills (Rimland & Fein, 1988). Since I started taking the medication I have lost my fixation, but I have not lost my visualization skill. Some of my best work has been done while on the medication.

My opinion is that savants lose their skill because they lose the fixated attention. Card counting (shown in the *Rain Man* movie) is no mystery to me. I think savants visualize the cards being dealt onto a table in a pattern, like a series of clocks or a Persian rug pattern. To tell which cards are still in the deck, they simply look at their patterns. The only thing that prevents me from card counting or calendar calculation is that I no longer have the concentration to hold a visual image completely steady for a long period of time. I speculate that socialized savants still retain their visualization skills. I still have the perfect-pitch skill, even though I don't use it. If I had greater concentration, I could sing back much longer songs after hearing them once.

In my own case the strongest visual images are of things that evoked strong emotions, such as important big jobs. These memories never fade and they remain accurate. However, I was unable to recall visual images of the houses on a frequently traveled road until I made an effort to attend to them. A strong visual image contains all details, and it can be rotated and made to move like a movie. Weaker images are like slightly out-of-focus pictures or may have details missing. For example, in a meat-packing plant I can accurately visualize the piece of equipment I designed but I am unable to remember things I do not attend to, such as the ceiling over the equipment, bathrooms, stairways, offices, and other areas of little or no interest. Memories of items of moderate interest grow hazy with time.

I tried a little memory experiment at one of my jobs. After being away from the plant for 30 days, I tried recalling a part of the plant that I had attended to poorly, and another part I had attended to intently. I had not designed either of these places. The first place was the plant conference room, and the other was the entrance to the room that housed my equipment. I was able to draw a fairly accurate map of the office, but I made major mistakes on conference-room furniture and ceiling covering. The room I visualized was plain and lacked detail. On the other hand, I visualized the entrance door to the equipment room very accurately, but made a slight mistake on the door-handle style. The visualized door had much greater detail then the visualized conference room. The conference room was not attended to even though I negotiated with the plant managers in that room.

Talents need to be nurtured and broadened out into something useful. Nadia, a well-known autistic case, drew wonderful perspective pictures as a child (Seifel, 1977). When she gained rudimentary social skills, she stopped drawing. Possibly the talent could have been revived with encouragement from teachers. Seifel (1977) describes how Nadia drew pictures on napkins and waste papers. She needed proper drawing equipment. Treffert (1989) reported on several savants who did not lose their savant skills when they became more social. Use of savant skills was encouraged.

At the age of 28, my drafting drastically improved after I observed a talented draftsman named David. Building the house taught me how to understand blueprints, but now I had to learn to draw them. When I started drawing livestock facilities I used David's drawings as models. I had to "pretend" I was David. After buying a drafting pencil just like David's, I laid some of his drawings out and then proceeded to draw a loading ramp for cattle. I just copied his style, like a savant playing music, except my ramp was a different design. When it was finished I couldn't believe I had done it.

DEFICITS AND ABILITIES

Five years ago I took a series of tests to determine my abilities and handicaps. On the Hiskey Nebraska Spatial Reasoning test, my performance was at the top of the norms. On the Woodcock–Johnson Spatial Relations test, I only got an average score because it was a timed speed test. I am not a fast thinker; it takes time for the visual image to form. When I survey a site for equipment at a meat-packing plant, it takes 20 to 30 minutes of staring at the building to fully imprint the site in my memory. Once this is done, I have a "video" I can play back when I am working on the drawing. When I draw, the image of the new piece of equipment gradually emerges. As my experience increased, I needed fewer measurements to properly survey a job. On many remodeling jobs, the plant engineer often measures a whole bunch of stuff that is going to be torn out. He can't visualize what the building will look like when parts of it are torn out and a new part is added.

As a child I got scores of 120 and 137 on the Wechsler. I had superior scores in Memory for Sentences, Picture Vocabulary, and Antonyms–Synonyms on the Woodcock–Johnson. On Memory for Numbers I beat the test by repeating the numbers out loud. I have an extremely poor long-term memory for things such as phone numbers unless I can convert them to visual images. For example, the number 65 is retirement age, and I imagine somebody in Sun City, Arizona. If I am unable to take notes I cannot remember what people tell me unless I translate the verbal information to visual pictures. Recently I was listening to a taped medical lecture while driving. To remember information such as the drug doses discussed on the tape I had to create a picture to stand for the dose. For example, 300 mg is a football field with shoes on it. The shoes remind me that the number is 300 feet, not yards.

I got a second-grade score on the Woodcock–Johnson Blending subtest where I had to identify slowly sounded-out words. The Visual Auditory Learning subtest was another disaster. I had to memorize the meaning of arbitrary symbols, such as a triangle means "horse," and read a sentence composed of symbols. I could only learn the ones where I was able to make a picture for each symbol. For example, I imagined the triangle as a flag carried by a horse and rider. Foreign languages were almost impossible. Concept Formation was another test with fourth-grade results. The name of this test really irks me, because I am good at forming concepts in the real world. My ability to visualize broad unifying concepts from hundreds of journal articles has enabled me to outguess the "experts" on many livestock subjects. The test involved picking out a concept such as "large, yellow" and then finding it in another set of cards. The problem was, I could not hold the concept in my mind while I looked at the other cards. If I had been allowed to write the concept down, I would have done much better.

LEARNING TO READ

Mother was my salvation for reading. I would have never learned to read by the method that requires memorization of hundreds of words. Words are too abstract to be remembered. She taught me with old-fashioned phonics. After I laboriously learned all the sounds, I was able to sound out words. To motivate me, she read a page and then stopped in an exciting part. I had to read the next sentence. Gradually she read less and less. Mrs. David W. Eastham in Canada taught her autistic son to read in a similar manner, using some Montessori methods. Many teachers thought the boy was retarded. He learned to communicate by typing, and he wrote beautiful poetry. Douglas Biklen at Syracuse University has taught some nonverbal autistic people to write fluently on the typewriter. To prevent perseveration on a single key and key targeting mistakes the person's wrist is supported by another person.

A visualized-reading method developed by Miller and Miller (1971) would also have been helpful. To learn verbs, each word has letters drawn to look like the action. For example, *fall* would have letters falling over, and *run* would have letters that looked like runners. This method needs to be further developed for learning speech sounds. Learning the sounds would have been much easier if I had a picture of a choo-choo train for *ch* and a cat for hard *c* sound. For long and short vowels, long *a* could be represented by a picture of somebody praying. This card could be used for both *pr* and long *a* by having a circle around *pr* on one card and the *a* on another.

At first, reading out loud was the only way I could read. Today, when I read silently, I use a combination of instant visualization and sounding words. For example, this phrase from a magazine—"stop several pedestrians on a city street"—was instantly seen as moving pictures. Sentences that contain more abstract words like *apparent* or *incumbent* are sounded out phonetically.

As a child, I often talked out loud because it made my thoughts more "concrete" and "real." Today, when I am alone designing, I will talk out loud about the design. Talking activates more brain regions than just thinking.

MENTOR

"A skilled and imaginative teacher prepared to enjoy and be challenged by the child seems repeatedly to have been a deciding factor in the success and educational placement of high-functioning, autistic children" (Newson, Dawson, & Everard, 1982). Bemporod (1979) also brings forth the mentor concept. My mentor in high school was Mr. Carlock, my high school science teacher. Structured behavior modification methods that work with small children are often useless with a high-functioning older child with normal intelligence.

I was lucky to get headed on the right path after college. Three other high-functioning autistics were not so fortunate. One man has a Ph.D. in math and he sits at home. He needed somebody to steer him into an appropriate job. Teaching math did not work out; he should have obtained a research position that required less interaction with people. The other lady has a degree in history and now works doing a boring telephone-sales job. She needs a job where she can fully utilize her talents. She also needs a mentor to help her find an appropriate job and help open doors for her. Both these people needed support after college, and they did not receive it. The third man did well in high school and he also sits at home. He has a real knack for library research. If some interested person worked with him, he could work for a newspaper researching background information for stories. All three of these people need jobs where they can make maximum use of their talents and minimize their deficits.

Another autistic lady I know was lucky. She landed a graphic-arts job where she was able to put her visualization talents to good use. Her morale was also boosted when her paintings received recognition and were purchased by a local bank. Her success with the paintings also opened up many social doors. In my own case, many social doors opened after I made scenery for the college talent show. I was still considered a nerd, but now I was a "neat" nerd. People respect talent even if they think you are "weird." People became interested in me after they saw my drawings and pictures of my jobs. I made myself an expert in a specialized area.

High-functioning autistics will probably never really fit in with the social whirl. My life is my work. If a high-functioning autistic gets an interesting job, he or she will have a fulfilling life. I spend most Friday and Saturday nights writing papers and drawing. Almost all my social contacts are with livestock people or people interested in autism. Like the Newson *et al.* (1982) subjects, I prefer factual, nonfictional reading materials. I have little interest in novels with complicated interpersonal relationships. When I do read novels, I prefer straightforward stories that occur in interesting places with lots of description.

The mentor needs to be somebody who can provide support on several different fronts. Employment is only one area. Many high-functioning autistics need to learn about budgeting money, how to make claims on health insurance, and nutritional counseling. As the person becomes more and more independent the mentor can be phased out, but the mentor may still be needed if the autistic loses his job or has some other crisis.

WHO HELPED ME RECOVER

Many people ask me, "How did you manage to recover?" I was extremely lucky to have the right people working with me at the right time. At age 2, I had all the typical autistic symptoms. In 1949, most doctors did not know what autism was, but fortunately a wise neurologist recommended "normal therapy" instead of an institution. I was referred to a speech therapist who ran a special nursery school in her home. The speech therapist was the most important professional in my life. At age 3, my mother hired a governess who kept me and my sister constantly occupied. My day consisted of structured activities such as skating, swinging, and painting. The activities were structured, but I was given limited opportunities for choice. For example, on one day I could choose between building a snowman or sledding. She actually participated in all the activities. She also conducted musical activities, and we marched around the piano with toy drums. My sensory problems were not handled well. I would have really benefited if I had had an occupational therapist trained in sensory integration.

I went to a normal elementary school with older, experienced teachers and small classes. Mother was another important person who helped my recovery. She worked very closely with the school. She used techniques that are used today in the most successful mainstreaming programs to integrate me into the classroom. The day before I went to school, she and the teacher explained to the other children that they needed to help me.

As discussed earlier, puberty was a real problem time. I got kicked out of high school for fighting. I then moved on to a small country boarding school for gifted children with emotional problems. The director was an innovative man and considered a "lone wolf" by his psychologist colleagues. This is where I met Mr. Carlock. Another extremely helpful person was Ann, my aunt. I visited her ranch during the summer.

In high school and college, the people that helped me the most were the creative, unconventional thinkers. The more traditional professionals such as the school psychologist were actually harmful. They were too busy trying to psychoanalyze me and take away my squeeze machine. Later when I became interested in meat-packing plants, Tom Rohrer, the manager of the local meat-packing plant, took an interest in me. For three years I visited his plant once a week and learned the industry. My very first design job was in his plant. I want to emphasize the importance of a gradual transition from the world of school to the world of work. The packing plant visits were made while I was still in college. People with autism need to be gradually introduced to a job before they graduate. The autistics I discussed earlier could have excellent careers if they had a local businessperson take an interest in them.

AUTISM PROGRAMS

During my travels I have observed many different programs. It is my opinion that effective programs for young children have certain common denominators that are similar regardless of theoretical basis. Early, intense intervention improves the prognosis. Passive approaches don't work. My governess was sometimes mean, but her intense, structured intervention prevented me from withdrawing. She and my mother just used their good instincts. Good programs do a variety of activities and use more than one approach. A good little children's program should include flexible behavior modification, speech therapy, exercise, sensory treatment (activities that stimulate the vestibular system and tactile desensitization), musical activities, contact with normal children, and lots of love. The effectiveness of different types of programs is going to vary from case to case. A program that is effective for one case may be less effective for another.

REFERENCES

Ayres, J. A. (1979). *Sensory integration and the child.* Los Angeles: Western Psychological Services.

Bauman, M. (1989). The anatomy of autism. In *Conference Proceedings, Autism Society of America* (pp. 10–12). Washington, DC: Autism Society of America.

Bauman, M., & Kemper, T. L. (1985). Histoanatomic observations of the brain in early infantile autism. *Neurology, 35,* 866–874.

Bemporad, J. R. (1979). Adult recollections of a formerly autistic child. *Journal of Autism and Developmental Disorders, 9,* 179–197.

Bhatara, V., Clark, D. L., Arnold, L. E., Gunsett, R., & Smeltzer, D. J. (1981). Hyperkinesis treated with vestibular stimulation: An exploratory study. *Biological Psychiatry, 61,* 269–279.

Biklen, D. Communication unbound: Autism and praxis. *Harvard Educational Review, 60,* 291–314.

Casler, L. (1965). Effects of extra tactile stimulation on a group of institutionalized infants. *Genetic Psychology Monographs, 71,* 137–175.

Chambers, W. W. (1947). Electrical stimulation of the interior cerebellum of the cat. *American Journal of Anatomy, 80,* 55–93.

Condon, W. S. (1985). Sound-film microanalysis: A means of correlating brain and behavior. In F. Duffy

& N. Geschwind (Eds.), *Dyslexia: A neuroscientific approach to clinical evaluation*. Boston: Little, Brown.

Condon, W., & Sander, L. (1974). Neonate movement is synchronized with adult speech. *Science, 183,* 99–101.

Courchesne, E. (1989). Implications of recent neurobiologic findings in autism. In *Conference Proceedings, Autism Society of America* (pp. 8–9). Washington, DC: Autism Society of America.

Courchesne, E., Courchesne-Yeung, R., Press, G. A., Hesselink, J. R., & Jernigan, T. L. (1988). Hypoplasia of cerebellar vermal lobules VI and VII in autism. *New England Journal of Medicine, 318,* 1349–1354.

Crispino, L., & Bullock, T. H. (1984). Cerebellum mediates modality-specific modulation of sensory responses of midbrain and forebrain in rats. *Proceedings, National Academy of Science–Neurobiology, 81,* 2917–2920.

Denenberg, V. H., Morton, J. R., Kline, N. J., & Grota, L. J. (1962). Effects of duration of infantile stimulation upon emotionality. *Canadian Journal of Psychology, 16*(1), 72–76.

Ehrlich, A. (1959). Effects of past experience on exploratory behavior in rats. *Canadian Journal of Psychology, 13*(4), 248–254.

Einstein, A., & Einstein, M. W. (1987). *The collected papers of Albert Einstein* (A. Beck & P. Havens, Trans.). Princeton, NJ: Princeton University Press.

Farah, M. J. (1989). The neural basis of mental imagery. *Trends in Neuroscience, 12,* 395–399.

Gillberg, G., & Schaumann, H. (1981). Infantile autism and puberty. *Journal of Autism and Developmental Disorders, 11,* 365–371.

Grandin, T. (1980). Observations of cattle behavior applied to the design of cattle handling facilities. *Applied Animal Ethology, 6,* 19–31.

Grandin, T. (1983). Letters to the editor: "Coping strategies." *Journal of Autism and Developmental Disorders, 13,* 217–221.

Grandin, T. (1984). My experiences as an autistic child. *Journal of Orthomolecular Psychiatry, 13,* 144–174.

Grandin, T. (1987). Animal handling. In E. O. Price (Ed.), *Farm animal behavior, veterinary clinics of North America* (Vol. 3, pp. 323–338). Philadelphia: W. B. Saunders.

Grandin, T. (1989). *Effect of rearing environment and environmental enrichment on the behavior and neural development of young pigs*. Doctoral dissertation, University of Illinois.

Grandin, T., & Scariano, M. (1986). *Emergence: Labelled autistic*. Novato, CA: Arena.

Grandin, T., Dodman, N., & Shuster, L. (1989). Effect of naltrexone on relaxation induced by lateral flank pressure in pigs. *Pharmacology, Biochemistry and Behavior, 33.*

Holton, G. (1971–1972). On trying to understand scientific genius. *American Scholar, 41,* 102.

Hutt, S. J., Hutt, C., Lee, D., & Ounsted, C. (1965). A behavioral and electroencephalographic study of autistic children. *Journal of Psychiatric Research, 3,* 181–197.

Kanner, L. (1971). Follow-up study of eleven autistic children originally reported in 1943. *Journal of Autism and Childhood Schizophrenia, 1,* 112–145.

Kumazawa, T. (1963). Deactivation of the rabbit's brain by pressure application to the skin. *Electroencephalography and Clinical Neurology, 15,* 660–671.

Lepscky, I. (1982). *Albert Einstein*. New York: Barrons.

McCray, G. M. (1978). Excessive masturbation in childhood: A symptom of tactile deprivation. *Pediatrics, 62,* 277–279.

McGimsey, J. F., & Favell, J. E. (1988). The effects of increased physical exercise on disruptive behavior in retarded persons. *Journal of Autism and Developmental Disorders, 18,* 167–179.

Melzack, R., & Burns, S. K. (1965). Neurophysiological effects of early sensory restriction. *Experimental Neurology, 13,* 163–175.

Melzack, R., Konrad, K. W., & Dubrobsky, B. (1969). Prolonged changes in the central nervous system produced by somatic and reticular stimulation. *Experimental Neurology, 25,* 416–428.

Miller, A., & Miller, E. E. (1971). Symbol accentuation, single-track functioning and early reading. *American Journal of Mental Deficiency, 76,* 110–117.

Newson, E., Dawson, M., & Everard, P. (1982). *The natural history of able autistic people: Their management and functioning in a social context.* Nottingham, England: University of Nottingham Child Development Unit.

Ornitz, E. (1985). Neurophysiology of infantile autism. *Journal of the American Academy of Child Psychiatry, 24,* 251–262.

Park, D., & Youderian, P. (1974). Light and number: Ordering principles in the world of an autistic child. *Journal of Autism and Childhood Schizophrenia, 4,* 313–323.

Powers, M. D., & Thorworth, C. A. (1985). The effect of negative reinforcement on tolerance of physical contact in a preschool autistic child. *Journal of Clinical Psychology, 14,* 299–303.

Ratey, J. J., Mikkelsen, E., Sorgi, P., Zuckerman, S., Polakoff, S., Bemporad, J., Bick, P., & Kadish, W. (1987). Autism: The treatment of aggressive behaviors. *Journal of Clinical Pharmacology, 7,* 35–41.

Ray, T. C., King, L. J., & Grandin, T. (1988). The effectiveness of self-initiated vestibular stimulation in producing speech sounds in an autistic child. *Journal of Occupational Therapy Research, 8,* 186–190.

Rekate, H. L., Grubb, R. L., Aram, D. M., Hahn, J. F., & Ratcheson, R. A. (1985). Muteness of cerebellar origin. *Archives of Neurology, 42,* 697–698.

Rimland, G., & Fein, D. (1988). Special talents of autistic savants. In L. K. Obler & D. Fein (Eds.), *The exceptional brain.* New York: Guilford.

Ritvoe, E., Freeman, B. J., Scheibel, A. B., Duong, T., Robinson, H., Guthrie, D., & Ritvoe, A. (1986). Lower Purkinje cell counts in the cerebella of four autistic subjects. *American Journal of Psychiatry, 143,* 862–866.

Rumsey, J. M., Duara, R., Grady, C., Rapoport, J. L., Margolin, R. A., Rapoport, S. I., & Cutler, N. R. (1985). Brain metabolism in autism. *Archives of General Psychiatry, 42,* 448–455.

Schopler, H. R. (1965). Early infantile autism and the receptor process. *Archives of General Psychiatry, 13,* 327–337.

Seifel, L. (1977). *Nadia: A case of extraordinary drawing ability in an autistic child.* New York: Academic Press.

Sheehan, D. V., Beh, M. B., Ballenger, J., & Jacobsen, G. (1980). Treatment of endogenous anxiety with phobic, hysterical and hyperchondriacal symptoms. *Archives of General Psychiatry, 37,* 51–59.

Simons, D., & Land, P. (1987). Early tactile stimulation influences organization of somatic sensory cortex. *Nature, 326,* 694–697.

Simons, J., & Sabine, O. (1987). *The hidden child.* Kensington, MD: Woodbine House.

Takagi, K., & Kobagasi, S. (1956). Skin pressure reflex. *Acta Medica et Biologica, 4,* 31–37.

Treffert, D. A. (1989). Extraordinary people: Understanding the savant syndrome. Ballantine Books, New York.

Volkmar, F. R., & Cohen, D. J. (1985). The experience of infantile autism: A first person account by Tony W. *Journal of Autism and Developmental Disorders, 15,* 47–54.

Walters, R. G., & Walters, W. E. (1980). Decreasing self-stimulatory behavior with physical exercise in a group of autistic boys. *Journal of Autism and Developmental Disorders, 10,* 379–387.

White, G. B., & White, M. S. (1987). Autism from the inside. *Medical Hypothesis, 24,* 223–229.

II

Social Issues

7

Manifestations of Social Problems in High-Functioning Autistic People

LORNA WING

This chapter is concerned with disorders within the autistic continuum (Wing, 1988), and not only classic autism as described by Kanner (1943, 1973). The continuum is roughly equivalent to the "pervasive developmental disorders" as defined in the *Diagnostic and Statistical Manual of Mental Disorders* (third edition, revised) of the American Psychiatric Association (1987). The concept, in the form to be described here, was derived from an epidemiological study of a population of children in a former London borough (Camberwell) carried out by Wing and Gould (1979). The continuum comprises disorders involving the presence, in any form, of the triad of impairments of social interaction, communication, and imagination, together with a marked preference for a rigid, repetitive pattern of activities. (For the sake of brevity, in this chapter the terms *autism* and *autistic* will be used to refer to the whole continuum unless qualified as "classic" or "typical" autism, or as "Kanner syndrome" or "Asperger syndrome.")

The literature contains little in the way of systematic studies of the social impairments in higher-functioning children or adults with autism, as distinct from other features such as problems affecting cognition and language. The descriptions given here will be based on the few available studies, some published accounts of individual histories (Bemporad, 1979; DesLauriers, 1978; Grandin & Scariano, 1986; Park, 1982, 1983, 1986), and my own experience with autistic people I have known over many years. Some comments will be made concerning childhood and adolescence, but the main focus will be on adult life. This is the time when the

---

LORNA WING • MRC Social Psychiatry Unit, Institute of Psychiatry, University of London, London SE5 8AF, England.

High-Functioning Individuals with Autism, edited by Eric Schopler and Gary B. Mesibov. Plenum Press, New York, 1992.

hopes and expectations raised by good progress in childhood are put to the test, and the consequences of the social impairments are most obvious.

It is in the high-functioning group that the central role of the triad of social impairments can be seen most clearly. The other abnormalities found in autistic disorders, such as impairment of the formal aspects of language (vocabulary, syntax, semantics), motor stereotypies, or abnormal responses to sensory stimuli may be minimal or absent—at least after the early years—and the characteristic social and communication problems and the underlying repetitiveness and rigidity of thought and action may be the only features of autism that can be observed.

THE NATURE OF SOCIAL IMPAIRMENT

The idea that autistic children have potentially normal intelligence, but do not relate to others nor use their skills because they are emotionally disturbed as a result of deviant upbringing, is opposed by the weight of the evidence that has accumulated over the years (see, e.g., DeMyer, Hingtgen, & Jackson, 1981). A major focus of current scientific work is the identification of the abnormalities of neurological and psychological function underlying autistic behavior.

Psychological Theories

Regardless of whether it was considered to be a primary or secondary phenomenon, the importance of the abnormality of social behavior in autism has been recognized ever since Kanner published his original paper in 1943 (see the multiauthored book on the subject edited by Schopler & Mesibov, 1986).

In their epidemiological study, Wing and Gould (1979) found that impairments of social interaction, reciprocal social communication, and socially oriented imaginative, pretend play (the triad of social impairments) virtually always occurred in association with each other and with an inflexible, repetitive pattern of activities. It seems likely that these are different facets of some more fundamental abnormality. Various theories have been proposed as to the nature of this underlying dysfunction.

Hobson (1986a, b) has suggested that normal infants are innately programmed to be sensitive to and to comprehend other people's emotional states from direct observation of their physical expression, and that autistic children are impaired in this function. He hypothesized that this leads to a failure to appreciate other people's concepts, as well as their feelings, and thus impairs the development of the child's own ability to abstract and to symbolize. This, in turn, produces the characteristic difficulty in using language appropriately within the social context and impairment of the development of imaginative activities. This formulation is similar to Kanner's original description of autism as an "innate lack of affective contact with others."

Baron-Cohen, Leslie, and Frith (1985) and Leslie and Frith (1988) saw the basic problem as cognitive rather than affective (emotional) in origin. They postulated an impairment of development of the understanding that mental events are different from external events. This skill underlies the emergence of pretense (Leslie, 1987); the ability to recognize that other people have thoughts, feelings, and beliefs; and the capacity for reflection on one's own ideas. They refer to this problem as the absence or impairment of the "theory of mind" that normally develops in early childhood. Baron-Cohen (1988, 1989) suggested that, in autism, this is a specific developmental delay that gives rise to the severe difficulties in social interaction, reciprocal communication, and the capacity for pretense, making up the triad of impairments referred to above.

Hermelin and O'Connor (1985) proposed that the basic impairment in autism can best be regarded as a "logico-affective" abnormality, thus combining the cognitive and the emotional theories.

The discussions concerning the experimental results and the theories continue. Resolution of this semantic debate will come only when the location and nature of the underlying brain dysfunction are finally established.

Clinical Observations

Parents and others in close contact with high-functioning autistic people, especially adolescents and adults, recognize that the social problems are not due to an absence of feelings. The raw materials for basic emotions such as anger, fear, or joy are there in abundance. Neither, in the majority, is there a lack of desire for human interaction. Those in the higher-functioning group, as they grow older, become aware that other people are of interest and want to join in, make friends, and enjoy human company (see, e.g., Clara Park's description of her daughter, 1982, 1983, 1986). The problems appear to arise from an overwhelming difficulty in acquiring and understanding the multitudinous rules of social life and developing empathy with others.

Both affective and cognitive abnormalities can be observed in the high-functioning group that lead to difficulties of social understanding. For example, a mother of a young high-functioning adult (Jo Ann Jeffries, personal communication) only recently discovered that he assumed she knew he was very attached to her without any need for him to express this in words or actions. Elizabeth Newson (personal communication) illustrated another aspect of the problem by quoting a young man who said, with great sadness, "people give each other messages with their eyes, but I do not know what they are saying."

The rigidity and repetitiveness of thought and action also contribute to the social gaucheness, as with the autistic child who, at the end of his first day at a school with rather formal standards of behavior, returned home and addressed his parents as Mr. and Mrs. Brown. The lack of understanding of other people's thoughts and feelings is at the root of the combination of egocentricity and innocence that is so characteristic of autistic people of any level of ability.

The presence of the triad of social impairments in high-functioning people with autistic disorders, without the confounding effects of associated mental retardation, should provide the opportunity for examining the triad's essential nature. Issues of diagnosis and classification arise with those who have social impairment in its most subtle form, especially if their developmental abnormalities do not fit the pattern of classic autism (Schopler, 1985; Schopler & Rutter, 1988; Wing, 1981, 1986, 1988). Nevertheless, interest in high-functioning people is growing, and further research into the social problems should yield interesting results.

TYPES OF SOCIAL IMPAIRMENT

In their epidemiological study of children in Camberwell, a former London borough, Wing and Gould (1979) found that impairment of the capacity to engage in reciprocal social interaction could be manifested in three main ways. The most severe form was aloofness and indifference to other people. Children with this type of social impairment showed no interest in or concern for others, except as dispensers of food and drink or providers of physical comfort or stimulation (such as tickling or rough-and-tumble play).

Some children were socially passive. They rarely or never made spontaneous approaches, but amiably accepted interactions initiated by others and would take a passive role in games devised by sociable children. Copying other people's actions without real understanding was common in this group.

The third type of social impairment observed among the study children was described as "active but odd." The children concerned approached adults and sometimes their age peers, but did this in a repetitive, bizarre, one-sided fashion, often to indulge their own circumscribed interests. Their behavior was not modified by the responses of the people they approached.

In a study of adolescents and young adults, Shah (1988) described a fourth style of social interaction. Those concerned were polite, apparently aware of other people, and able to initiate and give and take in conversational exchanges. Nevertheless, there was a stilted, even mechanical quality to their social behavior. It seemed as if they had learned the rules of social interaction by intellectual effort rather than by instinct.

These different manifestations of social impairment are not discrete entities. They shade into each other, and some children can show different ways of responding in different situations and at different ages (Kanner, 1973; Wing, 1988). Furthermore, autistic people from the same family may have different interaction styles (see, e.g., Bowman, 1988). Despite the contrasts in behavior at the extreme ends of the scale, a strong case can be made that the various manifestations are in the same continuum (Wing, 1988), though proof or refutation of this hypothesis depends upon advances in knowledge of neurophysiology and neuropathology.

SOCIAL INTERACTION IN CHILDHOOD

In the early years, children in the autistic continuum who will be high functioning may show any of the first three forms of social impairment mentioned above.

Kanner (1973) described 11 children who became independent as adults (out of 96 he had diagnosed as classically autistic), all of whom had the characteristic aloofness and indifference when very young. Kanner felt there was nothing in the behavior of the 11 children in their early years to indicate their eventual prognosis.

Asperger (1944) wrote an account of some children and adolescents who were passive or active-but-odd in their social interaction, who had good grammar and large vocabularies but were repetitive in speech and odd in social communication, whose activities were centered around one or two circumscribed interests and who were poorly coordinated in movement. Asperger recognized that this group shared many features with Kanner autism, and Schopler (1985) and Wing (1981, 1986, 1988), among others, argued that Asperger syndrome is part of the autistic continuum. Most of the subjects in his group have overall intelligence in the normal range, though a minority are mildly retarded. As infants and young children, their abnormal development may not have been obvious to their parents, though detailed retrospective questioning usually reveals that their style of social interaction was always passive or odd (Wing, 1981). Some children who begin life with classic Kanner syndrome develop, over the years, the features of Asperger syndrome (Wing, 1988). Asperger reported that the majority of his group achieved good job performance in adult life despite continuing difficulties with social relationships, although he gave no figures.

PROGNOSIS FOR INDEPENDENCE IN ADULT LIFE

Rimland (1964) pointed out that although classically autistic children have similar patterns of overt behavior in their early years, they tend to separate out into subgroups developing along different paths from about 5 or 6 years of age. Experience gained from the Camberwell study (Wing, 1988; Wing & Gould, 1979) suggested that, by middle childhood, it was possible to distinguish the predominant style of social interaction for each child and to obtain reliable scores on psychological tests, so that a tentative prognosis regarding future development was possible.

Considering Kanner's and Asperger's papers together, it would appear that the young children with passive or odd interaction were more likely to be high functioning as adults than were the aloof group. The findings from the Camberwell study supported this conclusion, as shown in Table 7-1.

The table shows the outcome in adult life of the 20 children in the study (17 boys and 3 girls) with intelligence quotients on standardized tests, on one or both occasions of testing, of 70 or above (i.e., in the borderline or normal range). As can be seen, 5 out of the 18 who were followed up in 1988 (when their ages ranged from 18 to 33 years) had jobs, and 1 was working well for payment in a sheltered setting, giving a total of 6 (or 33%) who were, at that time, gainfully employed. Three of those in open employment had been in and out of work, mainly because of difficulties arising when they were required to adapt to changes. The 7 individuals (39%) living at home or in small adult communities helped in domestic and other practical

Table 7-1. Outcome in Adult Life (Adults in the Camberwell Study with IQ 70+ and Age Range 18–33 Years)

Social impairment in early life	Open employ-ment	Sheltered work	In small sheltered community	In own home	Disturbed —in special service	Not known	Total
Aloof	—	1	2	—	1	—	4
Passive	5	—	2	1	1	1	10
Odd	—	—	—	2	3	1	6
Total	5	1	4	3	5	2	20

tasks and were well settled. Two of these could play the piano to a high standard. However, 5 (28%) were presenting major problems because of their disturbed and physically aggressive behavior and were being cared for in specialized service settings (in one case, in prison for causing grievous bodily harm). Out of the whole group, only 4 (22%) had been aloof in their early years. All those who were working in open employment (28%) had been passive as young children. By the time of follow-up, only 2 remained aloof in their social interactions—one being placed in a sheltered community and the other in a special service because of very aggressive behavior. The rest were passive (7 people) or odd (9 people). Only 4 had received education specifically designed for autistic children; one was the young man in sheltered work, two were in small sheltered communities, and one was living at home with his parents.

SOCIAL INTERACTION IN ADULT LIFE

The behavior and adjustment of high-functioning autistic adults will be discussed in relation to each of the four types of social impairment shown in adult life.

The Aloof Subgroup

As already mentioned, this is the least common subgroup among high-functioning autistic people, although it is the most frequent type of social impairment among those of lower ability (Wing, 1988; Wing & Gould, 1979). The high-functioning adults in this subgroup tend to show a combination of aloofness and passivity rather than being completely aloof and indifferent.

Most have a history of typical Kanner syndrome, and in the United Kingdom, they are likely to have attended a special school. An uneven profile of psychological functions, with at least one specific skill at a high level, is characteristic. Language use is limited, but comprehension is better than speech. The rigid, repetitive activities are usually still marked, and the person concerned manages to cope with life by means of autistic routines. Diagnosis presents the fewest problems in this subgroup, and most (though by no means at all) are recognized as autistic in childhood.

Despite the special skills, full independence is difficult to achieve because of the resistance to change, the marked lack of sociability, and often eccentricity of dress and poor self-care unless supervision is available.

Those who become independent, at least as far as work is concerned, have skills that are useful in a job, as well as understanding and support from their families and from sympathetic employers. The work has to follow a fixed pattern; any unexpected changes are likely to cause distress due to inability to adapt. For example, a young adult in this subgroup who lived at home with his widowed mother worked at filling shelves in a supermarket. He was distressed when the positions of some goods were changed, and nearly lost his job. However, he was able to cope when, at his mother's suggestion, he was provided with a diagram of the store on which projected changes could be marked so that he was prepared in advance. Occupations necessitating social interaction and social skills are obviously unsuitable.

The social life of the adults in this sub-group is limited, but underneath the apparent lack of interest in people, there may be feelings of loneliness and sadness. Parents and siblings usually do their best to help, but if the person concerned has no family, the support and friendship of an experienced counselor is needed though not easy to find.

The autistic man, Raymond, played by Dustin Hoffman in the film *Rain Man* is an excellent example of this subgroup.

The Passive Subgroup

Passive autistic people are often amiable, gentle, and easily led. Some begin life with the typical autistic aloofness, but others are passive from infancy onwards and may fit all the criteria for Asperger syndrome. In the United Kingdom, they are more likely than the aloof subgroup to have been educated in a mainstream school.

The profiles of psychological skills tend to be less uneven than for the aloof people, so they are better able to keep up with schoolwork. They may need to be prompted to keep up standards of self-care, but the ability to copy others helps some to look respectable and neatly dressed.

Social approaches are accepted, but there is not much response or show of feelings. The passivity makes the characteristic autistic egocentricity rather less obvious in this subgroup compared with the others. Their activities are, as in all autistic people, limited and repetitive, but these are pursued with rather less of the usual determination. However, if pressed too hard to change their routine, or if sudden demands are made, even the most gentle and passive autistic person can react with unexpected distress or anger.

If the passivity is present from infancy, the diagnosis of autism is more likely to be missed than in the aloof subgroup. Especially for those who are high functioning, recognition of autism by others depends more on observation of the absence of the social and creative aspects of normal development than of the presence of positive abnormalities such as motor stereotypies, visual avoidance, and intense resistance to change.

In the Camberwell study, a history of passive social interaction appeared to be favorable for the achievement of independence in work even if not in daily living, although the numbers were too small for certainty. The general amenability is an advantage, but the tendency to lack drive holds some back from finding work. As usual, success is most likely in a job with a low level of pressure, a steady and predictable routine, and a sympathetic employer. Where the diagnosis of autism has never been recognized, the parents and teachers of a passive autistic young adult may be disappointed to find that he or she cannot keep a job at the level that would have been predicted from their schoolwork.

In general, once they find suitable work, people in this subgroup make good and reliable employees, but sometimes their social passivity and naïveté can lead to great problems. One young man, Robert (not in the Camberwell study), had a job in which he had to count and put away large amounts of money. Another employee, recognizing an innocent when he saw one, told Robert to keep back regularly a certain sum, which they shared between them. Inevitably, the theft was discovered and both were arrested, charged, and tried. Fortunately, the court understood that Robert had no idea of the implications of his actions and had simply obeyed directions without question. He was put on probation, but he lost his job. Robert had never been diagnosed as autistic until his parents sought psychiatric help for him after this episode. If his handicap had been known, and his gullibility anticipated, the problems might have been avoided. Following diagnosis, he was found a place in a sheltered workshop where the staff have special experience with autistic adults, and he is enjoying the work and the leisure program.

The Active-but-Odd Subgroup

People in this subgroup do not lack drive, but they use it to pursue their own idiosyncratic interests. In early childhood, they can show any of the first three types of social impairment described earlier. Some begin as evidencing classic Kanner syndrome; others follow the developmental course described by Asperger; and yet others, though socially impaired, do not as young children fit neatly into either of these groups.

The profiles of psychological skills also vary. While some individuals have the characteristic picture of higher visuospatial abilities, others have better verbal scores. However, this is mainly due to a wide vocabulary and subtests requiring memory for facts; comprehension of meaning is usually poorer than other aspects of speech. There may be specific learning disorders in, for example, numerical skills.

There is often a history of difficulty with school placement. The apparently good verbal skills mislead parents and teachers into too-high expectations. The problems are compounded by the social naïveté, the odd, persistent approaches to others, and a strong tendency for lack of cooperation when work is required that does not interest the child.

The diagnosis of autism is often missed, especially if the social interaction is odd rather than aloof from early on. These individuals tend to talk a lot and to look at people too long and hard rather than avoiding eye contact, thus not fitting the stereotyped view of autistic behavior. There may appear to be a teasing, malicious quality in the peculiar social approaches of some of those in this subgroup that gives rise, erroneously, to the view that the behavior is "deliberate" rather than the result of impairment. Children of this kind may have been moved from one type of school to another in the hope of finding one in which they can cope.

Circumscribed interests in particular subjects are common in this subgroup; the best outcome is achieved if these can be utilized in employment. An interest in dinosaurs helped one young man to a back-room post in a museum, and a young woman whose passion was reading encyclopedias worked in a library.

Sometimes the special interests are a hindrance, as with the man who was fasinated by astrology. He worked as a messenger, but each time he delivered a note he would not hand it over until he had given the recipient his or her horoscope for that day. His employment did not last long.

The Subgroup with Stilted Social Interaction

On first meeting people in this subgroup, there are few if any clues to the underlying subtle handicap. Recognition comes only with knowledge of their pattern of social relationships and their lifestyle.

Shah (1988) found that adults of this kind had a variety of early histories of social impairment, ranging from the aloofness of Kanner syndrome to active-but-odd interaction. The features of Asperger syndrome are particularly frequent. These individuals tend to be within the normal range of ability, and some have peaks of performance in one or two areas (such as visuospatial, mathematical, or musical skills) that may determine their working career.

In terms of behavior, individuals with this type of autism usually manage very well at work, being models of politeness and conventionality, if sometimes with a somewhat pompous and long-winded style of speech. Since their employment is mostly of the kind where the rules are clear-cut and relationships can be purely formal, they do not have much difficulty in fitting in. I personally know of such individuals in, for example, accountancy, the lower grades of the civil service, work with computers, and assembly work in factories.

Problems arise in more intimate relationships within the family, where spontaneity, empathy, and the provision of emotional support are required. People in this subgroup, like all those with autistic disorders, find it difficult to respond to the emotional needs of others. They have poor judgment as to the relative importance of different demands on their time and, characteristically, pursue their circumscribed interests—which may be work taken home, or separate hobbies—to the exclusion of everything and everyone else. At home, if too many demands are made that break the regular routine, there may be quite childish temper tantrums, even physical aggression, in marked contrast to the well-mannered, polite front seen at work.

Sometimes the diagnosis of autism is made in early childhood, but it is very often missed. Parents and teachers may be aware that the child is rather unusual, but do not know why. Most of the children attend mainstream schools although, in the United Kingdom, parents may place them in small private schools because they recognize their child's special needs.

Independence is achieved in most cases, and many do well if they are able to find the type of work that suits their abilities and interests. It is mainly in the social sphere that the presence of the underlying impairments can be detected by the experienced observer.

This subgroup shades into the eccentric end of the wide range of normal behavior, which raises theoretical questions concerning the nature of pathology and normality. (Asperger [1944] commented that his syndrome represented "the extreme end of the normal male personality." Whatever its scientific merit, this statement is a guaranteed party conversation opener.) In practice, the subtle type of social impairment comes to the attention of psychologists or psychiatrists only if the people concerned have difficulties in their lives and they, or people close to them, request help.

PROBLEMS AFFECTING ALL SUBGROUPS

Autistic children who are also mentally retarded are protected from many of the stresses of everyday life by their parents and by their teachers in special schools. Even if, because of a policy of integration, they are placed in mainstream schools, special help is provided in various ways. High-functioning autistic children, especially if their problems are not diagnosed, often have to manage as best they can with their age peers in an ordinary class.

Relationships with teachers can be difficult. Many autistic children, especially those fitting Asperger's descriptions, pursue their own interests in as well as out of school and ignore all their teachers' attempts to make them attend to the subjects in hand.

Normal children are quick to recognize oddity and may mercilessly bully autistic children, who in most cases are unable to defend themselves physically or verbally. Teaching staffs need to exercise good leadership and supervision if such problems are to be avoided. On the other hand, some autistic children in mainstream schools have special skills, such as musical or mathematical gifts, that command admiration and respect in their peers. The passive, amenable children may be popular because they are easily led; this can present other sorts of problems if they are led into mischief rather than constructive activities.

Problems concerning occupations in adult life have already been mentioned. These can be solved for some high-functioning adults (see, e.g., Temple Grandin's account of her remarkable success in her chosen profession, Grandin & Scariano, 1986). Finding appropriate leisure pursuits is often a more difficult challenge. It is helpful if this aspect of life is considered during the school years. Physical activities such as swimming, walking, jogging, or horse riding are a source of pleasure for some. In other cases, the circumscribed interests fill any leisure time, but for some the hours outside work are empty, boring, and lonely.

Despite the social impairment, some high-functioning people, even among those who appear aloof, long to have friends. They may have little concept of what friendship involves, but they know they want some kind of positive relationship with someone of their own age outside the family (Newson, Dawson, & Everard, 1982). In some cases, this problem is solved by joining a group dedicated to a specialized interest that appeals to the autistic person, such as stamp collecting, recording railway engine numbers, bird-watching, or playing chess. Occasionally, two autistic people will form a relationship with each other based on a shared circumscribed interest.

Some high-functioning adults have no interest in sex, but others wish to have a partner, to marry, and to have a family. Their social gaucheness is a major impediment to achieving these goals (see DesLaurier's, 1978, account of a high-functioning young man). They are conscious of their failure and will often ask for advice or for a book to read that will tell them how to attract a girlfriend or boyfriend.

Marriage is extremely unlikely except for those, mostly men, in the autistic continuum who have the social impairment in its most subtle form, and who are successful in their work. In my clinical experience, the success or otherwise of such marriages depends upon the personality and emotional needs of the partner. The unequal partnership can sometimes work well, but if full sharing of practical and emotional responsibilities is required, then major problems arise.

All kinds of psychiatric conditions can be superimposed on the autistic developmental disorder from adolescence onward (Gillberg, 1983, 1984; Gillberg & Steffenburg, 1984; Wing, 1981, 1983). This fact has relevance in the context of this chapter because the stresses arising from the social impairment can precipitate such illnesses. High-functioning autistic people are vulnerable to such problems, because they often have some insight and more is expected of them than of the severely handicapped groups. It is also the case that psychiatric illnesses are more easily recognizable in those with enough speech to convey their symptoms.

The condition seen most commonly is depression, often in response to recognition of poor performance in social situations, especially failure to find a friend or marriage partner. Severe anxiety states can also occur, especially in those in whom anxiety levels have always been high (see, e.g., Bemporad's, 1979, account of an autistic adult's recollection of his childhood). Obsessional conditions with, for example, hand-washing rituals are occasionally seen. It is difficult to know if these are exacerbations of autistic repetitive routines, but in some cases they more closely resemble classic obsessional states.

Undifferentiated psychoses with delusions and occasionally what seem to be hallucinations are sometimes seen in response to stress. They tend to resolve once the stress is identified and removed, though they can go on to become chronic.

HELP AND SUPPORT

The needs and ways of helping high-functioning autistic people will be discussed by other authors in other chapters of this volume. In the present context, a few points particularly relevant to the problem of social impairment can be emphasized.

It should always be remembered by those in close contact with autistic people—especially those with higher levels of ability—that their lack of understanding of the subtle rules of social interaction and communication does not necessarily indicate an absence of feeling or of a desire for a relationship. There have been considerable advances in methods of education for autistic people, especially in practical and academic skills. Further exploration is needed of methods of measurement of the ability to recognize and express socioemotional cues (Rutter *et al.*, 1988), and of techniques of teaching the many ways in which people show their own feelings and recognize such feelings in others. Clara Park (1986) discussed the difficulties (and the fascination) of this aspect of teaching. One of the impediments to developing this area is that much of human communicative behavior occurs without conscious attention and comprises sequences of complex movements that cannot be captured and specified for an autistic person to copy and apply in practice. Nevertheless, the efforts must continue, using photographs, videos, role-playing, and any other techniques that can be devised. Among the many facets of social interaction, modulation of vocal pitch and volume is important. The booming, monotonous voice, perhaps oddly high or low pitched, of many autistic people marks them out from others in a social gathering.

High-functioning autistic people may come into contact with adult psychiatric services as a result of their social problems or because of superimposed psychiatric illnesses. There is often confusion over diagnosis because the underlying autistic developmental disorder is not recognized. The inappropriate treatment and counseling that frequently results could be avoided if adequate information concerning disorders in the autistic continuum were to be included in the training of psychologists, psychiatrists, and other relevant professional workers working in the field of adult mental illnesses.

In the Camberwell study, the few autistic adults who achieved occupational independence all had intelligence quotients on at least one occasion of testing of 70 or above, but the majority of people functioning at this level remained dependent. It is to be hoped that specialized help during childhood will be available to all and will improve the prognosis. Investigations are needed to identify the reasons why some high-functioning autistic children become severely disturbed in adolescence and early adult life, and to find ways to prevent this waste of potential ability.

Helping an autistic person of any level of ability requires patience, understanding, affection, and a sense of humor. The rewards are the evidence of progress, however slow, and the knowledge that underneath the uncommunicative surface the affection is reciprocated, even if it is in an immature and partial way.

REFERENCES

American Psychiatric Association. (1987). *Diagnostic and statistical manual of mental disorders* (3rd ed.—Revised). Washington, DC: Author.

Asperger, H. (1944). Die "autistischen Psychopathen" im Kindesalter. *Archiv fur Psychiatrie und Nervenkrankheiten, 117,* 76–136.

Baron-Cohen, S. (1988). Social and pragmatic deficits in autism: Cognitive or affective? *Journal of Autism and Developmental Disorders, 18,* 379–402.

Baron-Cohen, S. (1989). The autistic child's theory of mind: A case of specific developmental delay. *Journal of Child Psychology and Psychiatry, 30,* 285–297.

Baron-Cohen, S., Leslie, A. M., & Frith, U. (1985). Does the autistic child have a "theory of mind"? *Cognition, 21,* 37–46.

Bemporad, J. R. (1979). Adult recollections of a formerly autistic child. *Journal of Autism and Developmental Disorders, 9,* 179–198.

Bowman, E. P. (1988). Asperger's syndrome and autism: The case for a connection. *British Journal of Psychiatry, 152,* 377–382.

DeMyer, M., Hingtgen, J., & Jackson, R. (1981). Infantile autism reviewed: A decade of research. *Schizophrenia Bulletin, 7,* 388–451.

DesLauriers, A. M. (1978). The cognitive–affective dilemma in early infantile autism: The case of Clarence. *Journal of Autism and Developmental Disorders, 8,* 219–228.

Gillberg, C. (1983). Psychotic behaviour in children and young adults in a mental handicap hostel. *Acta Psychiatrica Scandinavica, 68,* 351–358.

Gillberg, C. (1984). Autistic children growing up: problems during puberty and adolescence. *Developmental Medicine and Child Neurology, 26,* 125–129.

Gillberg, C., & Steffenburg, S. (1987). Outcome and prognostic factors in infantile autism and similar conditions: A population-based study of 46 cases followed through puberty. *Journal of Autism and Developmental Disorders 17,* 273–287.

Grandin, T., & Scariano, M. M. (1986). *Emergence: Labelled autistic.* Tunbridge Wells, England: Costello.

Hermelin, B., & O'Connor. N. (1985). Logico-affective states and non-verbal language. In E. Schopler & G. Mesibov (Eds.) *Communication Problems in Autism.* New York: Plenum.

Hobson, R. P. (1983). The autistic child's recognition of age-related features of people, animals and things. *British Journal of Developmental Psychology, 1,* 343–352.

Hobson, R. P. (1986a). The autistic child's appraisal of expressions of emotion. *Journal of Child Psychology and Psychiatry, 27,* 321–342.

Hobson, R. P. (1986b). The autistic child's appraisal of emotions: a further study. *Journal of Child Psychology and Psychiatry, 27,* 671–680.

Kanner, L. (1943). Austic disturbances of affective contact. *Nervous Child, 2,* 217–250.

Kanner, L.)1973). *Childhood psychosis: Initial studies and new insights.* New York: Winston/Wiley.

Leslie, A. M. (1987). Pretense and representation: The origins of "theory of mind." *Psychological Review, 94,* 412–426.

Leslie, A. M., & Frith, U. (1988). Autistic children's understanding of seeing, knowing and believing. *British Journal of Developmental Psychology, 6,* 315–324.

Newson, E., Dawson, M., & Everard, P. (1982). *The natural history of able autistic people: Management and functioning in a social context.* London: Department of Health and Social Security.

Park, C. C. (1982). *The siege*. New York: Atlantic–Little, Brown.

Park, C. C. (1983). Growing out of autism. In E. Schopler & G. Mesibov (Eds.), *Autism in adolescents and adults*. New York: Plenum.

Park, C. C. (1986). Social growth in autism: A parent's perspective. In E. Schopler & G. Mesibov (Eds.), *Social Behavior in Autism*. New York: Plenum.

Rimland, B. (1964). *Infantile autism: The syndrome and its implications for a neural theory of behavior*. New York: Meredith.

Rutter, M., LeCouteur, A., Lord, C., Macdonald, H., Rios, P., & Folstein, S. (1988). Diagnosis and subclassification of autism: Concepts and instrument development. In E. Schopler & G. B. Mesibov (Eds.), *Diagnosis and assessment in autism* (pp. 239–259). New York: Plenum.

Schopler, E. (1985). Editorial: Convergence of learning disability, high level autism and Asperger's syndrome. *Journal of Autism and Developmental Disorders, 15*, 359–360.

Schopler, E., & Mesibov, G. B. (Eds.). (1986). *Social behavior in autism*. New York: Plenum.

Schopler, E., & Rutter, M. (1988). Autism and pervasive developmental disorders: Concepts and diagnostic issues. In E. Schopler & G. B. Mesibov (Eds.), *Diagnosis and assessment in autism*. New York: Plenum.

Shah, A. (1988). *Visuo-spatial islets of abilities and intellectual functioning in autism*. Unpublished doctoral dissertation, London.

Wing, L. (1981). Asperger's syndrome: A clinical account. *Psychological Medicine, 11*, 115–130.

Wing, L. (1983). Social and interpersonal needs. In E. Schopler & G. B. Mesibov (Eds.), *Autism in adolescents and adults*. New York: Plenum.

Wing, L. (1986). Clarification on Asperger's syndrome (letter to the editor.) *Journal of Autism and Developmental Disorders, 16*, 513–515.

Wing, L. (1988). The continuum of autistic characteristics. In E. Schopler & G. B. Mesibov (Eds.), *Diagnosis and assessment in autism*. New York: Plenum.

Wing, L., & Gould, J. (1979). Severe impairments of social interaction and associated abnormalities in children: Epidemiology and classification. *Journal of Autism and Developmental Disorders, 9*, 11–29.

8

Treatment Issues with High-Functioning Adolescents and Adults with Autism

GARY B. MESIBOV

INTRODUCTION

Following its identification by Leo Kanner in 1943, autism was viewed as an emotional handicap caused by inadequate mothering. Few questioned this assumption for several decades. This conception of autism led to many inappropriate interventions based on psychoanalytic principles. Among the most inappropriate and destructive of these were the group and individual therapeutic interventions directed toward these children and their families (Schopler & Mesibov, 1984). Many of the families that participated in these programs vividly remember them and their associated feelings of guilt and ineptitude.

Most current interventions with autistic people and their families are based on educational approaches acknowledging the organic basis of autism (Dawson, 1989; Schopler & Mesibov, 1987). Although the current professional climate is healthier and more productive than it was in the 1950s and 1960s, bitter memories make everyone vigilant whenever new treatments appear to resemble the older psychodynamic techniques. Although such vigilance assures us that those earlier practices will not be reinstated, there is a negative side effect as well. The recent rejection of psychoanalytic approaches has caused professionals to dismiss as well all treatments vaguely resembling these interventions, even if they are, in reality, different. The understandable, though sometimes unfortunate, association of all group and individual intervention approaches with psychoanalytic theory has precluded possibly productive treatments for high-functioning autistic people.

GARY B. MESIBOV • Division TEACCH, Department of Psychiatry, The University of North Carolina at Chapel Hill, Chapel Hill, North Carolina 27599-7180.

High-Functioning Individuals with Autism, edited by Eric Schopler and Gary B. Mesibov. Plenum Press, New York, 1992.

This chapter proposes that individual and group work can be useful with high-functioning adolescents and adults with autism. Although these treatment modalities should be conceptualized differently from the psychoanalytic approaches they resemble, they can nevertheless make an important contribution if used properly and validated empirically. This chapter will trace principles that can be followed in individual and group counseling, describe potential applications of these intervention approaches, and provide empirically validated case study examples of treatment effectiveness.

INDIVIDUAL TREATMENT

Individual treatment approaches in autism unfortunately have been dominated by psychoanalytic theory. The best known of the psychoanalytic theorists in autism, Bruno Bettelheim (1967), was a strong advocate of individual therapy. His writings on autism, however, stress separation of children from parents, rather than describing the specific techniques implemented in individual sessions with the children.

DesLauriers (1978) advocated Pheraplay, a type of play therapy. Viewing autism as a sensory impairment, DesLauriers's technique provides sensory-stimulating experiences that are strong enough to overcome the basic sensory deficits of autism. The goal of Pheraplay is to develop sensory awareness in the context of enjoyable interpersonal interactions.

Rapoport (1942) described an individual treatment approach based on the psychoanalytic theories of Melanie Klein. The goal of this treatment is to establish a relationship in which the child feels dependent and safe. Techniques described by the Rapoport group are similar to those used with schizophrenic youngsters. There are no reports of the effectiveness of these interventions with either the autistic or the schizophrenic group.

Mahler, Boss, and DeFries (1949) treated several autistic youngsters within a psychoanalytic framework. Although there were no supporting data, Mahler *et al.* claimed that the autistic children were "lured" out of their autistic shells (Mahler, 1952). The Mahler group expressed optimism about the possible outcomes for autistic children following their therapeutic approaches; their optimism generally has not been supported by any data nor shared by other professionals.

Although these early attempts at individual treatment for autistic children were generally ineffective, the problem could be the psychoanalytic orientation, rather than the individual counseling. Our experience across the state of North Carolina with close to 100 high-functioning adolescent and adult clients suggests that individual counseling can be valuable for adolescents and adults with autism if appropriate goals are pursued in reasonable ways.

In the TEACCH program we maintain our focus on appropriate goals by conceptualizing individual counseling as one of many techniques for improving adaptation (Schopler, 1990). We see improved adaptation as coming in one of two ways for our clients: skill development of the client and environmental modifications to accommodate deficits. Skill enhancement, to the extent possible, is a popular strategy for assisting handicapped people by developing the abilities that are important for effective functioning. Given the scope and organic basis of the autistic deficit, however, we must acknowledge that not all skills can be enhanced to the extent necessary. Environmental adaptations are therefore important to make these undeveloped deficits less essential.

One-to-one counseling relationships can provide autistic people with the structure, guidance, information, and support that they need to function more effectively in society. These relationships can help develop skills and guide the necessary environmental adjustments. Those working individually with high-functioning autistic adolescents and adults must learn about their clients' perspectives of the world, establish trust, and develop rapport. One-to-one counseling sessions can achieve these vital objectives and then confront common issues of daily living.

Learning about Their Perspectives

Individuals with autism are often like visitors from a foreign culture, viewing the world in different ways from the rest of us. As a young man with autism, Jim Sinclair, writes in Chapter 14 of this book, "After reading Temple Grandin's autobiography (Grandin & Scariano, 1986), someone once asked me if I thought a cattle chute would have helped me. I said I didn't need a cattle chute, I needed an orientation manual for extraterrestrials. Being autistic does not mean being inhuman. But it does mean being alien." An effective counselor tries to understand each autistic person's "culture" and worldview. Once that understanding is achieved, the counselor tries to reconcile that culture with the realities of our "normal" society. Successful outcomes occur when compromises are achieved, both assisting autistic people to fit more easily into society (skill development) and adjusting society's expectations of them (environmental adaptations).

An example is Tom, a young autistic man who talks incessantly. He has difficulty separating essential from nonessential details; his conversations drift back and forth from important and interesting ideas to dull and nonessential facts. Many interventions have been designed to limit his conversations by abbreviating what he is allowed to say. These have been ineffective, however, because the man resents being cut off in midsentence and does not understand the distinctions that are being made. Gradually his counselor began exploring his "cultural" perspective and realized how hard it is for him to separate essential from nonessential information. The counselor also recognized from personal experience how difficult it was for others to suffer through Tom's ever-expanding statements. A recent compromise has improved the situation: Tom's open-ended conversations are now limited to specific blocks of time (15 or 20 minutes) each day when he can talk about topics he enjoys in the way he likes to discuss them. At other times he tries to end his statements the moment they exceed two sentences (or a total of 25 words).

Establishing Rapport and Developing a Sense of Trust

One essential goal in a counseling relationship with an autistic person is the development of trust. Although autistic people have difficulty forming interpersonal relationships, once established, these relationships become meaningful and important to them. A counselor who has good rapport with autistic clients has many opportunities to guide and assist them.

Rapport and trust can be established by showing genuine interest in the person with autism and those things that person values. Too often we try to squelch the narrow, idiosyncratic range of interests that are characteristic of high-functioning autistic people, a strategy that is neither effective nor fair. Imagine the effects of refusing to talk about topics of interest in a relationship with a nonhandicapped friend. A balance is needed between inviting autistic clients to share generally accepted ideas with us and joining them in narrow subjects of interest to them: train or airline schedules, birthdays, area codes, modes of transportation, locks, geography, the weather, witchcraft, or specific historical events, among others. Whatever their interests, each of these topics is a way of relating and making social interactions more intriguing to them. These topics should be pursued rather than stifled.

Relating to autistic people around their concerns and interests opens up new opportunities by establishing the counselor as an interesting and desirable person, providing a vehicle for teaching conversational skills, and enhancing motivation. Each of these is difficult to achieve otherwise when counseling people with autism. Entering into their culture earns us their trust and provides us with opportunities to teach them about our culture and expectations.

Once rapport and trust are established, a counselor can focus on other objectives: organizing their thinking, integrating ideas emphasizing relationships between events, and solving everyday problems by developing effective strategies and coping mechanisms.

Analyzing and Organizing Their Thinking

Helping autistic people to analyze and organize their thinking improves their understanding of the environment and its expectations. Even high-functioning autistic people have difficulty making sense out of the world and their own place in it. Their focus on details prevents them from understanding relationships between events and their meaning. Autistic people are classic examples of people who often cannot see the forest for the trees.

A focus on specific details without analyzing overall contexts can be problematic. An autistic woman working in a bakery regularly bumps into people as she walks to the oven to prepare the bread. She always follows the same route at the same speed, failing to react to anyone in her way. An autistic man working in a library notices trivial changes like a new clock, but did not realize that one of the major filing systems had been completely reorganized. Another young man notices tiny differences in buses, depending on the year they were made, but does not understand that 18-year-old peers expect different responses from him than his 7-year-old brother.

Another example of this problem is the confusion many autistic people have with time perspectives. Events happening 15 years ago seem as important and vivid to some autistic people as yesterday's activities. Emphasizing the irrelevance of yesterday's events and the importance of focusing on the present can be helpful on those occasions.

Emotions are a complex part of being human and are especially difficult for autistic people to analyze, understand, and interpret. Concrete and literal, they often lack the analytic skills and flexible strategies needed to comprehend emotional issues. Understanding one's own emotions is difficult enough; the difference between feeling sad and feeling depressed is subtle and elusive. Other people's emotions are even more challenging, requiring the consideration of another's perspective simultaneously with one's own.

Emotions are especially difficult for people who cannot consider two concurrent perspectives and thus focus on one aspect of a situation rather than the whole. A counselor's role is to help autistic people to clarify their own feelings and see those of others as well. A better understanding of emotionality makes many situations more comprehensible and leads to more effective interpersonal functioning.

One client in his thirties expressed a desire to be married. The counselor thought this strange from a man who rarely talked to women and had never dated. Although the man stated his need as finding a marriage partner, counseling sessions clarified the emotions of the young man as wanting companionship and some form of intimacy. These goals were more achievable in the short run for a young man who had never even dated.

In addition to misinterpreting his own feelings and needs, this same young man had trouble with other people's perspectives. As soon as a woman showed any interest in him—even if it was only to smile politely and say "hello"—he would follow her around and might even show up unannounced at her home. He had trouble seeing why his actions surprised these women and why they might be nervous when a large, male caller appeared unexpectedly at the door late at night. Explaining the women's perspective became the role of the counselor, who also identified and practiced more suitable ways of finding companionship and achieving intimacy.

Emphasizing Relationships between Events

Counselors also can explain relationships between events and especially between autistic clients' own behaviors and their consequences. A supportive relationship with a counselor makes feedback less threatening and more comprehensible. Because of their difficulty in integrating ideas and seeing relationships, these clients benefit from specific feedback about these connections.

Many autistic adults have employment difficulties because they do not fully understand the impact of their behaviors on others. One man lost a job because he "teased" a female employee about her weight. Although he saw this as good-natured, she found it offensive and demanded his termination. The employer complied because the other employee was more valuable to him than the autistic man. Although his job coach had several conversations with the client while the conflict was progressing, he was unable to communicate the seriousness of the situation and how the comments to the woman might become a reason to terminate his employment.

Explanations of how their own behavior can be counterproductive and of what others expect can lead to an understanding of how autistic people can be more effective. These explanations also reduce anxiety in social situations. One client once received a flower as a gift from an acquaintance. An avid conservationist, his immediate response was a lecture about the undesirable environmental impact of picking flowers. When told this was a gesture of friendship from a nice person, he responded that if she were nice, she would want to know she was destroying the environment.

Although progress was slow because of the subtleties involved, the counselor was eventually able to explain the issues to the man. His trust in his counselor made him receptive to suggestions about the subtle social aspects of this interaction. Although he will undoubtedly have similar difficulties in the future, the man was eventually able to understand why a positive gesture of friendship could be more important than the environmental implications of picking one flower. His inability to identify priorities from among the many concrete details of everyday life contributed to his confusion in understanding the consequences of his behavior.

Coping with Everyday Problems

Controlling behavior is another crucial hurdle for high-functioning autistic people. Excessive talking, temper tantrums, interrupting others, and arguing when corrected are behaviors that often cause problems. Reinforcing the importance of controlling these behaviors, helping clients to identify when they are occurring, and discussing how they can be avoided are crucial goals for counseling sessions. Coping strategies also can be planned and practiced. If a client is having problems on the job or at school, the counselor can help to pinpoint the problems and generate potential solutions. Counselors also can role-play alternatives to nonproductive interactions with their autistic clients.

Although capable in many ways, high-functioning autistic people are sometimes emotionally labile and have temper tantrums when confused or frustrated. Many times, they are able to understand the inappropriateness of these emotional outbursts that perplex and embarrass them. Reassurance that these behaviors are common in autism is helpful, as are examples of their occurrence in others with similar disabilities. Concrete statements concerning emotional behaviors, with examples and explanations of why they occur, do not always eliminate them but can be helpful. These discussions, if appropriate for their developmental level, can make the autistic people involved feel better about themselves and their situations.

Relaxation is a coping strategy that has proven effective with many autistic people (Cautela & Groden, 1978). The concreteness, structure, and repetitiveness of this technique make it well-suited to the needs and abilities of people with autism. Counselors can help autistic people find the most appropriate relaxation procedures for their unique situations and learn how to use them in a variety of situations.

In summary, trusting relationships with counselors can be extremely beneficial for high-functioning adolescents and adults with autism. These relationships can help them to organize their environments, integrate ideas, and develop appropriate coping mechanisms to deal with the many problems they face. An effective counselor tries to understand each client's "culture" and to bring him or her closer to the rest of society. This should not be done, however, without accepting the clients' views of their own surroundings and how they attempt to meet their own needs.

SOCIAL SKILLS GROUP TRAINING

Individual counseling can be an important component of treatment programs for high-functioning individuals with autism. Alone, however, it is not sufficient to meet their needs. Several investigators (Mesibov, 1983; Rutter, 1970; Schopler & Mesibov, 1983) have documented a growing social awareness in autistic people during adolescence, especially among the higher-functioning group. Unfortunately, this is not accompanied by increased social skills (Rutter, 1970; Schopler & Mesibov, 1986). If we are to adequately meet the needs of this higher-functioning group, individual counseling must be supplemented by social skills training.

Division TEACCH at The University of North Carolina at Chapel Hill has emphasized social skills group training with high-functioning autistic clients since the early 1980s (Mesibov, 1984, 1986). Our social skills groups include high-functioning adolescents and adults who meet regularly to share experiences and learn new skills. Group meetings include structured learning lessons and social activities. Participants learn the skills necessary for effective social functioning and then practice them in natural social situations. The social skills groups follow a cognitive, social learning model; improving understanding of social expectations through specific teaching techniques such as role-playing and behavioral rehearsal, participating in social activities in natural social settings, and understanding social expectations through discussions and group activities are three important aspects of this model.

Our social skills program is another illustration of the two components of the TEACCH interventions in autism: skill development and environmental adaptation. Social skills are developed, to the extent possible, through teaching sessions and instructional activities. The group itself, however, is an environmental adaptation. It was developed for and is adjusted to the needs and interests of each individual member. Participation, therefore, is more fun than in other groups because of the focus on what group members enjoy and how they experience activities.

Although there are many reasons why autistic people have social difficulties, these groups focus on three aspects in particular: their lack of interest in social interactions, their difficulties in understanding social rules, and their lack of social opportunities.

Lack of Interest in Social Interactions

An important reason why autistic people have problems with most social interactions is their lack of interest. Autistic people are described as having a narrow range of interests (American Psychiatric Association, 1987)—which means, among other things, that most of what we do in social situations has little value for them. An important goal of the TEACCH social skills program is to devise social activities that group members will find interesting and enjoyable. There are general strategies we use to help motivate our group members: generating activities based on group members' interests, incorporating group games, having group competitions for prizes, and developing positive and predictable routines.

Although many of the topics that preoccupy autistic people seem narrow and limited, we try to adapt them into group activities. For example, if two group members have special interests in buses, a natural activity is to take bus rides. Group members interested in nature enjoy our hikes, those interested in music enjoy visits to a local record store, those interested in food like our trips to local restaurants, and those interested in birthdays or zip codes enjoy looking them up for each group member. In the course of a 15-week semester, we can generally incorporate activities around each member's specific interests.

Group games are motivating, especially those that we base on favorite TV shows such as "Wheel of Fortune" or "Jeopardy." We follow the structure of these shows, but make adjustments to meet additional interpersonal goals. For example, our game of "Jeopardy" consists of categories based on group members' interests and skills. Questions within these categories include favorite restaurants, favorite activities, strongest skills, favorite celebrities, and other personal information. To win these games, group members must develop an awareness of the other group members and their particular strengths and preferences. Although initial attempts at these games were slow because each group member projected his or her own interests onto all of the others, considerable progress has been made.

Simple competitions enhance these quiz-show games and increase motivation in other activities as well. We often divide our group into small teams of three or four people each and give a candy bar to winning team members at the end of an activity. The small prize heightens their awareness of one another and builds cooperation and cohesiveness within the group. Small groups work together in our quiz-show games, our sporting activities (e.g., relay races), our scavenger hunts, and several other activities. These small groups have been effective in fostering interpersonal awareness and cooperation.

Establishing predictable and understandable routines has been another way of making our Social Skills Group more appealing. Routines are reassuring to autistic people and, once established, make activities that are part of the routine more desirable in and of themselves. Positive routines that we have established over the years are our semiannual trips to Camp Dogwood, Halloween and Christmas parties, an end-of-spring picnic, trips to the state fair, and our popular adventures in local restaurants. Consistent, enjoyable, and appropriate activities have enhanced the value of our group.

Difficulties in Understanding Social Rules

Another social problem for autistic people that our groups address is the difficulty in understanding social rules. For autistic people the problem is twofold: They have trouble reading social cues, and by nature our social rules are elusive. Because of their social deficits and problems when concepts are not specific and concrete, the area of social relationships is especially problematic for individuals with autism.

Our intervention techniques are designed to make social situations and expectations as clear as possible for our group members. We often generate social rules where they are not ordinarily specified, even if they are less than perfect. Autistic people need rules in situations where actions are guided by judgment and subtle cues from other people. Although concrete rules often do not work as well as good judgment, they are better and more adaptable for autistic people than having no rules at all.

In developing reasonable guidelines, we identify the situations that are most difficult for our clients and generate the best rules we can create. Group members are instructed to greet new people by looking at them, smiling, and saying that they are happy to meet them. We also suggest and practice the use of questions as a way of maintaining conversations (of course, some are perseverative questioners and do not need this instruction). Suggested conversation topics are families, sports, radio and television shows, and current events, among others. We practice taking turns in conversations and make this more concrete by passing a microphone from speaker to speaker. The visual cue of a microphone can be helpful in reminding the person of whose turn it is to talk.

Although the rules we generate are not always perfect, they are preferable to the alternative, which is asking autistic people to function without any structure or simply prohibiting a class of behaviors. If our rules are not effective, they can always be revised. An example is the autistic woman who had spent many years in a residential institution. Upon moving into a community-based group home, she sometimes told off-color jokes in public forums with strangers. This woman did not understand the social conventions involving these kinds of situations. She needed some structure (or rules) to understand when this behavior was acceptable. One possibility would have been to prohibit off-color jokes in all situations. This would represent an undesirable restriction, however, because many adults participate in this activity, which enhances their enjoyment of others. As an alternative, we developed rules for where and when these jokes are appropriate.

We started by assessing her understanding of the difference between an off-color joke and a more widely accepted one. These distinctions are often difficult for people with autism. In this particular situation, however, the problem was not her inability to make this distinction. She was, in fact, able to explain graphically her jokes and the anatomical parts of the body they represented.

After establishing her understanding of what she said, our next approach was to define limiting conditions. We suggested to her that off-color jokes are only to be shared among friends. She quickly pointed out that I had previously told her that most people in the world are her friends, so that she does not have to worry about asking for help. Further clarification was obviously needed, so we defined friends as people one has regular (more than 10 times) contact with. This seemed to provide the structure she needed without limiting her any more than necessary.

The new rule was effective for about three weeks. One night, the group home manager heard the woman talking with her mother on the telephone. She began to tell her mother that since she was a friend who she had seen more than 10 times, she wanted to tell her a joke. Our rule was immediately revised (while the mother was on the telephone) to define friends as people we have regular contact with and who are under 50 years of age.

Our rule—imperfect though it might be—has served this woman well. She is able to share off-color humor like the rest of us, but with some structure and the limitations she needs to maintain common social expectations. The process of defining subtle social rules is an ongoing one, often requiring revisions and changes. It is an important process that is very helpful for high-functioning people with autism.

Lack of Social Opportunities

The third goal of our social skills program is to provide social experiences for our participants. When we began this program several years ago, we viewed these experiences as a way to practice social skills in real-life settings. This is still an important reason for our outings because of the well-documented difficulties autistic people have with generalization when new behaviors are not practiced in the actual settings where they will be performed (Cohen & Donnellan, 1987; Falvey, 1986; Schopler & Mesibov, 1986). There are, however, two additional benefits to these community outings: They are interesting to our group members, and provide social opportunities generally lacking in their lives. As with other aspects of our social skills program, we try to select the social activities that will be the most interesting and meaningful.

Group members enjoy our visits to restaurants, minor league baseball games, bowling alleys, and the state fair, as well as our popular trips to Camp Dogwood. Camp Dogwood was built by the Lions Club to serve blind adults, but two weekends each year it is available to us for boating, horseback riding, baseball, basketball, soccer, Frisbee, bingo, and whatever else we can think of. These weekends are the most popular activities that we do with our group members.

As we participate in these activities together, we note a significant increase in the conversational skills of our group members. Meaningful, interesting, and enjoyable, these shared experiences provide common threads for social conversations. Although our clients are limited because of their communication deficits, these activities have taught us about a specific aspect of their limitations that can be remediated: They do not have a lot of things to talk about with other people because their experiences and interests are typically not shared by other people. Common experiences like Camp Dogwood and our community activities are important ways of increasing communication.

Another reason for these community-based activities is that they provide ongoing social opportunities for our group members. Although our initial hope was that better social skills would increase their social opportunities—and this has happened to a certain extent—the unfortunate reality is that their deficits continue to limit their social possibilities. Providing an ongoing group assures that our high-functioning autistic people will have regular social contacts that are satisfying and meaningful. This is another indication that improving skills alone is not enough; our group members need environmental adaptations as well.

Our social skills groups have been effective and useful. Making activities interesting, clarifying rules, and providing social experiences have been productive targets for our intervention efforts. In addition, several ongoing strategies have further enhanced our efforts: using nonhandicapped peers, developing game rules designed to further our interpersonal goals, and accepting some of the inherent social difficulties of our clients instead of trying to change every aspect of their interpersonal functioning.

Many investigators have found nonhandicapped peers to be helpful in teaching social behaviors to individuals with autism (McHale, Olley, Marcus, & Simeonsson, 1981; Strain & Cooke, 1976; Wooten & Mesibov, 1986). Our experience has been consistent with theirs. Nonhandicapped peers are more responsive than other handicapped youngsters and can be directed more easily to respond in specific ways. Nonhandicapped peers also bring an enthusiasm and energy to our social skills programs that is often lacking when handicapped students are the only ones involved. This enthusiasm is often contagious and can be the impetus for enhanced enjoyment and participation in social activities.

Because our social skills groups include mostly high-functioning adults, our nonhandicapped peers are college students. They are usually undergraduates interested in learning more about developmental disabilities (Mesibov, 1984, 1986). These students are excellent peers for our group members and also benefit themselves from these opportunities. Many of our finest staff working with autistic people in North Carolina had their initial experiences in our social skills program.

Another general strategy we pursue is modifying rules of the games we play to clarify and facilitate the social interactions we desire. For example, in playing soccer we have only two or three people on a team so that the participants can be more aware of what is happening. Points are awarded for successful passes to teammates as well as for goals in order to encourage teamwork and cooperation. Our game of "Jeopardy," as mentioned earlier, includes categories based on each of the group members. Other games and activities, like basketball and football, are adapted in similar ways.

A final ingredient of our social skills program is our acceptance of some differences inherent in autism. Our goal is not to eliminate all vestiges of autism or to make our group members look normal. Instead, we want them to be appropriate enough so that they do not offend others and to be able to enjoy a wide range of activities. This distinction is subtle yet critical. It allows us to focus on enriching clients' lives, rather than on their deficits. Our focus on enhancement, rather than normalcy, also helps us establish realistic goals and prevents us from assuming the role of the nagging parent or spouse. Environmental adaptation is as important to us as skill development.

In summary, individual counseling and group training opportunities have enhanced our work with high-functioning adolescents and adults with autism. Although abused by some psychoanalysts during earlier years, these interventions have been valuable additions to our treatment efforts. Professionals working with high-functioning individuals with autism might consider their clients' needs and ways in which individual counseling and group opportunities can facilitate the achievement of worthwhile goals. There seems to be an important place for these interventions, based on current practices and our own experiences.

REFERENCES

American Psychiatric Association. (1987). *Diagnostic and statistical manual* (3rd ed.—Revised). Washington, DC: Author.

Bettelheim, B. (1967). *The empty fortress*. New York: Free Press.

Cautela, J. R., & Groden, J. (1978). *Relaxation: A comprehensive manual for adults, children, and children with special needs*. Champaign, IL: Research Press.

Cohen, D. J., & Donnellan, A. M. (Eds.). (1987). *Handbook of autism and pervasive developmental disorders*. New York: Wiley.

Dawson, G. (Ed.). (1989). *Autism: Nature, diagnosis, and treatment*. New York: Guilford.

DesLauriers, A. M. (1978). Play, symbols, and the development of language. In M. Rutter & E. Schopler (Eds.), *Autism: A reappraisal of concepts and treatment* (pp. 313–326). New York: Plenum.

Falvey, M. A. (1986). *Community-based curriculum: Instructional strategies for students with severe handicaps*. Baltimore: Paul Brookes.

Grandin, T., & Scariano, M. (1986). *Emergence: Labelled autistic*. Novato, CA: Arena.

Mahler, M. S. (1952). On child psychosis and schizophrenia. *Psychoanalytic Study of the Child, 7,* 286–305.

Mahler, M. S., Ross, J. R., DeFries, Z. (1949). Clinical studies in benign and malignant cases of childhood psychosis (schizophrenia-like). *American Journal of Orthopsychiatry, 19,* 295–305.

McHale, S. M., Olley, J. G., Marcus, L. M., & Simeonsson, R. J. (1981). The effectiveness of nonhandicapped peers as tutors for autistic children. *Exceptional Children, 48,* 263–264.

Mesibov, G. B. (1983). Current perspectives and issues in autism and adolescence. In E. Schopler & G. B. Mesibov (Eds.), *Autism in adolescents and adults* (pp. 37–53). New York: Plenum.

Mesibov, G. B. (1984). Social skills training with verbal autistic adolescents and adults: A program model. *Journal of Autism and Developmental Disorders, 14,* 395–404.

Mesibov, G. B. (1986). A cognitive program for teaching social behaviors to verbal autistic adolescents and adults. In E. Schopler & G. B. Mesibov (Eds.), *Social behavior in autism* (pp. 265–303). New York: Plenum.

Rapoport, J. (1942). Therapeutic process in a case of childhood schizophrenia. *Nervous Child, 1,* 188–198.

Rutter, M. (1970). Autistic children: Infancy to adulthood. *Seminars in Psychiatry, 2,* 435–450.

Schopler, E. (1990). Principles for directing both educational treatment and research. In C. Gillberg (Ed.), *Diagnosis and treatment of autism*. New York: Plenum.

Schopler, E., & Mesibov, G. B. (Eds.). (1983). *Autism in adolescents and adults*. New York: Plenum.

Schopler, E., & Mesibov, G. B. (Eds.). (1984). *The effects of autism on the family*. New York: Plenum.

Schopler, E., & Mesibov, G. B. (Eds.). (1986). *Social behavior in autism*. New York: Plenum.

Schopler, E., & Mesibov, G. B. (Eds.). (1987). *Neurobiological issues in autism*. New York: Plenum.

Strain, P. S., & Cooke, T. P. (1976). An observational investigation of two elementary-age autistic children during free play. *Psychology in the Schools, 13,* 82–91.

Wooten, M., & Mesibov, G. B. (1986). Social skills training for elementary school autistic children with normal peers. In E. Schopler & G. B. Mesibov (Eds.), *Social behavior in autism* (pp. 305–319). New York: Plenum.

9

Social Perception in High-Level Autism

R. PETER HOBSON

INTRODUCTION

What does it mean to perceive, relate to, know about, even *be* a "person"? Time and again since Kanner's (1943) original paper on autistic disturbances of affective contact, children with autism have been described as treating others as if they were things more like pieces of furniture than sentient human beings. We are led to ask: What is so special about persons, how does the normal infant (and child) come to recognize people *as* people, and what has gone so badly awry in autism? These are questions I shall be trying to address in the course of this chapter.

I have chosen the title "social *perception* in high-level autism" because I wish to survey the very foundations of social relations and social understanding, and here it is necessary to deal with perceptually anchored psychological abilities and propensities. If one wishes to take a developmental and evolutionary perspective, however, it is hazardous to disjoin perception from action and feeling, even from knowledge. When a normal infant perceives what we as adults call the mother's nipple and turns towards it, seizes it with its mouth, and starts to suck rhythmically, the infant's perception of the breast entails at once an orientation, a bringing of the stimulus under a sensory–motor classificatory system, a motivated action, and in all probability, affectively charged experiences. Piaget's (e.g., 1972) idea that the infant assimilates an aspect of the perceptual world to a "sucking scheme" is intended to capture something of the dynamics as well as the cognitive structure of such events. What we actually observe is the infant relating to the breast in a particular way. Or again, an older infant who recognizes a rattle and shakes it expresses a practical understanding that this object is a shakable, noise-making

---

R. PETER HOBSON • Developmental Psychopathology Research Unit, Tavistock Clinic and University College, London NW3 5BA, England.

High-Functioning Individuals with Autism, edited by Eric Schopler and Gary B. Mesibov. Plenum Press, New York, 1992.

object; it is possible for him or her to perceive a rattle *as* a rattle only to the extent that he or she has some understanding of what a rattle is, and can bring the object under an appropriate "description" (Hamlyn, 1978). Very early in development, therefore, biologically based forms of perceptually anchored activity and awareness, perhaps with the backing of innate categories of understanding (Kant, 1929), constitute a basis for the infant to apprehend and classify objects and events in the world; later in development, conceptual understanding has a direct bearing on the way a child perceives an object *as* a "this" or a "that." Thus, to refer to a child's perception of things and events is to presuppose a constitutional and developmental background in which diverse aspects of the individual's transactions with the world play an essential role.

It may be worthwhile to ground these rather abstract considerations by returning to the specific domain of social perception. Since we are concerned with the foundations of experience and understanding, I shall refer to some theoretical perspectives on normal infancy. Baldwin (1902) suggested that the child is endowed with an "organic" (instinctive) capacity for sympathy with others, and can differentiate persons from things by responding to "suggestions of personality" in other people. This approach was also espoused by Darwin (1877), who wrote, "An infant understands to a certain extent, and as I believe at a very early period, the meaning or feelings of those who tend him, by the expression of their features" (pp. 293–294, cited in Murray & Trevarthen, 1985). For Baldwin and Darwin, therefore, an initial demarcation of the personal and nonpersonal spheres of experience is accomplished through an infant's more or less innate perceptual–affective propensities. In recent times, J. J. Gibson (1979) has been most influential in highlighting the importance of basic "meaning-sensitive" faculties. With respect to the social environment, Gibson (1977) wrote: "The other animals of the environment afford, above all, a rich and complex set of interactions, sexual, predatory, nurturing, fighting, play, cooperating, and communicating. What other persons afford, for man, comprise the whole realm of social significance" (p. 68). The individual's propensities and capacities to perceive such "affordances" and attune to perceptually anchored social events may be essential determinants of interpersonal experience and thus provide a necessary foundation for the development of knowledge about the nature of persons. Innately determined forms of social perception may constitute a basis for early modes of social understanding.

What kinds of evidence have a bearing on these theoretical proposals, and what might be their relevance for an understanding of autism? I shall consider some selected phenomena from normal infant development before turning to the case of autism.

ASPECTS OF INFANT SOCIAL–PERCEPTUAL DEVELOPMENT

I shall be overselective in considering only specific facets of infant social development. My concern is with perceptually grounded prerequisites for what might be called *personal relatedness*. For the present, I shall define personal relatedness in a question-begging way as those forms of interpersonal behavior and experience that are necessary prerequisites for a child to acquire knowledge that other people are subjects of experience with their own feelings, attitudes, thoughts, and so on. I shall not have space to dwell upon less "perceptual" but nonetheless critical aspects of personal relatedness, such as the temporal patterning and "activation contours" of interpersonal events (Stern, 1985), the infant's own innately determined propensities for bodily expressive patterns (e.g., Hiatt, Campos, & Emde, 1979; Malatesta, 1981), and the representational structures that may serve to organize early social experience (e.g., Isaacs, 1948). I merely emphasize the importance of these topics for characterizing normal personal relatedness and for specifying the impairments of autistic children.

Thus, my focus in this chapter is upon those of an infant's capacities that concern the perception of meaning in other people's bodily expressions. It is against such capacities that we might measure the severity and extent of autistic children's social-perceptual disabilities. For both theoretical and practical reasons, I shall take the perception of emotionally expressive behavior as a paradigm case. The theoretical reason is that such perception is likely to have special importance for establishing "intersubjectivity" between individuals (Habermas, 1970; Hobson, 1989a, b, 1990a, b; Trevarthen, 1979). The practical reason is that a major part of the recent experimental work on social perception in autistic children, as well as an important tradition in research on infants, has been concerned with the perception and understanding of emotional expressions. In what follows, therefore, I shall attempt to highlight normal infants' capacities for emotion-related social perception, and to indicate the route by which infants come to experience themselves as both connected to and differentiated from other people *as* people with their own psychological orientations to the world.

Recognizing Emotions

The first task is to analyze what is involved in recognizing emotions (Klinnert, Campos, Sorce, Emde, & Svejda, 1983; Nelson, 1987; Oster, 1981; Walker-Andrews, 1988). As we have seen, to recognize meaning is to have some level of understanding of that which is perceived. A minimal degree of understanding would entail that infants abstract the invariant features of given emotional expressions across individuals who might differ in, for example, age, sex, and identity. Then the infant might be able to appreciate which expressions of emotion are associated with each other (e.g., how an angry face is likely to accompany an angry vocalization) or which expressions are accompanied by which kinds of action (e.g., an angry face with attacking behavior). Another mode of recognition is manifest when infants demonstrate differential affective responsiveness to expressions of emotion in others. A yet further level of understanding, perhaps more controversially "perceptual" in nature, is when an infant can use the emotional expressions of others to appraise environmental events—for example, in assessing the dangerousness of a situation by reading a caretaker's face (Klinnert *et al.*, 1983). Finally, there comes a point when the child arrives at an explicit understanding that expressions are indeed expressive of the subjective emotional life of persons, that is, people whose feelings are similar in kind but often different in content to the child's own emotional states. By this time, to perceive other human beings *is* to recognize them as persons.

When it comes to reviewing the evidence concerning infants' capacities for perceiving emotion in others (see also, e.g., Walker-Andrews, 1988), it is salutary to note the contradictory claims that are a feature of the past and recent literature. One source of disagreement is the range of methodologies applied to the study of infant social capacities, from closely controlled but highly contrived experiments on infants' attentiveness to drawings or slides of faces, to interpersonal but nevertheless "staged" imitation studies, to more naturalistic recordings of mother–infant interaction. Although the evidence from early observational and quasi-experimental studies of infants' responses to facial expressions was rather conflicting (e.g., Ahrens, 1954; Buhler & Hetzer, 1928; Spitz & Wolf, 1946), more recent evidence suggests that infants discriminate photographed facial expressions from around 3 or 4 months, but may not recognize them according to their emotional characteristics until after the middle of the first year of life—and even then, not surprisingly, the infants show minimal signs of differential relatedness to such artificial stimuli (e.g., Caron, Caron, & Myers, 1982; La Barbera, Izard, Vietze, & Parisi, 1976; Young-Browne, Rosenfeld, & Horowitz, 1977). The situation becomes more interesting when one considers infants' reactions to less static forms of expression, especially vocalizations, and investigates their sensitivity to face–voice combinations that more nearly capture something of the dynamic, multimodal qualities of human expressiveness. Even for neonates, certain vocal expressions may have an emotional impact: Simner (1971) and Sagi and Hoffman (1976) found that in the first few days of life, infants became distressed at the sound of another infant's cry but not at equally loud nonhuman sounds. Certainly by 5 months of age, infants can differentiate amongst different dynamic face–voice expressions shown on videotape (Caron, Caron, & MacLean, 1988).

How soon do infants recognize the correspondence between vocal and facial expressions of particular emotions, and therefore manifest some grasp of emotional meaning? Walker (1982) reported four experiments demonstrating that infants of 5 and 7 months can detect information that is invariant across the acoustic and optic presentations of given affective expressions. Infants were presented with two filmed facial expressions side-by-side, accompanied by a single vocal expression characteristic of one of the facial expressions. Thus, for example, infants saw two moving facial images of a woman speaking continuously, one with a happy face and the other with a sad face, and they heard a vocalization broadcast from a point between the two faces. The infants increased their looking time to the facial expression corresponding to the emotion expressed by the voice, even if the face and voice were out of synchrony (although this lessened the effect). However, such selective attentiveness was not recorded when the faces were presented upside down. Walker concluded that the infants perceived the faces and voices to have a common meaning.

Even in studies that have been concerned with infants' recognition of meaning in relatively abstracted emotions, therefore, subjects as young as 7 months or so have demonstrated quite impressive social-perceptual capacities. How do infants perceive emotion in more real-life, interpersonal settings?

Emotion Perception in Contexts of Personal Relatedness

A first step toward naturalistic studies has been to investigate infants' perception of real-life people under rather artificial, controlled conditions. The studies of neonatal imitation conducted by Field and her colleagues (Field *et al.*, 1983; Field, Woodson, Greenberg, & Cohen, 1982) are particularly challenging. For example, when infants under 2 days old were presented with a model who posed fixed happy, sad, and surprised facial expressions, they tended to show widened eyes and wide mouth opening in response to the model's surprised face, lip widening to the happy face, and tightened mouth with protruding lips accompanied by a furrowed brow to the sad expression. Haviland and Lelwica (1987) reported that somewhat older infants, around 10 weeks of age, showed nonrandom behavior patterns indicative of induced emotional responses to their mothers' face-plus-voice affective expressions. The infants not only manifested facial expressions of affect, but also patterns of coordinated gaze that were not presented by the mothers, so it seemed that this behavior indicated the infants' emotional states rather than specific matching behavior. Even very early in life, therefore, infants not only can discriminate amongst the "live" affective expressions of others, but can respond as if the presented expressions are meaningful. In some circumstances at least, the infants appear to experience corresponding emotional states of their own.

Even more striking evidence for the organization of interpersonal-affective perception and communication comes from studies of perturbations in mother–infant interactions. Following up early reports of infants' responses to still-faced mothers (Carpenter, Tecce, Stechler, & Friedman, 1970; Tronick, Als, Adamson, Wise, & Brazelton, 1978), Cohn and Tronick (1983) instructed mothers of 3-month-old infants to interact with depressed expressions during three-minute periods of face-to-face exchanges. Infants responded by becoming more negative and showed increased protest and wariness, reactions that tended to continue for a brief period after mothers switched to normal interaction. A similar picture emerged from the studies of Murray and Trevarthen (1985), who not only exposed infants to their mothers' blank-faced staring, but also devised a condition in which they used a videotape feedback system to present the mother's behavior after a delay of 30 seconds. In the latter condition, infants manifested signs of distress, with turning away from the mother's image accompanied by brief looks. Thus, the infants displayed coherently organized and complex expressions of affect and attention that were systematically sensitive to the form and direction of the mother's behavior. These findings vividly illustrate how affective perception and communication are multifaceted and finely organized in time both within the infant and between the infant and his or her mother.

The next question is whether infants can recognize the meaning of emotional expressions not only in the context of face-to-face interactions, but also with regard to another individual's relatedness to a commonly perceived environment. I shall take the study by Sorce, Emde, Campos, and Klinnert (1985) to serve as an illustration of the phenomenon of "social referencing" (Campos & Stenberg, 1981; Feinman, 1982; Klinnert *et al.*, 1983). Infants aged 12 months were placed on the shallow side of a visual cliff (which takes the form of an apparent sudden drop beneath a transparent surface), and the mother and an attractive toy were positioned across the deep side. The results concerned those infants who, on noticing the drop-off, spontaneously looked to the mother's face. When the mother posed a happy face, 14 out of 19 infants crossed to the deep side; when the mother posed a fearful expression, none of the infants ventured across. When the mother posed an angry expression, only 2 out of 18 infants proceeded across the cliff, and 14 actively retreated by moving back to the shallow side. In this and in other comparable circumstances (Feinman & Lewis, 1983; Klinnert, 1984; Walden & Ogan, 1988), infants around 1 year of age seem to have the capacity to seek out their mother's affective expression, relate this to a current situation, and react accordingly with feeling and action. The infants appear to recognize that another person's expression has meaning with reference to an environment common to themselves and the other person.

It seems probable that social referencing emerges sometime in the second half of an infant's first year of life. This is a period of dramatic changes in the quality of the infant's social relatedness. From age 9 months or so, an infant comes to give, show, and point things out to others, often looking back and forth between the object and the mother's eyes; requests help to obtain objects; initiates games such as peekaboo; imitates household activities and conventional actions; and manifests a range of additional social accomplishments (e.g., Bretherton & Bates, 1979; Bretherton, McNew, & Beeghly-Smith, 1981; Harding & Golinkoff, 1979; Reddy, 1990; Trevarthen & Hubley, 1978). As Bretherton *et al.* (1981) have discussed, such developments imply that infants have come to recognize the psychological similarity, as well as the separateness, of self and others. They have come to perceive others as subjects of experience with their own psychological orientations toward the world and toward themselves, and to recognize human beings as persons with whom things can be shared (Hobson, 1989a). As I have indicated, the course of early infant development suggests that this sophisticated level of "person perception" might have precursors and perhaps prerequisites in prior forms of emotion-related social perception.

Further Aspects of Social Perception

I now wish to make brief reference to certain additional aspects of normal social perception that are relevant for the subsequent discussion. The first point concerns the infant's earliest propensities to attend to aspects of other human beings, whether these involve visual, tactile, or auditory characteristics. There is a great deal of evidence to suggest that infants are predisposed to show selective attentiveness to a variety of objects and events with humanlike qualities (see, e.g., Field & Fox, 1985; Lamb & Sherrod, 1981). The second point concerns the infant's capacity to recognize specific individuals as familiar, a capacity that has very early manifestations (Field, 1985; Zucker, 1985) but flowers with the formation of specific attachments to individual people who provide a secure base from which to explore, who act as sources of comfort, and separations from whom often prompt distress (e.g., Bretherton, 1985). Clearly, an infant perceives such attachment figures as very special people.

Then we need to note that there are additional features of people that infants appear to perceive in the first year of life. Notable amongst these are the categories of age and sex. Infants as young as 6 or 7 months are able to discriminate age-related and sex-related features of human faces in photographs (Fagan, 1972, 1976; Fagan & Singer, 1979). Toward the end of their first year, infants respond more positively to the approach of unfamiliar children than to that of adults (Brooks & Lewis, 1976), and when watching videotapes of figures represented by dots of light, they seem able to differentiate the sexes according to cues of body movement alone (Aitken, 1977; Kujawski, 1985). There is also evidence that 6-month-olds can categorize male and female voices (Miller, 1983). Such findings offer support for the ideas of those ethologists and proponents of the "ecological" approach to perception who emphasize the perceptual bases for recognizing such meaningful human attributes as "babyishness" and gender (e.g., Hess, 1970; McArthur and Baron, 1983; Runeson & Frykholm, 1986; Shaw & Pittenger, 1977).

Finally, it is pertinent to make one further remark about normal infants' capacities to achieve visual co-orientation with others. I have already noted how from 9 months of age, infants may point to things and monitor the direction of their caretaker's gaze. There is evidence to suggest that even younger infants have some mechanism by which they can follow another person's line of visual regard (Butterworth & Grover, 1990; Churcher & Scaife, 1982; Scaife & Bruner, 1975). The point to note is that such a mechanism might operate independently of the infant's recognition of other people as subjects of experience (Hobson, 1989b).

Summary

I have dwelt at some length on the manifestations of a normal infant's developing capacities to discriminate and recognize meaning in other people's bodily and especially affective expressions. I have implied that there are links with the infant's developing awareness and perception of persons as subjects of experience. More specifically, I have tried to highlight important features of and prerequisites for what Trevarthen (1979) has called primary intersubjectivity, the earliest meeting or perhaps meshing of minds in infancy, which leads on to the more differentiated forms of psychological sharing and coordination appearing toward the end of the first year.

Here it is relevant to note that there are philosophical arguments to support the claim that a normal child's concept of persons *as* persons with mental life arises out of the child's experience of biologically based and often affectively coordinated personal relatedness with others (Hamlyn, 1974; Hobson, 1990b).

Now that we have an outline of some essential features of social perception in normal infants—especially their abilities to perceive emotion in others, but also their early capacities to attend to people; to differentiate individuals according to familiarity, age, and sex; to follow other people's line of regard; and, finally, to orientate to other people's psychological orientations to the world—we are in a position to compare these abilities with what we know of autistic children's development.

SOCIAL PERCEPTION IN AUTISM

As I observed at the beginning of the chapter, many authors have remarked how in the presence of an autistic child, they have felt themselves to be treated like pieces of furniture. I believe that a proper understanding of autism requires that we analyze the nature and source of this uniquely abnormal "feel" that is a feature of relations with autistic people. Following Kanner (1943), I take the view that there are impairments in basic capacities for bodily intercoordination between the autistic child and other people, and more specifically, impairments in the capacities needed to achieve interpersonal affective contact and participation in the emotional lives of others. I would argue that autism is best viewed as an interpersonal impairment, an abnormality in what can and cannot transpire *between* the young autistic child and others (Hobson, 1991a). This functional impairment may have many kinds of etiology (e.g., a range of physical afflictions causing limbic system dysfunction in the child; Damasio & Maurer, 1978) or predisposing conditions (e.g., congenital blindness; Hobson, 1990a; Keeler, 1958; Wing, 1969), but it has a relatively constant expression across autistic individuals. In most cases, the disorder in interpersonal relations has specific kinds of implications for the children's cognitive and linguistic as well as social development—and especially for their understanding of persons with mental life (Hobson, 1989a).

If this approach has some validity, it behooves us to reexamine the detail contained in clinical descriptions of autistic children and, measuring these accounts against the standard pattern of normal infant and child development, review the quality and levels of communicative disability. Kanner's (1943) own description provides rich detail of autistic children's relative lack of personal relatedness; an abnormality that seems to be rooted in the children's deficient attentiveness to, perceptiveness toward, and comprehension of the bodily expressions of others, and one that has sequelae for the children's restricted understanding of people as agents with their own subjective experiences. For example, Kanner recorded that one of his patients, Elaine (case 11, aged 7), was said to have made no personal appeal for help or sympathy in her early years:

> Her expression was blank, though not unintelligent, and there were no communicative gestures. . . . She does not look into one's face. . . . She has no relation to children, has never talked to them, to be friendly with them, or to play with them. She moves among them like a strange being, as one moves between the pieces of furniture of a room. (pp. 240–241)

Or again, of 5-year-old Paul (case 4), he wrote:

> There was, on his side, no affective tie to people. He behaved as if people as such did not matter or even exist. It made no difference whether one spoke to him in a friendly or a harsh way. He never looked up at people's faces. When he had any dealings with persons at all, he treated them, or rather parts of them, as if they were objects. (pp. 227–228)

Elaine did not look *into* one's face, and to Paul it made no *difference* whether one spoke to him in a friendly or a harsh way. Our attention is drawn to autistic children's lack of affective engagement with the expressive bodily features and behavior of other people.

Of course one could multiply descriptions like these—for instance, Bosch (1970) gives five illuminating case histories, including that of a child who would get people's sexes mixed up—and I cite these excerpts because our familiarity with and detached attitude toward the "phenomena" of autism may have blunted our sensitivity to the profundity and developmental significance of the children's impaired personal relatedness. For all the areas of overlap between autistic and nonautistic retarded or even normal children, what makes autistic children "autistic" is the *quality* of their (relative) unengagement with others.

It is obvious but nonetheless noteworthy that such unengagement has implications for the child's *experience* of others, and therefore implications for the understanding and knowledge that is built upon this experience. Intelligent autistic adults' accounts of their own early lives afford further insight here. For example, one exceptionally articulate autistic man described how he had always been different from other boys, "as it were, on a lonely island in their midst" (Bosch, 1970, p. 39). Another 31-year-old patient originally diagnosed by Kanner conveyed how he had no idea how to go about making interpersonal contact, how he could not empathize with others (Bemporad, 1979). Even more strikingly, an intelligent young autistic adult interviewed by Cohen (1980) described how the first years of his life were devoid of people

> I really didn't know there were people until I was seven years old. I then suddenly realized that there were people. But not like you do. I still have to remind myself that there are people . . . I never could have a friend. I really don't know what to do with other people, really. (p. 388)

EXPERIMENTS WITH AUTISTIC INDIVIDUALS

The scientific challenge is to devise appropriate methodologies to examine the nature and specificity of the children's abnormal social behavior and restricted social experience and understanding. The basic scientific technique, of course, is to compare and contrast autistic children and appropriately matched nonautistic children, and to trace the patterns of association and dissociation amongst the children's social, cognitive, conative, and linguistic abilities and disabilities. One aim, easier to formulate than to achieve, is to discern cause-and-effect relations amongst the children's disabilities from a developmental perspective. We need to determine in which senses the children's social-affective impairments are basic—"basic" to which other aspects of the disorder—and in which senses they are derived from psychological abnormalities of different kinds (e.g., cognitive) and/or from physical abnormalities that must be specified at lower levels of description such as the neurological or the physiological.

Once again, I shall need to be selective in illustrating the progress that has been made in specifying autistic children's abnormalities in social perception, and once again I shall focus upon emotion recognition. The underlying hypothesis that the following experiments were designed to test is one that posits a fundamental impairment in autistic children's nonverbal communicative capacities, on what might be called an infantile level. That is, autistic children are hypothesized to suffer a relative lack of propensities and abilities in interpersonal perception and interpersonal relations that even 1-year-olds normally manifest. If this hypothesis is correct, then there might be far-reaching implications for the children's understanding of persons and for critical aspects of their cognitive development. For the sake of exposition, I shall begin by outlining the evidence that there *are* deficits in emotion perception amongst autistic individuals, and then review studies that have seemed to yield contradictory results.

Evidence for Emotion-Recognition Deficits in Autism

The first formal, published experimental study on emotion-recognition deficits in autism was one in which I employed videotapes as a way of capturing the aliveness of emotional expressions (Hobson, 1986a, b). The purpose of the experiment was to examine some minimal criteria for autistic and matched nonautistic children's understanding of the meaning of different bodily expressions of emotion, such as a happy face, or gesture, or vocalization. The criteria were that the children should recognize how the different expressions of a particular emotion are associated with each other, and be able to judge which facial expressions a person might show when he or she encounters particular environmental events. Thus, a child's task was to choose schematically drawn (and subsequently photographed) emotionally expressive faces to accompany videotape-and-picture displays of emotion gestures, audiotaped vocal expressions of emotion, and finally videotape-and-picture versions of situational contexts that might precipitate different emotions. In a subsequent experiment, subjects chose drawn gestures for videotaped faces and voices. There was also a test to evaluate subjects' ability to coordinate drawings of four objects—a car, a bird, a dog and a train—with corresponding videotaped and audiotaped scenes. By employing materials in different sensory modalities, it was hoped to avoid the possibility that meaning-independent perceptual strategies might be sufficient to accomplish the matching tasks. It will be noted that the approach has some affinity with work conducted on emotion recognition in normal infants, and that the task requires abilities at the interface of perceptual and conceptual judgement. It may also be recalled that normal 6-month-olds seem to recognize the match across facial and vocal expressions of emotion.

In all, there were 23 autistic and 23 individually matched normal children, and a subgroup of 11 of the autistic children were also matched with nonautistic retarded children. The children were matched according to their performance on Raven's (1960, 1965) Progressive Matrices, a test of nonverbal cognitive function. Given that emotion-recognition abilities are thought to depend upon the holistic and nonverbal functions of the right cerebral hemisphere (Buck, 1982; Tucker, 1981), matching by Raven's matrices should reduce the likelihood that generalized impairments in nonverbal intelligence might be responsible for group differences in task performance. Having said this, it is important to note that autistic children perform better on Raven's matrices than they do on other tests of cognitive function, especially those that involve language (e.g., Bartak, Rutter, & Cox, 1975). Unless it is established that the children can meet basic task demands, therefore, there is a danger that autistic subjects matched in this way will show spuriously poor performance on a range of other tasks. It is also probable that if verbally mediated strategies are being employed, these nonverbally able but relatively verbally disabled autistic subjects might be at a disadvantage.

The results were as follows. As it turned out, all subjects approached ceiling performance on the objects videotape. It was striking how quick the autistic children were to choose the correct drawing for the videotaped events, even when this involved (for example) choosing the drawing of a train for an out-of-focus tubular form flickering across the television screen. Here the results clearly demonstrated that the autistic children could comply with the basic task demands of attentiveness, memory, cross-modal matching and so on. On the other hand, the ceiling effects rendered this a screening task rather than a control task, in that it was not possible to evaluate whether one group would have been superior to the other on more difficult items. On the emotions task, by contrast, there were clear group differences in that the autistic children performed less well than the matched normal children on all parts of the task, and less well than the matched nonautistic retarded children on all but the "contexts" condition. A further comparison between a subgroup of the autistic children and normal children of similar verbal mental age (MA) also yielded significant group differences. It was evident from the hesitant manner in which the autistic children approached the task that they were frequently perplexed or uncertain in their responses. Yet few of the autistic children were responding at random, indicating that they were able to understand the nature of the task and could appreciate meaning in some of the task materials. Similar results were obtained from the task involving a choice of drawn gestures for videotaped faces and voices.

The next step (Hobson, Ouston, & Lee, 1988a) was to tighten the experimental procedures by individually matching autistic and nonautistic retarded subjects according to age and verbal ability—this greatly decreased the possibility that the autistic children's verbal disability might be causing the previously observed group differences—and by employing emotion and nonemotion tasks that were comparable in level of difficulty. The range of emotional expressions tested was also increased to include surprise and disgust, and the standardized facial expressions of Ekman and Friesen (1975) were employed instead of photographs of myself. The task itself was limited to that of coordinating faces and expressive voices; not only grunts, groans, and so on, but also emotionally intoned passages of prose. There was a range of nonemotion sound-to-picture matching tasks, and the items here comprised different exemplars within relatively homogeneous categories of sound-generating objects or events (six kinds of vehicles, of birds, of electric appliances, of gardening tools, of moving water, and of walking, respectively). The results were that relative to nonautistic retarded control subjects, the autistic subjects performed less well on the emotion tasks than on the nonemotion tasks. On the other hand, when the two verbal MA-matched groups (equated for performance on the British Picture Vocabulary Scales [BPVS]) (Dunn, Dunn, & Whetton, 1982) were compared on the emotion tasks considered in isolation, the group difference was not significant.

Closely similar results were obtained from a follow-up study in which the same subjects were asked to give free-response labels for a subset of the same task materials (Hobson, Ouston, & Lee, 1989). Once again, autistic subjects differed from nonautistic retarded (and also normal) subjects in being relatively poor at naming feelings vis-à-vis naming nonpersonal objects. These findings have been complemented by those of Tantam, Monaghan, Nicholson, and Stirling (1989), who reported that autistic children performed less well than nonautistic retarded children matched for nonverbal MA in choosing the odd one out amongst facial expressions of emotion and in choosing labels for such expressions, there being some indication that this latter group difference was still apparent when subjects of similar verbal MA were compared. Macdonald *et al.* (1989) studied very high-ability autistic adults and nonverbal MA-matched control subjects for the ability to name the emotions in expressive speech (either normally produced or electronically filtered), and to name facial-affect photographs as well as to match them with contexts that might elicit each emotion. The autistic subjects were significantly poorer than control subjects on each of these tasks, results that could not be attributed to discrepancies in subjects' verbal ability.

It may be worthwhile to juxtapose the findings reported so far with those that have emerged from studies of normal infants. It is obvious that the methodologies employed with high-functioning autistic individuals have been selected for use with children well beyond infancy, and both the materials presented and the response measures employed are very different from those that have been used with infants. Nevertheless, the processes underlying normal infants' performance on emotion-recognition tasks may well be relevant for understanding the sources of contrast between autistic and control subjects in performance on the present tasks. We have noted how there is evidence that by 6 months of age or so, normal infants not only can discriminate amongst different expressions of emotion, but also can coordinate the meanings common to different modes of expression and respond to these with appropriate, affectively toned behavior. Clinical evidence suggests that even high-functioning autistic children often fail to demonstrate affective responses toward others, and appear uncomprehending toward other people's feelings. The experimental evidence points to specific impairments in the children's capacities to discriminate facial, gestural, and vocal emotional expressions, and to recognize how different expressions are coordinated with each other. The case is growing for the possibility that autistic children may not perceive or be attuned to emotional meanings in the bodily expressions of others, and that this might be very important for their limitations in affective understanding. It is now important to pursue these ideas further. For instance, how *do* autistic individuals perceive faces?

This matter was investigated in another of our experiments (Hobson, Ouston, & Lee, 1988b). On this occasion, groups of BPVS-matched, relatively high-functioning autistic and nonautistic retarded adolescents and young adults were tested for their ability to recognize emotion and personal identity in photographed faces and parts of faces. The tasks were to sort the faces according to the same emotions when these appeared in different people, and to sort them according to people's identities when the same people appeared with different emotions. For both conditions, there was a set of photographs of full faces, another showing faces with blanked-out mouths, and another showing faces with blank mouths and foreheads, so designed that even the latter photographs retained some feel of the emotions in the faces. The principal result was that there was a significant second-order interaction of diagnosis by condition (emotion, identity) by form of face (full face, blank mouth, blank mouth and forehead). Essentially, the performances of the two groups were similar on the identities task, with scores declining steadily as the photographs to be sorted became increasingly blanked out. On the task of matching emotions, by contrast, the autistic subjects were adept in matching full-face emotions, but their performance declined more precipitately than did that of control subjects as the cues to emotion were progressively reduced. They seemed relatively unable to use the "feel" in the faces to guide performance.

The question arose whether the autistic children might be succeeding in sorting the full-face emotions by employing a different strategy than that used by control subjects—indeed, whether they might hardly be recognizing emotions at all. Two further findings were relevant here. Firstly, correlations between individual subjects' scores on the identity and emotions tasks were lower for nonautistic than for autistic subjects. This suggested that while nonautistic subjects might have employed different processes or strategies for emotion than for nonemotion face recognition, autistic subjects might have been sorting the expressive faces in a "nonemotional" way. Secondly, an additional task was administered in which subjects repeated both full-face sorting tasks, only this time the target faces and the photographs to be sorted were presented upside down. Somewhat startlingly, although in keeping with Langdell's (1978) report of autistic children's proficient recognition of peers in upside-down photographs, the autistic subjects were significantly more successful than control subjects in matching both identities and emotions in the upside-down faces. Tantam *et al.* (1989) have also reported that autistic children were unusual in performing well in choosing labels for emotions in upside-down faces, relative to their performance on other emotion-recognition tasks. Whatever these results mean, they serve to caution against too facile an interpretation of emotion-recognition abilities when autistic subjects succeed in sorting still photographs of faces.

Once again, the contrast with findings from experiments with normal infants is worth bearing in mind. Even in infancy, normal children are sensitive to emotional meanings in upright but not upside-down faces. Although comparisons with much older individuals must be made with caution, it does appear unlikely that autistic children's profiles of ability and disability are simply the result of developmental delay.

One singular feature of other people's emotional expressions is that they have the power to "grab you." They do not seem to be so arresting for many autistic children. This matter of the salience of expressions was the focus of the next experiment, conducted by a colleague, Jane Weeks, and me (Weeks & Hobson, 1987). The experiment involved 15 autistic and 15 nonautistic retarded subjects, individually matched for chronological age, sex, and performance on three subtests of the Verbal scale of the WISC-R: Information, Similarities, and Vocabulary. We presented a picture-sorting task in which subjects were shown a pair of target photographs of the head and shoulders of individuals who differed in three, two, or one of the following respects: sex, age, facial expression of emotion, and the type of hat they were wearing. When given similar photographs to sort, the majority of nonautistic children sorted according to people's facial expressions (happy versus unhappy) before they sorted according to type of hat (floppy versus woolen), but most autistic children gave priority to sorting by type of hat. Even with such small groups of subjects, and with regard to such a crude, indirect test of attentiveness to emotion, the group difference was significant in the predicted direction. Moreover, when in the course of the experiment the number of contrasting features in the target photographs was progressively reduced, all 15 nonautistic children sooner or later sorted by emotional expression without being told to do so, but only 6 of the 15 autistic children did this ($p = 0.0003$, Fisher's exact test). Unbeknownst to us at the time of our experiment, Jennings (1973) had conducted a similar but unpublished study that yielded results closely comparable to our own. In effect, therefore, these results have been replicated. From experimental as well as clinical evidence, it seems that facial expressions of emotion do *not* have the same degree of salience—and very likely, not the same degree of emotional impact—for autistic as for nonautistic individuals.

Points of Controversy

It is not surprising that some experimental studies have yielded results that cast doubt on the existence of specific emotion-recognition deficits in autism. From an experimental perspective, the two principal points of controversy are, first, whether the evidence for such deficits merely reflects autistic children's impaired language ability, and second, whether or not there is something specific about *emotion*-recognition deficits vis-à-vis deficits in other aspects of autistic children's perceptual and conceptual function. The sources of evidence here are studies that have matched autistic and nonautistic subjects according to verbal ability and/or have compared subjects' performance on emotion-related vis-à-vis emotion-unrelated forms of tasks (Braverman, Fein, Lucci, & Waterhouse, 1989; Ozonoff, Pennington, & Rogers, 1990; Prior, Dahlstrom and Squires, 1990; also Hertzig, Snow, & Sherman, 1989; Szatmari, Bartolucci, Krames, Flett, & Tuff, 1989). Although this is not the place to examine each of these studies in detail (see Hobson, 1991b), I shall indicate some considerations to be borne in mind when evaluating the findings from such experiments.

There are now a number of published studies in which verbal MA-matched autistic and nonautistic subjects have been found to differ on certain forms of emotion-recognition tasks only to a nonsignificant degree (Braverman *et al.*, 1989; Hobson, Ouston, & Lee, 1988a, b, 1989; Prior *et al.*, 1990). There are three points to note here. Firstly, verbal MA-matched autistic and nonautistic subjects *have* differed significantly—and strikingly—in their levels of performance on emotion-related tasks that have employed other kinds of methodology (especially Jennings, 1973; Weeks & Hobson, 1987). Secondly, there are instances in which similar *levels* of emotion-related task performance among autistic and nonautistic subjects seem to have obscured different processes or strategies underlying task performance in the different diagnostic groups (Hobson *et al.*, 1988b; Macdonald *et al.*, 1989; also Hobson & Lee, 1989; to be discussed later). Thirdly, even verbal MA-matched autistic and nonautistic subjects have differed in their profiles of performance on emotion-related vis-à-vis emotion-unrelated control tasks (Hobson & Lee, 1989; Hobson, Ouston, & Lee, 1988a, b, 1989; and some parts of Hertzig *et al.*, 1989). The significant group-by-task interactions have often been quantitatively small, but this finding needs to be weighed against the fact that they have occurred in the predicted direction (i.e., with autistic subjects performing significantly less well on the emotion-related tasks) on a number of very different kinds of tasks. In addition, most experimental materials are very crude representations of real-life, dynamic, emotionally expressive interpersonal events, so that the representations might be "recognized" by relatively nonemotion-specific perceptual and cognitive strategies. Most of the studies that have reported a lack of emotion-specific group contrasts have either employed control tasks that were restricted in range or unsuitable in level of difficulty (Hertzig *et al.*, 1989; Prior *et al.*, 1990), or have compared relatively small groups of autistic children with much younger normal rather than age-matched nonautistic retarded subjects, so that the effects of both age and IQ on subjects' performance in either the emotion-related and/or control tasks might have obscured the influence of autism per se (Braverman *et al.*, 1989; Ozonoff *et al.*, 1990).

There is a further, more theoretical issue that is often overlooked. As we have seen, nonsignificant group differences in emotion-recognition scores vis-à-vis scores on tests of verbal ability have been a frequent, though by no means universal, feature of the studies. The question is, what do such findings signify? One possibility is that limitations in verbal ability constrain subjects' performance for reasons that are incidental to the emotional content of the tasks; another is that real-life emotion recognition is in part dependent on verbal ability or on some related cognitive function; another is that language and emotion-recognition abilities are relatively independent of one another, but in certain tasks (and not others) they appear to be equally impaired in autistic individuals. We have also noted the possibility that abnormal perceptual or conceptual strategies might compensate for autistic children's emotion-recognition disabilities, especially when highly artificial and often nondynamic stimulus materials are presented. I shall not dwell on these possibilities (see also Hobson *et al.*, 1988a), but instead emphasize something else: It needs to be considered how far autistic individuals' verbal disabilities might stem from, rather than lead to, their emotion-recognition disabilities, insofar as the latter constrain the child's experience of a shared world with others within which common understandings and a common language are developed. If this were so, it would be unsurprising if, to some degree, verbal ability and emotion-recognition ability were correlated with one another. Shortly I shall consider a further experiment that bears upon this possibility.

It remains arguable whether autistic individuals' impairments on tests of emotion recognition might reflect secondary consequences of social inattentiveness arising from nonperceptual sources such as active social avoidance or deficits in so-called theory of mind (see later discussion). For the present, I merely note that this is an important issue that requires careful evaluation in the light of clinical as well as experimental evidence.

Further Aspects of Social Perception in Autism

I shall now give brief consideration to additional aspects of social perception in autism. To begin with, I shall mention the suggestive but by no means conclusive evidence that autistic children may have difficulty in perceiving the age and sex categories of other people. The principal evidence comes from videotape studies of a similar design to the cross-modal emotion-recognition studies described earlier (Hobson, 1987); the results were that autistic children were markedly less consistent than nonverbal MA-matched normal and retarded control subjects in choosing drawings and then photographs of the faces of a man, a woman, a boy, and a girl for such individuals depicted on videotape in characteristic gestures, vocalizations, and contexts. The major limitation to this study was that once again, most subjects achieved near-ceiling performance on the nonpersonal control task, so that the specificity of the findings is open to question. It is also perfectly possible that the autistic children's lower verbal abilities contributed to their poor performance. Further suggestive evidence comes from another study (Hobson, 1983) in which nonverbal MA-matched autistic and nonautistic retarded children differed in their propensity to sort pictures of people, animals, and nonpersonal things according to age-related characteristics. Although the autistic children were somewhat more consistent than the nonautistic children in sorting geometrical figures, and although both groups of subjects sorted drawings of things according to whether they were new or worn out, the autistic children were markedly less consistent than control subjects in sorting photographs of people, and also photographs of dogs, into those that were young and those that were adult. However, the photographs of people and animals differed from the drawings of things both in quality of representation and in the amount of contrast between the young and old exemplars, and so again the experiment did not establish the degree of specificity in this abnormality. It is clear that further, more adequately controlled studies are needed. The issues are important for theoretical as well as practical reasons, in that a normal child's knowledge of what age differences and sex categories *mean* might partly depend upon biologically based propensities to perceive and relate to old and young, and males and females, in different ways, as illustrated in the studies of infants cited earlier. The possibility arises that such differentiation in personal relatedness is part of what is missing in autism.

The next matter concerns the autistic child's recognition of particular individuals. Although it is evident that autistic children have some kind of ability to recognize individual people, for example by their facial characteristics (Hobson *et al.*, 1988b; Langdell, 1978; Volkmar, Sparrow, Rende, & Cohen, 1989), it is not established which kinds of personal qualities are being "recognized" here. Recent studies of attachment and separation reactions in autistic children (Shapiro, Sherman, Calamari, & Koch, 1987; Sigman & Mundy, 1989; Sigman & Ungerer, 1984) indicate that some forms of relationship exist for this group of children. According to rather crude measures such as degree of distress and proximity to a familiar adult in these contexts, for example, autistic and nonautistic retarded children appear to be rather similar. What remains to be determined is how far and in what respects familiar individuals *matter* to autistic children, compared with the manifold ways that parents matter to normal or to nonautistic retarded children. Clinical as well as experimental evidence suggests that autistic children's relationships matter, but it also indicates how greatly the quality and depth of such relationships may diverge from those of nonautistic people.

Finally, it is pertinent to consider the degree to which autistic children are impaired and/or delayed in coming to perceive other people as subjects of experience, beings with whom experiences can be shared (Hobson, 1989a, b). The evidence is that they are abnormal in this regard. In particular, autistic children may make requests for objects and actions and may understand other people's pointing gestures that convey instructions, but unlike normal 1-year-olds, they rarely make gestures such as showing, giving, or pointing in order to share awareness of an object's existence or properties, or comprehend such gestures when these are made by others (Baron-Cohen, 1989; Curcio, 1978; Landry & Loveland, 1988; Loveland & Landry, 1986; Mundy, Sigman, Ungerer, & Sherman, 1986; Sigman, Mundy,

Sherman, & Ungerer, 1986; Wetherby & Prutting, 1984). There is also some indication that they might be abnormal in their propensity to engage in other aspects of social referencing (Mundy *et al.*, 1986; Sigman & Mundy, 1989). By way of contrast, autistic children do have the ability to understand something of other people's visuospatial perspectives (Hobson, 1984; Leslie & Frith, 1988). As noted earlier, this latter ability might be derived through processes that are relatively independent of children's experiences of intersubjectivity. Overall, therefore, we face the possibility that autistic children are seriously impaired in perceiving and conceiving of other human beings as persons with minds.

In summary, there is very tentative evidence to suggest that even high-functioning autistic individuals may have deficits in perceiving age- and sex-related characteristics of people, firmer evidence to suggest that they are able to identify particular individuals and accord them special importance, and highly suggestive evidence that they are impaired in recognizing persons *as* persons with whom experiences can be shared.

IMPLICATIONS FOR COGNITIVE DEVELOPMENT

I have space only to signpost what I believe to be the far-reaching implications of autistic children's impaired social perception, and perhaps especially their impaired affective contact with others (Kanner, 1943), for the children's cognitive and linguistic development. It is perhaps worth noting that despite the claims of Baron-Cohen (1988), Leslie and Frith (1990), and other advocates of the view that autistic children lack an innately determined "theory of mind," there are few predictions or explanations generated by that view that are not also generated by the present approach—for the simple reason that what these authors call the autistic child's impaired theory of mind is very close to what I have been calling the autistic child's deficient concept of persons (e.g., Hobson, 1982, 1989a). Where the two perspectives diverge is in the ways that they characterize the nature and developmental origins of a normal child's interpersonal understanding, and therefore in the ways they account for the background to (rather than the sequelae to) the social impairments in autism. The theory-of-mind approach is essentially cognitive, whereas I pay more attention to the significance of those kinds of perceptual-affective and motivational-'communicative' phenomena that are rooted in normal infancy (Hobson, 1991c). As a result, my theory has a somewhat broader scope—for example, in relation to age and sex perception and self-concept development—but to a large extent, the two theories agree when it comes to tracing the implications of autistic children's relative failure to understand the minds of others.

A possible exception to this general rule concerns autistic children's understanding of specifically emotion-related concepts, although here too a theory-of-mind account might predict impairments. In a recent study, my colleague Tony Lee and I examined whether autistic and nonautistic retarded adolescents and young adults, very closely matched on an individual basis for age and for scores on the

BPVS, differed in their relative scores on those items of the BPVS that independent raters judged to be emotion related and emotion unrelated in content (Hobson & Lee, 1989). The emotion-related items included word-picture combinations in which the words were *delighted, disagreement, greeting,* and *snarling,* as well as more obviously "emotional" words such as *horror* and *surprise*. Thus, the study sampled a range of concepts for which affective understanding might have particular importance, and evaluated subjects' understanding of these concepts with reference to scores on nonemotion BPVS items that were identical in level of absolute difficulty for nonautistic subjects. The results were that compared to control subjects, autistic individuals scored lower on emotion-related vis-à-vis emotion-unrelated items, an effect that could not be attributed to the "social content" or abstractness of the concepts being tested. Although evidence is emerging that autistic children do use some apparently emotion-related words (Tager-Flusberg, 1989), it remains to be established how much the use of such words (like the names of emotionally expressive faces) might be learned without truly interpersonal understanding.

These results attest to the probable implications of autistic children's impaired affective understanding for their profile of scores *within* a measure of language ability. As already mentioned, however, such impaired social-affective understanding might seriously interfere with the development of their general language abilities, as well as causing more marked "pragmatic" deficits when the children need to adjust linguistic forms with regard to the speech roles and orientations of other listeners (e.g., Baltaxe, 1977; Baron-Cohen, 1988; Fay & Schuler, 1980; Hobson, 1989a). In other words, social-affective impairments might make a substantial contribution to general language delay in autism, as well as having a bearing on the form of such language as develops.

Then there is the question of autistic children's profile of cognitive abnormalities, manifest not only on standard IQ tests such as the WISC (e.g., Bartak, Rutter, & Cox, 1975) but also in their impaired capacity for symbolic play (e.g., Riguet, Taylor, Benaroya, & Klein, 1981; Ungerer & Sigman, 1981; Wing, Gould, Yeates, & Brierley, 1977; Wulff, 1985) and in the concreteness and lack of flexibility of their thought processes (Kanner, 1943; Scheerer, Rothmann, & Goldstein, 1945). I believe that to a significant degree, such cognitive abnormalities can be traced to autistic children's difficulty in "disembedding" from a particular point of view and acquiring the capacity to adopt a variety of co-orientations to given objects or events—for example, to pretend a matchbox "is" a car (Hobson, 1990a; Leslie, 1987; also Dawson & Fernald, 1987). I further believe that in the normal case, 1-year-olds first recognize that different people (including themselves) have different orientations toward a shared world, and only subsequently do they learn to apply multiple co-orientations (as in symbolic play) all by themselves. In other words, what is first required is that the children recognize that people are subjects of experience. The proposal is that such awareness may require as its foundation certain basic forms of interpersonal coordination and "sharing," especially of an affective kind (Hobson, 1982, 1989a, 1990a), that are relatively lacking in autism.

If this is so, there will be implications for the autistic child's developing self-awareness (Hobson, 1990c). The reason is that such awareness is awareness of self *as* a person among other persons. To understand what a self is, one must be able to take attitudes toward oneself as if from other people's perspectives. It is this that autistic children find so difficult. The expressions of impaired self-awareness and incomprehension of personal roles probably include a relative lack of propriety as well as an absence of coyness in front of mirrors (Dawson & McKissick, 1984; Neuman & Hill, 1978; Spiker & Ricks, 1984), personal pronoun difficulties (Charney, 1981; Fay, 1979; Silberg, 1978), a deficient sense of property, and a lack of competition or focused self-defense and counterattack (Bosch, 1970), and problems in identifying with others (e.g., in certain forms of imitation). In addition, autistic children's difficulties in understanding such mental-state concepts as belief or knowledge (Baron-Cohen, Leslie, & Frith, 1985, 1986; Leslie & Frith, 1988; Perner, Frith, Leslie, & Leekam, 1989) might be ascribed to their lack of a concept of persons or "selves" who are able to hold beliefs. In summary, an understanding of certain mental states entails an understanding of selves; an understanding of selves depends upon an understanding of persons as subjects of experience; and for an understanding of persons, perceptual-affective development may play a critical role. All "social knowing" cannot be accomplished through perceptual processes (Baron, 1981), but perhaps it is at the perceptual level that we can discern an essential substratum of social knowledge, and moreover a substratum that is deficient or incomplete in the case of autism.

CONCLUSION

In this chapter I have attempted to review experimental evidence for impairments in social perception among autistic people, and have emphasized the importance of evaluating such evidence with reference both to clinical descriptions of autism and to the picture of normal infant development. Whereas from the early months of life, normal human beings "pay the closest attention to the optical and acoustic information that specifies what the other person is, invites, threatens, and does" (Gibson, 1979, p. 128), autistic individuals seem to lack something essential to such social perception, a something that is also essential for intersubjective communication. This "something" might include the kind of affect-related physiognomic perception characterized by Werner (1948), or perhaps comprise more specific abilities that underpin a normal infant's "organic" modes of sympathy with others (Baldwin, 1902). I have followed Kanner (1943) in suggesting that autism might best be viewed as an impairment of *inter*personal relations (Hobson, 1991a), but that in many cases at least, biological perceptual-affective incapacities in the children may be basic to the disorder. I have also indicated how a range of the cognitive and linguistic impairments that are characteristic of autism might arise on this basis, especially as mediated through autistic children's failure to grasp how other people are "persons" with minds of their own. In all of this, I have had to omit a great deal that is relevant for autistic children's deficits in these domains, perhaps most notably the evidence for abnormalities in their emotional expressiveness and in various facets of interpersonal coordination (e.g. Attwood, Frith, & Hermelin, 1988; Dawson, Hill, Spencer, Galpert, and Watson, 1990; Kasari, Sigman, Mundy, and Yirmiya, 1990; Ricks, 1975; Snow, Hertzig, & Shapiro, 1987; Volkmar, 1987; Wing, 1981; Yirmiya, Kasari, Sigman, & Mundy, 1989). I have also glossed over the important fact that many autistic people do achieve an impressive degree of interpersonal contact and make genuine interpersonal relationships—a fact that must find a place in our understanding of autism.

At the end of the day, I think it is salutary to return to one's experience of being with autistic children, and to parents' and clinicians' writings on such experience, and to ponder two questions: First, at what level or levels do autistic children relate to oneself as a person, bodily as well as mentally? Secondly, is it plausible that the children's nonverbal as well as verbal communicative disabilities stem from a basic cognitive disorder, or is it more plausible that primary interpersonal impairments derail autistic children's cognitive development—or do we need a more complex account of "cognitive" and "social-affective" impairments that may involve both developmental and nondevelopmental functional interdependencies? In my own view, as in the views of some other contemporary writers (e.g., Bemporad, Ratey, & O'Driscoll, 1987; Fein, Pennington, Markowitz, Braverman, & Waterhouse, 1986; Hermelin & O'Connor, 1985; Mundy & Sigman, 1989), early social-affective abnormalities may hold the key to much that is unique about autism. Whatever present and future experimental studies contribute to our knowledge of autism, however, autistic children's disabilities in social perception, social experience, and social understanding will remain central issues.

Acknowledgment

This chapter would not have been written but for 10 years of warm and patient support, generous guidance, and invaluable critical comment from Dr. Beate Hermelin.

REFERENCES

Ahrens, R. (1954). Beitrag zur Entwicklung des Physiognomie- und Mimikerkennens. *Zeitschrift fur Experimentelle und Angewandte Psychologie, 2,* 412–454.

Aitken, S. (1977). *Psychological sex differentiation as related to the emergence of a self-concept in infancy.* Honors thesis, University of Edinburgh.

Attwood, A., Frith, U., & Hermelin, B. (1988). The understanding and use of interpersonal gestures by autistic and Down's syndrome children. *Journal of Autism and Developmental Disorders, 18,* 241–257.

Baldwin, J. M. (1902). *Social and ethical interpretations in mental development.* New York: Macmillan.

Baltaxe, C. A. M. (1977). Pragmatic deficits in the language of autistic adolescents. *Journal of Pediatric Psychology, 2,* 176–180.

Baron, R. M. (1981). Social knowing from an ecological-event perspective: A consideration of the relative domains of power for cognitive and perceptual modes of knowing. In J. H. Harvey (Ed.), *Cognition, social behavior, and the environment* (pp. 61–89). Hillsdale, NJ: Lawrence Erlbaum.

Baron-Cohen, S. (1988). Social and pragmatic deficits in autism: Cognitive or affective? *Journal of Autism and Developmental Disorders, 18,* 379–402.

Baron-Cohen, S. (1989). Perceptual role-taking and protodeclarative pointing in autism. *British Journal of Developmental Psychology, 7,* 113–127.

Baron-Cohen, S., Leslie, A. M., & Frith, U. (1985). Does the autistic child have a "theory of mind"? *Cognition, 21,* 37–46.

Baron-Cohen, S., Leslie, A. M., & Frith, U. (1986). Mechanical, behavioural and intentional understanding of picture stories in autistic children. *British Journal of Developmental Psychology, 4,* 113–125.

Bartak, L., Rutter, M., & Cox, A. (1975). A comparative study of infantile autism and specific developmental receptive language disorder: I. The children. *British Journal of Psychiatry, 126,* 127–145.

Bemporad, J. R. (1979). Adult recollections of a formerly autistic child. *Journal of Autism and Developmental Disorders, 9,* 179–197.

Bemporad, J. R., Ratey, J. J., & O'Driscoll, G. (1987). Autism and emotion: An ethological theory. *American Journal of Orthopsychiatry, 57,* 477–484.

Bosch, G. (1970). *Infantile autism* (D. Jordan and I. Jordan, Trans.). New York: Springer-Verlag.

Braverman, M., Fein, D., Lucci, D., & Waterhouse, L. (1989). Affect comprehension in children with pervasive developmental disorders. *Journal of Autism and Developmental Disorders, 19,* 301–316.

Bretherton, I. (1985). Attachment theory: Retrospect and prospect. In I. Bretherton & E. Waters (Eds.), *Growing points of attachment theory and research.* Monographs of the Society for Research in Child Development, Serial No. 209, *50,* 3–35.

Bretherton, I., & Bates, E. (1979). The emergence of intentional communication. In I. C. Uzgiris (Ed.), *Social interaction and communication during infancy: New directions for child development, no. 4* (pp. 81–100). San Francisco: Jossey-Bass.

Bretherton, I., McNew, S., & Beeghly-Smith, M. (1981). Early person knowledge as expressed in gestural and verbal communication: When do infants acquire a "theory of mind"? In M. E. Lamb, & L. R. Sherrod (Eds.), *Infant social cognition: Empirical and theoretical considerations* (pp. 333–373). Hillsdale, NJ: Lawrence Erlbaum.

Brooks, J., & Lewis, M. (1976). Infants' responses to strangers: Midget, adult and child. *Child Development, 47,* 323–332.

Buck, R. (1982). Spontaneous and symbolic nonverbal behavior and the ontogeny of communication. In R. S. Feldman (Ed.), *Development of nonverbal behavior in children* (pp. 29–62). New York: Springer.

Buhler, C., & Hetzer, H. (1928). Das erste Verstandnis fur Ansdruck im ersten Lebensjahr. *Zeitschrift fur Psychologie, 107,* 50–61.

Butterworth, G., & Grover, L. (1990). Joint visual attention, manual pointing and pre-verbal communication in human infancy. In M. Jeannerod (Ed.), *Attention and performance XIII.* New York: Lawrence Erlbaum.

Campos, J. J., & Stenberg, C. R. (1981). Perception, appraisal and emotion: The onset of social referencing. In M. E. Lamb & L. R. Sherrod (Eds.), *Infant social cognition* (pp. 273–314). Hillsdale, NJ: Lawrence Erlbaum.

Caron, A. J., Caron, R. F., & MacLean, D. J. (1988). Infant discrimination of naturalistic emotional expressions: The role of face and voice. *Child Development, 59,* 604–616.

Caron, R. F., Caron, A. J., & Myers, R. S. (1982). Abstraction of invariant face expressions in infancy. *Child Development, 53,* 1008–1015.

Carpenter, G. C., Tecce, J. J., Stechler, G., & Friedman, S. (1970). Differential visual behavior to human and humanoid faces in early infancy. *Merrill–Palmer Quarterly of Behavior and Development, 16,* 91–108.

Charney, R. (1981). Pronoun errors in autistic children: Support for a social explanation. *British Journal of Disorders of Communication, 15,* 39–43.

Churcher, J., & Scaife, M. (1982). How infants see the point. In G. Butterworth & P. Light (Eds.), *Social cognition: Studies of the development of understanding* (pp. 110–136). Brighton, Sussex: Harvester.

Cohen, D. J. (1980). The pathology of the self in primary childhood autism and Gilles de la Tourette syndrome. *Psychiatric Clinics of North America, 3,* 383–402.

Cohn, J. F., & Tronick, E. Z. (1983). Three-month-old infants' reaction to simulated maternal depression. *Child Development, 54,* 185–193.

Curcio, F. (1978). Sensorimotor functioning and communication in mute autistic children. *Journal of Autism and Childhood Schizophrenia, 8,* 281–292.

Damasio, A. R., & Maurer, R. G. (1978). A neurological model for childhood autism. *Archives of Neurology, 35,* 777–786.

Darwin, C. (1877). A biographical sketch of an infant. *Mind, 2,* 285–294.

Dawson, G., & Fernald, M. (1987). Perspective-taking ability and its relationship to the social behavior of autistic children. *Journal of Autism and Developmental Disorders, 17,* 487–498.

Dawson, G., Hill, D., Spencer, A., Galpert, L., & Watson, L. (1990). Affective exchanges between young autistic children and their mothers. *Journal of Abnormal Child Psychology, 18,* 335–345.

Dawson, G., & McKissick, F. C. (1984). Self-recognition in autistic children. *Journal of Autism and Developmental Disorders, 14,* 383–394.

Dunn, L. M., Dunn, L. M., & Whetton, C. (1982). *British Picture Vocabulary Scale.* Windsor, England: NFER-Nelson.

Ekman, P., & Friesen, W. V. (1975). *Unmasking the face: A guide to recognizing emotions from facial cues.* Englewood Cliffs, NJ: Prentice-Hall.

Fagan, J. F. (1972). Infants' recognition memory for faces. *Journal of Experimental Child Psychology, 14,* 453–476.

Fagan, J. F. (1976). Infants' recognition of invariant features of faces. *Child Development, 47,* 627–638.

Fagan, J. F., & Singer, L. T. (1979). The role of simple feature differences in infants' recognition of faces. *Infant Behavior and Development, 2,* 39–45.

Fay, W. H. (1979). Personal pronouns and the autistic child. *Journal of Autism and Developmental Disorders, 9,* 247–260.

Fay, W. H., & Schuler, A. L. (1980). *Emerging language in autistic children.* London: Edward Arnold.

Fein, D., Pennington, B., Markowitz, P., Braverman, M., & Waterhouse, L. (1986). Toward a neuropsychological model of infantile autism: Are the social deficits primary? *Journal of the American Academy of Child Psychiatry, 25,* 198–212.

Feinman, S. (1982). Social referencing in infancy. *Merrill–Palmer Quarterly, 28,* 445–470.

Feinman, S., & Lewis, M. (1983). Social referencing at ten months: A second-order effect on infants' responses to strangers. *Child Development, 54,* 878–887.

Field, T. M. (1985). Neonatal perception of people: Maturational and individual differences. In T. M. Field & N. A. Fox (Eds.), *Social perception in infants.* Norwood, NJ: Ablex. pp. 31–52.

Field, T. M., & Fox, N. A. (Eds.). (1985). *Social perception in infants.* Norwood, NJ: Ablex.

Field, T. M. Woodson, R., Cohen, D., Greenberg, R., Garcia, R., & Collins, K. (1983). Discrimination and imitation of facial expressions by term and preterm neonates. *Infant Behavior and Development, 6,* 485–489.

Field, T. M., Woodson, R., Greenberg, R., and Cohen, D. (1982). Discrimination and imitation of facial expressions by neonates. *Science, 218,* 179–181.

Gibson, J. J. (1977). The theory of affordances. In R. Shaw & J. Bransford (Eds.), *Perceiving, acting and knowing* (pp. 67–82). Hillsdale, NJ: Lawrence Erlbaum.

Gibson, J. J. (1979). *The ecological approach to visual perception.* Boston: Houghton-Mifflin.

Habermas, J. (1970). Toward a theory of communicative competence. In H. P. Dreitzel (Ed.), *Recent sociology no. 2* (pp. 115–148). New York: Macmillan.

Hamlyn, D. W. (1974). Person-perception and our understanding of others. In T. Mischel (Ed.), *Understanding other persons* (pp. 1–36). Oxford: Blackwell.

Hamlyn, D. W. (1978). *Experience and the growth of understanding*. London: Routledge and Kegan Paul.

Harding. C. G., & Golinkoff, R. M. (1979). The origins of intentional vocalizations in prelinguistic infants. *Child Development, 50,* 33–40.

Haviland, J. M., & Lelwica, M. (1987). The induced affect response: 10-week-old infants' responses to three emotion expressions. *Developmental Psychology, 23,* 97–104.

Hermelin, B., & O'Connor, N. (1985). Logico-affective states and nonverbal language. In E. Schopler & G. B. Mesibov (Eds.), *Communication problems in autism* (pp. 283–310). New York: Plenum.

Hertzig, M. E., Snow, M. E., & Sherman, M. (1989). Affect and cognition in autism. *Journal of the American Academy of Child Psychiatry, 28,* 195–199.

Hess, E. H. (1970). Ethology and developmental psychology. In P. H. Mussen (Ed.), *Carmichael's manual of child psychology, vol. 1* (3rd ed., pp. 1–38). New York: Wiley.

Hiatt, S. W., Campos, J. J., & Emde, R. N. (1979). Facial patterning and infant emotional expression: Happiness, surprise and fear. *Child Development, 50,* 1020–1035.

Hobson, R. P. (1982). The autistic child's concept of persons. In D. Park (Ed.), *Proceedings of the 1981 International Conference on Autism* (pp. 97–102). Washington, DC: National Society for Children and Adults with Autism.

Hobson, R. P. (1983). The autistic child's recognition of age-related features of people, animals and things. *British Journal of Developmental Psychology, 1,* 343–352.

Hobson, R. P. (1984). Early childhood autism and the question of egocentrism. *Journal of Autism and Developmental Disorders, 14,* 85–104.

Hobson, R. P. (1986a). The autistic child's appraisal of expressions of emotion. *Journal of Child Psychology and Psychiatry, 27,* 321–342.

Hobson, R. P. (1986b). The autistic child's appraisal of expressions of emotion: A further study. *Journal of Child Psychology and Psychiatry, 27,* 671–680.

Hobson, R. P. (1987). The autistic child's recognition of age- and sex-related characteristics of people. *Journal of Autism and Developmental Disorders, 17,* 63–79.

Hobson, R. P. (1989a). Beyond cognition: A theory of autism. In G. Dawson (Ed.), *Autism: Nature, diagnosis, and treatment* (pp. 22–48). New York: Guilford.

Hobson, R. P. (1989b). On sharing experiences. *Development and Psychopathology, 1,* 197–203.

Hobson, R. P. (1990a). On acquiring knowledge about people, and the capacity to pretend: Response to Leslie. *Psychological Review, 97,* 114–121.

Hobson, R. P. (1990b). Concerning knowledge of mental states. *British Journal of Medical Psychology, 63,* 199–213.

Hobson, R. P. (1990c). On the origins of self and the case of autism. *Development and Psychopathology, 2,* 163–181.

Hobson, R. P. (1991a). What is autism? In J. Beitchman and M. Konstantareas (Eds.), Psychiatric Clinics of North America, Vol. 14, 1–17.

Hobson, R. P. (1991b). Methodological issues for experiments on autistic individuals' perception and understanding of emotion. *Journal of Child Psychology and Psychiatry, 32,* 1135–1158.

Hobson, R. P. (1991c). Against the theory of "Theory of Mind." *British Journal of Developmental Psychology, 9,* 33–51.

Hobson, R. P., & Lee, A. (1989). Emotion-related and abstract concepts in autistic people: Evidence from the British Picture Vocabulary Scale. *Journal of Autism and Developmental Disorders, 19,* 601–623.

Hobson, R. P., Ouston, J., & Lee, A. (1988a). Emotion recognition in autism: Coordinating faces and voices. *Psychological Medicine, 18,* 911–923.

Hobson, R. P., Ouston, J., & Lee, A. (1988b). What's in a face? The case of autism. *British Journal of Psychology, 79,* 441–453.

Hobson, R. P., Ouston, J., & Lee, A. (1989). Naming emotion in faces and voices: Abilities and disabilities in autism and mental retardation. *British Journal of Developmental Psychology, 7,* 237–250.

Isaacs, S. (1948). The nature and function of phantasy. *International Journal of Psycho-Analysis, 29,* 73–97.

Jennings, W. B. (1973). *A study of the preference for affective cues in autistic children.* Unpublished doctoral dissertation, Memphis State University.

Kanner, L. (1943). Autistic disturbances of affective contact. *Nervous Child, 2,* 217–250.

Kant, I. (1929). *Critique of pure reason* (N. K. Smith, Trans.). London: Macmillan.

Kasari, C., Sigman, M., Mundy, P., & Yirmiya, N. (1990). Affective sharing in the context of joint attention interactions of normal, autistic, and mentally retarded children. *Journal of Autism and Developmental Disorders, 20,* 87–100.

Keeler, W. R. (1958). Autistic patterns and defective communication in blind children with retrolental fibroplasia. In P. H. Hoch & J. Zubin (Eds.), *Psychopathology of communication* (pp. 64–83). New York: Grune and Stratton.

Klinnert, M. (1984). The regulation of infant behavior by maternal facial expression. *Infant Behavior and Development, 7,* 447–465.

Klinnert, M. D., Campos, J. J., Sorce, J. F., Emde, R. N., & Svejda, M. (1983). Emotions as behavior regulators: Social referencing in infancy. In R. Plutchik & H. Kellerman (Eds.), *Emotion: Theory, research and experience. Vol. 2: Emotions in early development* (pp. 57–86). New York: Academic Press.

Kujawski, J. (1985). *The origins of gender identity.* Doctoral dissertation, University of Edinburgh.

La Barbera, J. D. Izard, C. E., Vietze, P., & Parisi, S. A. (1976). Four- and six-month-old infants' visual responses to joy, anger, and neutral expressions. *Child Development, 47,* 535–538.

Lamb, M. E., & Sherrod, L. R. (Eds.). (1981). *Infant social cognition.* Hillsdale, NJ: Lawrence Erlbaum.

Landry, S. H., & Loveland, K. A. (1988). Communication behaviors in autism and developmental language delay. *Journal of Child Psychology and Psychiatry, 29,* 621–634.

Langdell, T. (1978). Recognition of faces: An approach to the study of autism. *Journal of Child Psychology and Psychiatry, 19,* 255–268.

Leslie, A. M. (1987). Pretense and representation: The origins of "theory of mind." *Psychological Review, 94,* 412–426.

Leslie, A. M., & Frith, U. (1988). Autistic children's understanding of seeing, knowing and believing. *British Journal of Developmental Psychology, 6,* 315–324.

Leslie, A. M., & Frith, U. (1990). Prospects for a cognitive neuropsychology of autism: Hobson's choice. *Psychological Review: 97,* 122–131.

Loveland, K. A., & Landry, S. H. (1986). Joint attention and language in autism and developmental language delay. *Journal of Autism and Developmental Disorders, 16,* 335–349.

Macdonald, H., Rutter, M., Howlin, P., Rios, P., LeCouteur, A., Evered, C., & Folstein, S. (1989). Recognition and expression of emotional cues by autistic and normal adults. *Journal of Child Psychology and Psychiatry, 30,* 865–877.

McArthur, L. Z., & Baron, R. M. (1983). Toward an ecological theory of social perception. *Psychological Review, 90,* 215–238.

Malatesta, C. Z. (1981). Infant emotion and the vocal affect lexicon. *Motivation and Emotion, 5,* 1–23.

Miller, C. L. (1983). Developmental changes in male/female voice classification by infants. *Infant Behavior and Development, 6,* 313–330.

Mundy, P., & Sigman, M. (1989). The theoretical implications of joint-attention deficits in autism. *Development and Psychopathology, 1,* 173–183.

Mundy, P., Sigman, M., Ungerer, J., & Sherman, T. (1986). Defining the social deficits of autism: The contribution of non-verbal communication measures. *Journal of Child Psychology and Psychiatry, 27,* 657–669.

Murray, L., & Trevarthen, C. (1985). Emotional regulation of interactions between two-month-olds and their mothers. In T. M. Field & N. A. Fox (Eds.), *Social perception in infants* (pp. 177–197). Norwood, NJ: Ablex.

Nelson, C. A. (1987). The recognition of facial expressions in the first two years of life: Mechanisms of development. *Child Development, 58,* 889–909.

Neuman, C. J., & Hill, S. D. (1978). Self-recognition and stimulus preference in autistic children. *Developmental Psychobiology, 11,* 571–578.

Oster, H. (1981). "Recognition" of emotional expression in infancy? In M. E. Lamb & L. R. Sherrod (Eds.), *Infant social cognition: Empirical and theoretical issues.* Hillsdale, NJ: Lawrence Erlbaum.

Ozonoff, S., Pennington, B. F., & Rogers, S. J. (1990). Are there emotion perception deficits in young autistic children? *Journal of Child Psychology and Psychiatry, 31,* 343–361.

Perner, J., Frith, U., Leslie, A. M., & Leekam, S. R. (1989). Exploration of the autistic child's theory of mind: Knowledge, belief and communication. *Child Development, 60,* 689–700.

Piaget, J. (1972). *The principles of genetic epistemology* (W. Mays, Trans.). London: Routledge and Kegan Paul.

Prior, M., Dahlstrom, B., & Squires, T.-L. (1990). Autistic children's knowledge of thinking and feeling states in other people. *Journal of Child Psychology and Psychiatry, 31,* 587–601.

Raven, J. C. (1960). *The Standard Progressive Matrice: Sets A, B, C, D and E.* London: H. K. Lewis.

Raven, J. C. (1965). *The Coloured Progressive Matrices: Sets A, Ab, B.* London: H. K. Lewis.

Reddy, V. (1990). Playing with others' expectations: Teasing and mucking about in the first year. In A. Whiten (Ed.), *The emergence of mindreading: Evolution, development and simulation of second order representations.* Oxford: Blackwell.

Ricks, D. M. (1975). Vocal communication in pre-verbal normal and autistic children. In N. O'Connor (Ed.), *Language, cognitive deficits and retardation* (pp. 75–80). London: Butterworths.

Riguet, C. B., Taylor, N. D., Benaroya, S., & Klein, L. S. (1981). Symbolic play in autistic, Down's, and normal children of equivalent mental age. *Journal of Autism and Developmental Disorders, 11,* 439–448.

Runeson, S., & Frykholm, G. (1986). Kinematic specification of gender and gender expression. In V. McCabe & G. J. Balzano (Eds.), *Event cognition: An ecological perspective* (pp. 259–273). Hillsdale, NJ: Lawrence Erlbaum.

Sagi, A., & Hoffman, M. L. (1976). Empathic distress in the newborn. *Developmental Psychology, 12,* 175–176.

Scaife, M., & Bruner, J. S. (1975). The capacity for joint visual attention in the infant. *Nature, 253,* 259–266.

Scheerer, M., Rothmann, E., & Goldstein, K. (1945). A case of "idiot savant": An experimental study of personality organization. *Psychological Monographs, 58,* (4 [whole no. 269]), 1–63.

Shapiro, T., Sherman, M., Calamari, G., & Koch, D. (1987). Attachment in autism and other developmental disorders. *Journal of the American Academy of Child and Adolescent Psychiatry, 26,* 485–490.

Shaw, R., & Pittenger, J. (1977). Perceiving the face of change in changing faces: Implications for a theory of object perception. In R. Shaw & J. Bransford (Eds.), *Perceiving, acting and knowing: Toward an ecological psychology.* Hillsdale, NJ: Lawrence Erlbaum.

Sigman, M., & Mundy, P. (1989). Social attachments in autistic children. *Journal of the American Academy of Child and Adolescent Psychiatry, 28,* 74–81.

Sigman, M., Mundy, P., Sherman, T., & Ungerer, J. (1986). Social interactions of autistic, mentally retarded and normal children and their caregivers. *Journal of Child Psychology and Psychiatry, 27,* 647–656.

Sigman, M., & Ungerer, J. A. (1984). Attachment behaviors in autistic children. *Journal of Autism and Developmental Disorders, 14,* 231–243.

Silberg, J. L. (1978). The development of pronoun usage in the psychotic child. *Journal of Autism and Childhood Schizophrenia, 8,* 413–425.

Simner, M. L. (1971). Newborn's response to the cry of another infant. *Developmental Psychology, 5,* 136–150.

Snow, M. E., Hertzig, M. E., & Shapiro, T. (1987). Expression of emotion in young autistic children. *American Academy of Child and Adolescent Psychiatry, 26,* 836–838.

Sorce, J. F., Emde, R. N., Campos, J., & Klinnert, M. D. (1985). Maternal emotional signaling: Its effect on the visual cliff behavior of 1-year-olds. *Developmental Psychology, 21,* 195–200.

Spiker, D., & Ricks, M. (1984). Visual self-recognition in autistic children: Developmental relationships. *Child Development, 55,* 214–225.

Spitz, R., & Wolf, K. (1946). The smiling response: A contribution to the ontogenesis of social relations. *Genetic Psychological Monographs, 34,* 57–125.

Stern, D. N. (1985). *The interpersonal world of the infant.* New York: Basic Books.

Szatmari, P., Bartolucci, G., Krames, L., Flett, G., & Tuff, L. (1989). *The perception of non-verbal social information among adolescents with pervasive developmental disorders.* Unpublished manuscript.

Tager-Flusberg, H. (1989). *An analysis of discourse ability and internal state lexicons in a longitudinal study of autistic children.* Paper presented at the meeting of the Society for Research in Child Development, Kansas City, MO.

Tantam, D., Monaghan, L., Nicholson, H., & Stirling, J. (1989). Autistic children's ability to interpret faces: A research note. *Journal of Child Psychology and Psychiatry, 30,* 623–630.

Trevarthen, C. (1979). Communication and cooperation in early infancy: A description of primary intersubjectivity. In M. Bullowa (Ed.), *Before speech* (pp. 321–347). Cambridge: Cambridge University Press.

Trevarthen, C., & Hubley, P. (1978). Secondary intersubjectivity: Confidence, confiding and acts of meaning in the first year. In A. Lock (Ed.), *Action, gesture and symbol: The emergence of language* (pp. 183–229). London: Academic Press.

Tronick, E., Als, H., Adamson, L., Wise, S., & Brazelton, T. B. (1978). The infant's response to entrapment between contradictory messages in face-to-face interaction. *Journal of American Academy of Child Psychiatry, 17,* 1–13.

Tucker, D. M. (1981). Lateral brain function, emotion, and conceptualization. *Psychological Bulletin, 89,* 19–46.

Ungerer, J. A., & Sigman, M. (1981). Symbolic play and language comprehension in autistic children. *Journal of the American Academy of Child Psychiatry, 20,* 318–337.

Volkmar, F. R. (1987). Social development. In D. J. Cohen & A. M. Donnellan (Eds.), *Handbook of autism and pervasive developmental disorders* (pp. 41–60). New York: John Wiley.

Volkmar, F. R., Sparrow, S. S., Rende, R. D., & Cohen, D. J. (1989). Facial perception in autism. *Journal of Child Psychology and Psychiatry, 30,* 591–598.

Walden, T. A., & Ogan, T. A. (1988). The development of social referencing. *Child Development, 59,* 1230–1240.

Walker, A. S. (1982). Intermodal perception of expressive behaviors by human infants. *Journal of Experimental Child Psychology, 33,* 514–535.

Walker-Andrews, A. S. (1988). Infants' perception of the affordances of expressive behaviors. In C. Rovee-Collier (Ed.), *Advances in infancy research, vol. 5* (pp. 173–221). Norwood, NJ: Ablex.

Weeks, S. J., & Hobson, R. P. (1987). The salience of facial expression for autistic children. *Journal of Child Psychology and Psychiatry, 28,* 137–151.

Werner, H. (1948). *Comparative psychology of mental development.* Chicago: Follett.

Wetherby, A. M., & Prutting, C. A. (1984). Profiles of communicative and cognitive–social abilities in autistic children. *Journal of Speech and Hearing Research, 27,* 364–377.

Wing, L. (1969). The handicaps of autistic children—a comparative study. *Journal of Child Psychology and Psychiatry, 10,* 1–40.

Wing, L. (1981). Language, social, and cognitive impairments in autism and severe mental retardation. *Journal of Autism and Developmental Disorders, 11,* 31–44.

Wing, L., Gould, J., Yeates, S. R., & Brierley, L. M. (1977). Symbolic play in severely mentally retarded and in autistic children. *Journal of Child Psychology and Psychiatry, 18,* 167–178.

Wulff, S. B. (1985). The symbolic and object play of children with autism: A review. *Journal of Autism and Developmental Disorders, 15,* 139–148.

Yirmiya, N., Kasari, C., Sigman, M., & Mundy, P. (1989). Facial expressions of affect in autistic, mentally retarded and normal children. *Journal of Child Psychology and Psychiatry, 30,* 725–735.

Young-Browne, G., Rosenfeld, H. M., & Horowitz, F. D. (1977). Infant discrimination of facial expressions. *Child Development, 48,* 555–562.

Zucker, K. J. (1985). The infant's construction of his parents in the first six months of life. In T. M. Field & N. A. Fox (Eds.), *Social perception in infants* (pp. 127–156). Norwood, NJ: Ablex.

III

Educational Issues

10

Outcome and Follow-Up Studies of High-Functioning Autistic Individuals

CATHERINE LORD and ANDRE VENTER

Almost 25 years ago, a series of follow-up investigations provided the first information about what happened to autistic children as they entered adolescence and adulthood (DeMyer *et al.*, 1973; Lockyer & Rutter, 1969, 1970; Lotter, 1974). These studies were important in indicating that language skills and intelligence were factors in predicting outcomes for autistic students and adults. For a number of reasons, it now seems time to take a serious second look at follow-up and outcome studies, particularly for high-functioning autistic individuals. Educational services have changed dramatically in the past 20 to 30 years. In the last 10 years, access to community living and supported employment has also become more widespread. In addition, while it seemed clear from the earlier studies that, compared to severely mentally handicapped autistic individuals, high-functioning children and adults were more likely to have some success academically and socially, so few high-functioning autistic people did well on social and academic measures that factors associated with good outcomes within this group were difficult to determine. The purpose of the present chapter is to provide a brief description of recent and earlier studies of high-functioning individuals across development and to discuss factors that predict later functioning.

FOLLOW-UP STUDIES

From Preschool to School

Follow-up studies of children diagnosed as autistic as preschoolers and then seen again in school age have shown fairly remarkable stability in diagnosis and in

CATHERINE LORD • Greensboro High Point TEACCH Center, 2415 Penny Road, High Point, North Carolina 27265. ANDRE VENTER • Department of Pediatrics, University of the Witwatersrand, Baragwanath Hospital, Post Office Bertsham 2013, Johannesburg, Republic of South Africa.

High-Functioning Individuals with Autism, edited by Eric Schopler and Gary B. Mesibov. Plenum Press, New York, 1992.

intelligence over six- or seven-year periods (Freeman, Ritvo, Needleman, & Yokota, 1985; Lord & Schopler, 1989a). In fact, high-functioning children (defined here as nonverbal IQ > 70) showed *lower* standard deviations in IQ at a follow-up assessment when grouped by earlier scores than did lower-functioning children (Lord & Schopler, 1989b). High-functioning autistic children showed equally strong relationships between scores at the initial assessment, and at follow-up seven years later, as children with nonverbal IQs between 55 and 69 and stronger relationships than children scoring below 55 as preschoolers. Correlations ranged from about .50 up to .86, depending on whether the test was changed and how young the children were when they were first assessed. In one study (Lord & Schopler, 1989a) of 48 children who received nonverbal IQ scores over 70 when they were under age 6, three-quarters (i.e., 36) of the children continued to score in the nonretarded range on tests (that were in most cases increasingly abstract) when they were 8 to 12 years old. In addition, of 103 children who had scored in the 55–70 range as preschoolers, about one-third (i.e., 36) scored in the nonretarded range at ages 8 to 12. Just over 10% (7 out of 62) of the children who had scored in the severely handicapped range also scored in the nonretarded range seven years later. Thus, when IQ scores for high-functioning children at school age were compared to their scores in preschool, there were more children who moved up in IQ than down.

The one group of children who had relatively high IQs during preschool and whose IQs dropped during school age were children who did not acquire language by age 6. In this particular study (Lord & Schopler, 1989a), language was defined as reaching a basal level on the Peabody Picture Vocabulary Test (Dunn, 1959), which consists of identifying eight consecutive pictures of common objects, equivalent to just over a 2-year-old level. Only 4 of the 48 children who, at age 3 or 4, had received nonverbal IQs over 70 were unable to carry out such a language activity by the age of 6 years. However, for this small number of high-functioning children who did not have receptive vocabularies at the 2-year-old level by age 6, IQs fell into the mentally handicapped range as they entered later childhood.

These children who showed IQ decreases at school age were identifiable as preschoolers by lower adaptive scores on the Vineland Social Maturity scale (Doll, 1965) than those received by other not-yet-verbal children with equivalent nonverbal IQs but who acquired some receptive language by age 6. The attribution of cause and effect is not clear, but it seems important that there is a small proportion of children who score well on nonverbal tests in preschool who, along with significant difficulties in language acquisition, show increasing cognitive problems as they get older. The same pattern was also apparent, for an even smaller proportion of children, in the matched group of nonautistic, language-impaired children who served as controls in this study (Lord & Schopler, 1989b).

Several treatment studies of high-functioning autistic preschoolers have shown dramatic increases in Full Scale IQ in response to either one-on-one behavioral treatments or exposure to integrated preschool programs (Harris, Handleman, Gordon, Kristoff, & Firentes, 1991; Lovaas, 1987). It is difficult to interpret these results, since matched control groups were not available. Thus, it is not possible to discern whether these results were similar to improvements noted in lower-functioning autistic children treated through parent-as-therapist programming. These children showed significant IQ increases as they became able to be tested on standard nonverbal tests, in contrast to earlier scores on more social- and language-oriented infant tests (such as the Bayley Scales of Mental Development).

In summary, autistic children who score above 70 on nonverbal tests as preschoolers are likely to remain relatively high functioning into school age, unless they show so little language development that by the time they are 6 years old, their receptive understanding of single words is less than that of a normally developing 2-year-old. In addition, there also seems to be a significant number of children who score in the mild-to-moderate range on IQ tests as preschoolers who will later perform in the nonretarded range on nonverbal and performance tests. Scores on adaptive measures, such as the daily living skills domain from the Vineland Adaptive Behavior Scales (VABS) (Sparrow, Balla, & Cicchetti, 1984), that are relatively close to nonverbal mental age may be useful predictors of this change. However, this suggestions needs confirmation by further research.

School Age to Adolescence

A recently published (though actually carried out in the late 1970s) follow-up of autistic children into later childhood described a group of 15 very high-functioning autistic children and a matched group of boys with severe receptive language disorders who had first been seen at a mean age of about 7 years (Cantwell, Baker, Rutter, & Mawhood, 1989). These children had initially shown nonverbal IQs well above the normal range, and all but one continued to fall in the normal range even when tested with the performance scales of the Wechsler Intelligence Scales—R (Wechsler, 1974). The autistic children showed progress in language, but only 1 of 15 reached the 72-month ceiling on the Reynell Comprehension Scale. Though originally matched to the autistic children on language level, the repetitive language-impaired children had made much more progress in all areas of language than had the autistic children. Overall, there were *no* marked changes in any of the four major areas of functioning (language, peer relations, stereotypic/repetitive behaviors, public behavior) for the autistic group, although the proportion with good peer relations and "adequate public behavior" increased from almost zero to about a third of the children for each area. At follow-up, the groups were not different in sensory abnormalities such as unusual responses to sound or appearing deaf, or in expressive language delay, immediate self-repetitions, grammar, using language to chat or converse, or intonation. However, the autistic children continued to have more stereotyped utterances, pronoun reversals, echolalia, and inappropriate remarks than the nonautistic children. For three aspects of language—thinking aloud, not asking to take part, and not reporting outside contexts—the autistic group was actually described by their parents as being more handicapped or abnormal as they approached their teens than they had been as preschoolers and early school age children. The autistic children also showed an equal or greater number of incidents of stereotypic hand movements and self-injury during the follow-up than they had originally.

It is important to remember that this was a very short-term follow-up study; the children were seen for the second time only about two years after the initial assessment, so that extreme changes would not be expected. However, most notable was that the autistic children did not show the significant improvements across a variety of language measures shown by nonautistic children with equivalent language problems several years before. Simmons and Baltaxe (1975) described the language of seven high-functioning verbal autistic adolescents and found marked difficulties that they characterized in terms of prosody and semantics. Some of these adolescents had difficulties with dysfluencies and what the authors called "hesitations," which included repeating sounds or syllables in rapid succession. They also noted unusual intonation to be a common problem. In addition, many of the students had trouble with what would now be called pragmatics, that is, failing to switch codes from formal to informal, using vague references, and telescoping ideas. The authors found no relationship between Wechsler Full Scale IQ and auditory processing or measures of linguistic disturbance. However, they did find relationships between neuropsychological measures of auditory perception and linguistic performance.

We recently followed a group of 58 high-functioning autistic boys and girls into their teens and early twenties (mean age about 15 years) (Venter, Lord, & Schopler, 1991). For these children, their mean original IQ received under age 6—in most cases on a nonverbal test—was 80.24; at follow-up, it was 89.02. Thirty-nine of 58 subjects had useful speech before the age of 5. At follow-up, all of the subjects could speak, and all but four reached a basal level on the Peabody Picture Vocabulary Test, but six of them did not have sufficient language to take the Wechsler tests. Of 52 out of 58 subjects who were able to complete a full WISC-R or WAIS-R at follow-up, mean Full Scale IQ was 79.2, so that on the whole test, scores were quite stable. Test scores for nonverbal tests were very stable, and when tests with a verbal component were used, they were stable for most subjects. The correlation between early and later nonverbal IQs was .79 and between early IQ and Wechsler IQ was .67.

When mean scores were studied, research has generally shown slight *decreases* (i.e., 2–6 point shifts downward) as children approach adolescence (Lockyer & Rutter, 1969; Venter *et al.*, 1991). However, at least some of this effect may be due to the fact that at follow-up, adolescents are often given tests such as the WISC-R that require a greater variety of behaviors and more attention to verbal instructions than the nonverbal tests such as the Merrill–Palmer (Stutsman, 1948) or the Leiter International Performance Scales (Arthur, 1952) used at earlier ages.

All of the children continued to meet DSM-III-R and ICD-10 criteria for autism. Forty-nine of the 58 students had academic skills above the first-grade level at the later assessment. Thirty-nine of the students could decode above the third-grade level, but fewer than half of the 58 had reading comprehension above the third-grade level. In contrast, 34 spelled at or above the third-grade level; but only about half of the students could carry out all simple arithmetic computations up to multiplying a three-digit number by another three-digit number.

This study was primarily oriented toward looking at cognitive skills, but some simple measurements of language and adaptive skills were undertaken. While the students' cognitive levels as measured on standardized tests remained high, and they achieved some academic skills (although not to the degree that one would expect from their intelligence scores), problems and limitations in adaptive behaviors remained significant. Almost all of the students had mean scores on the Vineland Adaptive Behavior Scales that were well below half the children's chronological ages. Similarly, age equivalents and standard scores on measures of receptive vocabulary and a test of oral comprehension of discourse indicated continued, marked difficulties in receptive language not accounted for by overall ability.

Into Adulthood

Studies of very high-functioning autistic adults by Rumsey and colleagues (Rumsey & Hamburger, 1988, 1990; Rumsey, Rapoport & Scccry, 1985) have shown that, as adults, autistic individuals continue to have major social, behavioral and cognitive difficulties. These autistic adults had IQs in the average range, and on the Wide Range Achievement Test (Jastak & Jastak, 1978)—which measures computations, word reading, and spelling—they also performed in the average range. Six out of nine had high school degrees or the equivalent. They continued to have marked language difficulties, particularly in pragmatics and prosody (Rumsey *et al.*, 1985), and to have particular difficulties in problem solving (Rumsey & Hamburger, 1988). All showed major behavioral and social impairments.

Only one of the nine subjects lived independently; four were employed, but only two had obtained their jobs without substantial help.

In contrast, Szatmari, Bartolucci, Bremner, Bond, and Rich (1989) described a follow-up study of 16 adults who were identified on the basis of earlier records as autistic children and followed up to age 26. These young adults had a mean IQ in the average range. They had much better outcomes than described in any of the previous studies. Seven were university graduates, and six were in paid employment. Six scored above average in adaptive functioning, with only 4 out of 16 scoring more than two standard deviations below the mean in adaptive skills. One was married; three were dating regularly. Four of the young adults were felt to have had truly good outcomes in terms of independence, employment, and psychiatric status.

The results of our recent follow-up studies (Venter *et al.*, 1991) fell between the earlier follow-up studies by Rumsey and Rutter and colleagues and that of Szatmari. Only 1 of 18 subjects over 25 years old had completed university. One other person had attended a university, but had left without a degree. None was married. At time of the study, 2 of the 18 lived on their own; now, several years later, two others are living independently and there are a total of six young adults living in apartments with minimal supervision. Of the 22 subjects who were 18 years or older at the time of follow-up, 6 were competitively employed, 13 were in sheltered or supervised employment or in special school programs, and 3 were unemployed and not in school. Since that time, eight other subjects have obtained competitive employment, although two others have lost jobs. All of the autistic young adults who are employed are in relatively low-level jobs in service industries, and all but one received special assistance in finding employment. Compared to Szatmari's group, of whom only 4 out of 16 scored below 70 on the VABS, 19 out of 22 subjects over 18 years of age scored at this level.

Recently, Gillberg and Steffenburg (1987) described the outcome of a heterogeneous sample of autistic children and adults in Sweden. This was a sample (Gillberg, Steffenburg, & Jakobsson, 1987) with an unusually high frequency of neurobiological findings (fragile-X syndrome, autistic siblings, hearing losses), compared to our sample and that of Szatmari. Gillberg and Steffenburg were particularly interested in the onset of seizures and deteriorations associated with adolescence. However, none of the subjects with IQ scores over 50 deteriorated, and only two had epilepsy. Similarly, 6 of our 58 subjects had epilepsy as children; one developed seizures for the first time during adolescence. None of the epileptic children showed deteriorations. However, two other subjects showed marked cognitive and intermittent behavioral deteriorations in their mid-teens. These deteriorations eventually plateaued, but left the students nearly two standard deviations below their earlier intellectual functioning, a phenomenon that remained stable for several years. Neither of these students had any evidence of seizures or any clinical neurological findings, even after extensive examinations.

Overall, we are left with a much more optimistic picture of the academic abilities and independent functioning possible for high-functioning autistic adolescents and adults than was available 20 years ago. There are still real inconsistencies in the data, as there is variability across geographical areas. Diagnostic differences, methods of subject ascertainment, and social class effects may have accounted for the differences among the adult follow-up studies, as well as possible differences in access to supported employment, adult education, and residential settings.

In fact, in our data, we found that employment and residential placement (as well as the type of school placement) was more predictable by where the student or young adult lived, given that these were all high-functioning individuals, than by any other factor—suggesting that the availability of support services is often one, if not the major factor in what happens to high-functioning autistic young adults. While there remain concerns about onset of seizures and deteriorations found in a small proportion of autistic subjects during adolescence, both conditions are rare (and perhaps independent) phenomena in high-functioning young adults who do not have diagnosable neurobiological conditions other than autism. However, given the rapid changes in medical technology and the relatively small size of all the present samples, this issue is certainly not resolved.

PREDICTION OF OUTCOME

From Preschool to School

When working with an autistic preschool child, the major questions about stability and predictability often are whether the child will acquire language—if the child is not yet verbal—and how predictive of his or her later skills is his or her current performance on cognitive tasks. Earlier research was interpreted to mean that relatively high nonverbal IQs predicted language acquisition in young children. However, when this question was explored more carefully (Lord & Schopler, 1989b), we were surprised to find that language skills in preschool children predicted nonverbal IQ more than the reverse. It is important to remember that our measure of language in this study was a very gross summary of whether or not the child had sufficient receptive vocabulary to receive a basal score on the PPVT. Within these constraints, however, we were able to determine that children who did not receive a score on the PPVT under age 6, but were able to do so at the later assessment four to six years later, were no different at the later assessment than children who had received a PPVT basal score at the earlier age. That is, while the children who had language at the earlier age had higher IQs at the earlier age, the children who gained language over this time period showed increases in nonverbal IQ not shown by the children who had already had sufficient language to take the PPVT as young preschool children. This sample was not limited to high-functioning children, so we must be careful in the extent to which we generalize from it. As noted earlier, the best predictor of language acquisition for children who had not yet received a basal score on the PPVT was an adaptive score on the Vineland Social Maturity Scale at the earlier assessment. This pattern held true for both autistic and nonautistic language-impaired children.

In fact, correlations between preschool and school-aged scores on IQ tests were consistent and strong for autistic and nonautistic children across IQ ranges and age ranges down to 3 years (Lord & Schopler, 1989a, b). The only exceptions were that, when nonverbal 3-year-olds were administered the Bayley, they tended to score much lower than they did on later tests. Also, as discussed earlier for the small number of children who scored well on nonverbal tests at age 3 or 4 who did not acquire language by ages 6 to 12, scores tended to decrease.

School Age to Adolescence

Intelligence scores have traditionally been both the most common predictor and the most common outcome variable in follow-up studies into adolescence. Early work by Rutter and colleagues (Lockyer & Rutter, 1969, 1970) showed correlations between Full Scale IQ scores over a 5- to 15-year period of .63, with correlations slightly higher for Verbal IQ and slightly lower for Performance IQ (Lockyer &

Rutter, 1969). DeMyer *et al.* (1973) found very similar results. In our most recent follow-up studies (Venter *et al.*, 1991), correlations between early IQ and later IQ ranged from .63 to .70, depending on whether Raven's or Wechsler tests and verbal or performance scores were used. Thus, early IQ remains a good predictor of intelligence at later ages.

A second characteristic that follow-up studies have attempted to predict has been adaptive functioning. This was the standardized measure employed in the original Rutter studies in the late 1960s. For a sample of 24 high-functioning subjects, these investigators found a correlation of .73 between early IQ and later Vineland Social Maturity Scales. In our larger, more recent sample using the VABS, which was deliberately constructed to be less of a measure of cognitive skills than the earlier Vineland, we found a correlation of .54 between early IQ and VABS in late adolescence and early adulthood. *Early* IQ was the strongest single predictor of adaptive skills in adolescence/adulthood. Current verbal IQ had an even higher correlation (.65) with the VABS standard score, but was exceeded by other language measures discussed below.

The other major outcome variable has consisted of general judgments of very poor, poor, and fair-to-good outcome in terms of the subjects' independence and need for supervision or special help in school, work, and residence. IQ has traditionally been looked upon as the best discriminator of outcome. However, careful inspection of earlier results suggests that what seems to be happening is that very low nonverbal IQs (that is, under 50) are associated generally with very poor outcome, whereas higher IQs are associated with outcomes from poor to good. In one paper (Rutter, Greenfeld, & Lockyer, 1967), the mean IQ for clients rated "good" was 83 in contrast to a mean IQ of 45 for those rated as very poor, but there were no significant IQ differences for the comparisons of adjacent outcomes (i.e., good versus fair, poor versus very poor).

Another variable that has been considered a strong predictor of later functioning in autism has been language. Language has been considered in a variety of ways; one of the most common has been to look at whether or not a child has communicative speech at the age of 5. Definitions for this term are not available; thus, we decided to define communicative speech in a child at age 5 as spontaneous production of at least five meaningful words intended to communicate per day and receiving at least a basal score (age equivalent 2 years 3 months) on the Peabody Picture Vocabulary Test of receptive single word knowledge. Thus, this was a rather minimal definition of speech at age 5. Other aspects of language that have been addressed have included response to sound, Peabody Picture Vocabulary Test scores, Verbal IQ, and language deviance as based on parental reports (LeCouteur *et al.*, 1989). In the earlier Lockyer and Rutter (1970) paper, speech at age 5 was found to be the best discriminator between good and fair outcome for subjects with IQs greater than 50 during adolescence. Similarly, we found that when PPVT test scores were available for our subjects prior to age 5, these replaced earlier IQ in multiple regressions and yielded even stronger correlations with adaptive skills at adolescence than had early IQ (r = .65). The language measure most correlated with current IQ was a nonstandardized test of oral comprehension of language, resulting in similar findings to those described by Lincoln, Courchesne, Kilman, Elmasian, and Allen (1988). Thus, while nonverbal IQ and language skills are certainly not independent phenomena in autism, each may yield different kinds of information about outcome, as well as different implications depending on the students' age.

There has been some concern that seizures in adolescents may be associated with deterioration and thus a very poor outcome. In the Rutter papers, 10 out of 63 children had seizures at infancy, with 8 of them developing seizures during adolescence. However, only two of these children had IQs greater than 60, and none showed marked regressions. In Gillberg and Steffenburg's (1987) follow-up study, none of the subjects who developed seizures or deteriorations had IQs above 50. As noted earlier, only one girl in our sample (Venter *et al.*, 1991) developed seizures during adolescence, though two nonepileptic students showed marked deteriorations at or around puberty. All of the children in our study who had seizures were in the lower half of our IQ distribution, but in other ways they were indiscriminable from the rest of the sample. Thus, the prognostic implications of early and/or later seizures may be different in high-functioning children than for the majority of autistic students.

The relationship between early factors and academic functioning is particularly interesting because in the late 1960s, the Rutter group found no significant correlation ($r = .26$) between initial IQ and Schonell reading scores for a group of relatively high-functioning students (Lockyer & Rutter, 1969). The autistic students were higher in reading accuracy than nonautistic matched controls. Thus, students with a mean chronological age of 15 years 7 months and an estimated verbal mental age (on the basis of Verbal IQ) of 11 years 5 months were generally found to have a reading accuracy age of 10 years 11 months, but reading comprehension at less than the 9-year-old level.

In contrast, in our sample collected in the late 1980s, we found a strong positive relationship ($r = .64$) between early IQ and an aggregate measure of achievement that included reading accuracy, reading comprehension, spelling, and computations. In addition, both speech before age 5 and the severity of restricted behaviors independently accounted for some of the variance in achievement. Current Verbal IQ was correlated .88 with the aggregate achievement scores, with both current social behavior and the PPVT scores also contributing to the variance. Early IQ and speech before age 5 both predicted spelling, math, and reading accuracy. Earlier language deviance, as well as speech before age 5 and nonverbal IQ, predicted reading comprehension. It was also interesting that current Performance IQ related to achievement in all areas except reading comprehension, which was related only to Verbal IQ and comprehension of oral language.

A final predictor variable that has been found to show some relationship with outcome in a number of studies has been a measure of symptom severity. Rutter, Greenfeld, & Lockyer (1967) found that subjects with a good outcome had fewer symptoms in all areas of autism. Similarly, DeMyer *et al.* (1973) also found a relationship between overall severity of autism and outcome. Both of these studies included subjects from a range of intellectual levels, so some of this effect might have been due to the relationship between IQ and severity of autism (Schopler, Reichler, & Renner, 1986). In our study, we found no effect of total number of symptoms as rated on a parent interview, but we did find relationships between severity of early language deviance and restrictive behaviors and later adaptive scores. We also found a relationship between early restricted behavior and achievement scores and current social behavior and academic achievement. It is tempting on the basis of these findings to speculate about possible transactional relationships among intelligence, language abnormalities (as opposed to deficits), and the intrusive effect of early high levels of resistance to change or repetitive behaviors in very young children. These effects could occur both in the sense of the problematic behaviors interfering on a minute-to-minute level with learning and also because of an overall effect on educational opportunities. However, more information is clearly needed.

Outcome and Adulthood

Szatmari *et al.* (1989) did not find an effect of symptom severity on the educational or vocational outcomes of the subjects in their particularly successful group. They also found no relationship between outcome and scores on a language comprehension test, but did find relationships between Full Scale IQ and adaptive behavior, and also between outcome and scores on the Wisconsin Card Sorting Test, a nonverbal test of problem solving that is highly correlated with Verbal IQ. Rumsey *et al.* (1985) had a much more socially handicapped sample than Szatmari *et al.*, though with equally high IQs. When contrasting the Rumsey *et al.* sample to subjects with IQs below 80, Szatmari *et al.* (1989) found that the subjects with IQs above 80 were much more likely to work competitively. These authors were also quite concerned about the effect that restricted and repetitive behaviors had on job placement. A number of their subjects had good technical skills but were unable to hold jobs, or jobs of much responsibility, because of interfering compulsive behaviors or difficulties with change. Szatmari *et al.* commented that many parents had spent a great deal of time helping their adult children find appropriate job placements and then supporting them in these jobs. In Gillberg and Steffenburg's (1987) sample, only one subject was employed.

In our study (Venter *et al.*, 1991) we found that the 6 out of 22 subjects over 18 years old who were employed had higher language scores—including Verbal IQ, PPVT, oral comprehension, and reading comprehension—than did the subjects who did not work. Four of the autistic adults employed at the time of the original study had been mainstreamed in high school, which seemed to indicate a possible relationship. However, since the study was originally done, eight other subjects have now found employment. These subjects were, in all cases but one, from North Carolina, and all came out of highly specialized school programs for autistic adolescents. Thus, what appeared to be a positive relationship between being mainstreamed in school and employment has now been reversed. This seems to be a good example of the complexity of the relationships among outcome, intervention, and various factors particular to the subjects. In this case, of the original six autistic subjects who were employed, all were very high functioning, and the fact that they had managed in regular high school despite having autism was indicative of their excellent verbal skills. However, with increased availability of supported employment programs and job coaches who can both find and provide support for initial placement, the skills adolescents learn in specialized programs—such as working to completion, following instructions, checking their work, and sustaining a task—and the connections between special adolescent classrooms and supported employment have made it more likely in the state of North Carolina that adolescents coming out of specialized programs will find themselves in supported employment than other students. Clearly this is a relationship more of convenience than of meaning; one would like to see supported employment programs available to all autistic persons. However, it seems important to recognize the reciprocal nature of the relationship between education and employment when interpreting outcome studies.

CONCLUSION

Follow-up and outcome studies have traditionally been very helpful both in identifying points of emphasis for programming and education and in giving parents and professionals a sense of what is to come. What is exciting about the most recent studies is that the acquisition of skills by high-functioning autistic people seems to be getting more predictable, in a positive way. That is, academic and adaptive skills seem to be somewhat higher for people than estimated 20 years ago, and to be more related to perhaps neurobiologically determined factors such as intelligence than previously estimated. Even the acquisition of language in young autistic students, particularly those with relatively good early adaptive scores and a lack of severe mental handicap, seems to be somewhat more predictable. These findings provide some support for a general clinical sense that improved services have made a real difference for high-functioning autistic individuals in the last 20 years, although there is much still to be done.

On the other hand, there are still many unknowns and many unresolved issues. While academic skills in high-functioning autistic adolescents and adults seem to have improved considerably for roughly comparable samples in the last 20 years, they are still not nearly as high as one would expect from the intellectual levels of these autistic people. There is room for improvement, particularly in teaching arithmetic and reading comprehension, two academic skills that are basic to independent functioning. Adaptive skills continue to be much less strong for autistic than more mentally handicapped but nonautistic populations, even in areas such as daily living skills where one would expect autistic adolescents and adults to have less difficulty than in socialization and communication. Again, such a finding might be taken as a challenge to teachers and clinicians to consider how best to ensure that autistic individuals can achieve as many of these skills as possible.

A clear role of language abilities and communication deviance in affecting outcome continues to be supported. It is frustrating to see that there are some children who seem to have relatively good nonverbal/performance skills as preschoolers who do not acquire even a minimal level of receptive language. Similarly, many high-functioning adults continue to have quite marked difficulties with language comprehension that seem likely to contribute to outcome. Figuring out more about the course of acquisition of comprehension might be helpful in providing us with ideas for future intervention.

The number of high-functioning students showing deteriorations during adolescence was quite small, but continued to be of concern since no clear source for these regressions was ever identified, and because of the significant loss of skill. In addition, a better understanding of how specific autistic symptoms contribute to later outcome in terms of academic and adaptive skills would be useful.

Recent studies have emphasized test scores and placement measures more than the earlier judgments of "outcome" in terms of psychiatric status. While the earlier judgments of outcome were sometimes difficult to interpret, it does seem important to consider the satisfaction and well-being of the autistic adults as part of outcome, as well as how they do on more easily definable standard measures. It is our impression, from the most recent follow-up studies, that many high-functioning autistic adults have far greater access to vocational opportunities and independence than in earlier years. Hopefully, with a better understanding of how these opportunities became available and how best to prepare the autistic students to maximize them,the "good outcome" will come to mean more and to apply to more and more of the autistic population.

REFERENCES

Arthur, G. (1952). *The Arthur Adaptation of the Leiter International Performance Scale.* Chicago: Psychological Service Center Press.

Cantwell, D. P., Baker, L., Rutter, M., & Mawhood, L. (1989). Infantile autism and developmental receptive dysphashia: A comparative follow-up into middle childhood. *Journal of Autism and Developmental Disorders, 19,* 19–32.

DeMyer, M. K., Barton, S., DeMyer, W. E., Norton, J. A., Allen, J., & Steel, R. (1973). Prognosis in autism: A follow-up study. *Journal of Autism and Childhood Schizophrenia, 3,* 199–245.

Doll, E. A. (1965). *Vineland Social Maturity Scale.* Circle Pines, MN: American Guidance Service.

Dunn, L. M. (1959). *Manual for the Peabody Picture Vocabulary Test.* Minneapolis: American Guidance Service.

Freeman, B. J., Ritvo, E. R., Needleman, R., & Yokota, A. (1985). The stability of cognitive and linguistic parameters in autism: A five-year prospective study. *Journal of the American Academy of Child Psychiatry, 24,* 459–464.

Gillberg, C., & Steffenburg, S. (1987). Outcome and prognostic factors in infantile autism and similar conditions: A population-based study of 46 cases followed through puberty. *Journal of Autism and Developmental Disorders, 17,* 273–288.

Gillberg, C., Steffenburg, S., & Jakobsson, G. (1987). Neurobiological findings in 20 relatively gifted children with Kanner-type autism or Asperger's syndrome. *Developmental Medicine and Child Neurology, 29,* 641–649.

Harris, S. L., Handleman, J. S., Gordon, R., Kristoff, B., & Firentes, F. (1991). Changes in cognitive and language functioning of preschool children in autism. *Journal of Autism and Developmental Disorders, 21,* 281–290.

Jastak, J. F., & Jastak, S. (1978). *The Wide Range Achievement Test: Manual of instructions—1978 revised edition.* Wilmington, DE: Jastak Associates.

LeCouteur, A., Rutter, M., Lord, C., Rios, P., Robertson, S., Holdgrafer, M., & McLennan, J. D. (1989). Autism Diagnostic Interview: A semi-structured interview for parents and caregivers of autistic persons. *Journal of Autism and Developmental Disorders, 19,* 363–387.

Lincoln, A. J., Courchesne, E., Kilman, B. A., Elmasian, R., & Allen, M. (1988). A study of intellectual abilities in high-functioning people with autism. *Journal of Autism and Developmental Disorders, 18,* 505–524.

Lockyer, L., & Rutter, M. (1969). A five- to fifteen-year follow-up study of infantile psychosis: III. Psychological aspects. *British Journal of Psychiatry, 115,* 865–882.

Lockyer, L., & Rutter, M. (1970). A five- to fifteen-year follow-up study of infantile psychosis: IV. Patterns of cognitive ability. *British Journal of Social and Clinical Psychology, 9,* 152–163.

Lord, C., & Schopler, E. (1989a). The role of age at assessment, developmental level, and test in the stability of intelligence scores in young autistic children. *Journal of Autism and Developmental Disorders, 19,* 483–499.

Lord, C., & Schopler, E. (1989b). Stability of assessment results of autistic and nonautistic language-impaired children from preschool years to early school age. *Journal of Child Psychology and Psychiatry, 30,* 575–590.

Lotter, V. (1974). Factors related to outcome in autistic children. *Journal of Autism and Childhood Schizophrenia, 4,* 263–277.

Lovaas, O. I. (1987). Behavioral treatment and normal educational and intellectual functioning in young autistic children. *Journal of Consulting and Clinical Psychology, 55,* 3–9.

Rumsey, J. M., & Hamburger, S. D. (1988). Neuropsychological findings in high-functioning men with infantile autism, residual state. *Journal of Clinical and Experimental Neuropsychology, 10,* 201–221.

Rumsey, J. M., & Hamburger, S. D. (1990). Neuropsychological divergence of high-level autism and severe dyslexia. *Journal of Autism and Developmental Disorders, 20,* 155–168.

Rumsey, J. M., Rapoport, M. D., & Sceery, W. R. (1985). Autistic children as adults: Psychiatric, social, and behavioral outcomes. *Journal of the American Academy of Child Psychiatry, 24,* 465–473.

Rutter, M., Greenfeld, D., & Lockyer, L. (1967). A five- to fifteen-year follow-up study of infantile psychosis: II. Social and behavioural outcome. *British Journal of Psychiatry, 113,* 1183–1199.

Schopler, E., Reichler, R. J., & Renner, B. R. (1986). *The Childhood Autism Rating Scale (CARS) for diagnostic screening and classification of autism.* New York: Irvington.

Simmons, J. Q., & Baltaxe, C. (1975). Language patterns of adolescent autistics. *Journal of Autism and Childhood Schizophrenia, 5,* 333–351.

Sparrow, S., Balla, D., & Cicchetti, D. (1984). Vineland Adaptive Behavior Scales. Circle Pines, MN: American Guidance Service.

Stutsman, R. (1948). Guide for administering the Merrill–Palmer Scale of Mental Tests. In L. M. Terman (Ed.), *Mental measurement of preschool children* (pp. 139–262). New York: Harcourt, Brace & World.

Szatmari, P., Bartolucci, G., Bremner, R. S., Bond, S., & Rich, S. (1989). A follow-up study of high-functioning autistic children. *Journal of Autism and Developmental Disorders, 19,* 213–226.

Venter, A., Lord, C., & Schopler, E. (1991). A follow-up study of high-functioning autistic children. *Journal of Child Psychology and Psychiatry, 32*(7).

Wechsler, D. (1974). Manual for the Wechsler Intelligence Scale for Children – Revised. San Antonio: San Antonio Psychological Corp.

11

A Comparison of Language Issues in High-Functioning Autism and Related Disorders with Onset in Childhood and Adolescence

CHRISTIANE A. M. BALTAXE and JAMES Q. SIMMONS III

INTRODUCTION

Speech, language, and communication in autism present a heterogeneous and complex picture that has fascinated clinicians and researchers since Kanner's (1943) original description of the syndrome. Deficits in these areas have been studied from the perspectives of normal language development, their relationship to cognition, and more recently, their relationship to socialization and affect (Baron-Cohen, 1988, 1989a; Hobson, 1986; Sigman, Mundy, Sherman & Ungerer, 1986). Important variables in these studies have included IQ, age, language acquisition history, and age of onset, as well as remedial and pharmacological intervention. While language function can vary considerably based on these variables, communication behaviors in autism appear to remain flawed in specific ways and constitute an essential aspect of the total diagnostic picture. Foremost are impairments in pragmatics, or the use of language in a social context. Fillmore (1981) characterized the are of pragmatics from a structural–functional perspective as "a three-termed relationship that unites (a) linguistic form and (b) the communicative functions that these forms are capable of serving, with (c) the contexts or settings in which those linguistic forms can have those communicative functions" (p. 144). Recent reviews of pragmatic deficits in autism are provided by Watson (1988) and Baron-Cohen (1988).

The purpose of this chapter is to (a) examine linguistic characteristics in higher-

---

CHRISTIANE A. M. BALTAXE and JAMES Q. SIMMONS III • Department of Psychiatry and Biobehavioral Sciences, UCLA School of Medicine, Los Angeles, California 90024.

High-Functioning Individuals with Autism, edited by Eric Schopler and Gary B. Mesibov. Plenum Press, New York, 1992.

functioning autistic individuals (IQ of 70 or more, with reasonably adequate language function),* (b) compare these characteristics with language behaviors seen in related disorders with onset in childhood and adolescence, and (c) consider their possible significance in the continuing controversy concerning the relationship of autism to these other disorders (Beitchman, 1983; Cantor, Evans, Pearce, & Pezzot-Pearce, 1982; Cantor, Pearce, Pezzot-Pearce, & Evans, 1981; Kanner, 1943, 1949; Kolvin, Ounsted, Humphrey, & McNay, 1971; Rutter & Schopler, 1987). With regard to these issues, the area of pragmatics is particularly relevant, but other aspects of communication need to be addressed as well.

The most extensive studies of language in psychiatric disorders of childhood and adolescence have centered on autism. Other related disorders have not received the same degree of attention, despite the presence of significant problems in communication. These disorders include, in particular, schizophrenia and schizotypal personality disorder with onset in childhood and adolescence, as well as pervasive developmental disorder, not otherwise specified. Language behaviors in these disorders become particularly relevant from the perspective of autism in the higher-functioning autistic individual because of the many apparent similarities and parallels. In order to provide a basis for comparison, a cursory summary of pragmatic deficits and other language problems in the higher-functioning autistic individual is provided below. We will then focus on identifying areas of communication deficits in these other disorders and compare them to those seen in higher-functioning autism. Historic perspectives, current diagnostic criteria pertaining to these disorders, developmental language histories, language perspectives from high-risk studies, specific language studies pertaining to older individuals, and language characteristics of autistic children who become schizophrenic will be examined for this purpose. Differences in the way communication is conceptualized diagnostically and in various research approaches will be highlighted. It is our claim that conceptual differences affect the way in which the relationship among these disorders is seen and interpreted.

LINGUISTIC CHARACTERISTICS IN HIGH-FUNCTIONING AUTISM

Most of the recent language research in autism appears to focus on pragmatics (Baron-Cohen, 1988; Watson, 1988). This research tends to overshadow research efforts in many other areas of speech and language that are also impaired. In the higher-functioning individual, these other areas include continuing problems in (a) comprehension as shown in verbal interaction as well as on formal language and IQ testing (Baltaxe & Simmons, 1981, 1983; Lord, 1985; Simmons & Baltaxe, 1975; Tager-Flusberg, 1981a); (b) semantics as manifested by peculiar word choices and difficulties with abstract language (Menyuk & Quill, 1985; Simmons & Baltaxe,

*It is estimated that no more than 20 to 30% of all individuals with autism fall into this category, and it is estimated that no more than 10% have nearly normal language function.

1975; Tager-Flusberg, 1981b); (c) speech production as evidenced by specific syntactic and morphological errors (Baltaxe & Simmons, 1977; Bartolucci, Pierce, & Streiner, 1980; Simmons & Baltaxe, 1975; Swisher & Demetras, 1985); (d) the residual use of echolalia (Prizant & Duchan, 1981; Prizant & Rydell, 1984; Simmons & Baltaxe, 1975; Schuler, 1979); (e) prosody for sentence intonation, emotional expression, and the expression of fine nuances in verbal communication (Baltaxe & Simmons, 1985, 1987, 1988; Baltaxe, Simmons, & Zee, 1984); and (f) dysfluencies as evidenced by hesitations, false starts, and reformulations (Baltaxe & Simmons, 1977; Simmons & Baltaxe, 1975). Research studies and clinical reports show that the above areas remain impaired in the higher-functioning autistic individuals, although the impairment may be less obvious. Pragmatic deficits, on the other hand, appear to be more visible in both their verbal and nonverbal forms. This chapter will also focus on pragmatic deficits in greater detail, since even in adolescence and adulthood these deficits appear to be prominent in linking autism and these other disorders with onset in childhood and adolescence.

The area of pragmatics has been characterized as the interface between social, cognitive, linguistic, and emotional development (Baltaxe & Simmons, 1988). Recent studies in pragmatics and language-disordered populations have covered a broad range of domains that has included discourse analysis, conversational rules, narrative abilities, cognitive and social skills prerequisite to or associated with communication, the communicative function of language as expressed in speech acts, and the use of language in the process of thinking, problem solving, and play behavior (Prutting, 1982; Rees, 1978). In comparing the conceptualizations and approaches to pragmatics among different practitioners and researchers, Snyder and Silverstein (1988) likened the fuzziness of the borders of pragmatics to the use of slightly different recipes by different master cooks preparing a specific dish.

Pragmatic studies in autism leave the same impression. No single study fully defines and encompasses the range of pragmatic abilities and disabilities in the disorder, but collectively these studies provide an interesting composite picture. There is general agreement that all autistic individuals suffer pragmatic impairments. But since existing studies use different variables in selecting and studying their populations (IQ, age, presence of language, pragmatic parameter examined, and approach used), it is not clear whether there actually exists a common core of such deficits. Some of the heterogeneity seen in these studies may well be a function of these individual variables.

Pragmatic deficits in autism appear to have precursors in infancy and early childhood. Some of the areas necessary for the development of adequate pragmatic behaviors appear deficient from the start. Examples are the abnormal cry behavior to indicate physical needs and emotional states in autistic infants (Ricks & Wing, 1975), poor eye contact in face-to-face interaction, early abnormalities in socialization, deficiencies in joint attention, and difficulties with reciprocal social play (Baron-Cohen, 1989a; Mundy & Sigman, 1989a; Ungerer & Sigman, 1981).

In later childhood and adolescence in the higher-functioning autistic individual, pragmatic deficits include difficulties with observing rules of politeness under varying social conditions, expressing appropriate emotions in a given context, imagination and humor, knowing when to switch from one social register to another, taking the listener's perspective when incorporating new and old information in a linguistic interchange, and simple and complex verbal problem-solving tasks (for review, see Baron-Cohen, 1988; Watson, 1988). Some of these problems have been interpreted as consequences of the autistic individual's difficulty with conceptual thinking and the ability to make inferences (Rumsey, Andreason, & Rappoport, 1986).

When some of the more "linguistic" deficits seen in comprehension, semantics, expression, prosody, and fluency are examined more closely, it might be argued that some of these are due to more basic problems in pragmatics and its precursors. Language-acquisition studies in young normal children have shown that they use socially determined cues and strategies for language comprehension, and that social behaviors and communicative meanings are closely tied to each other, especially in the early acquisition process (Lord, 1985; Menyuk & Quill, 1985). The autistic child who does not have appropriate eye contact or does not follow social cues and behaviors in a communicative interaction may not develop adequate comprehension strategies and may have difficulties in developing semantic meanings satisfactorily. Problems in expressive language might be explained similarly, as may some of the problems with prosody, particularly where affect and the fine nuances of language are concerned.

Baron-Cohen, in association with Leslie and Frith (Baron-Cohen, 1988, 1989b; Baron-Cohen, Leslie, & Frith, 1985; Leslie, 1987; Leslie & Frith, 1987, 1988), recently proposed a cognitive model as explanatory of the pragmatic deficits seen in autism. A basic assumption in this model concerns the ability to understand mental states in others. Such an ability is considered a necessary prerequisite to the metarepresentation of knowledge in an individual's mind. According to these authors, autistic individuals have difficulty in understanding other people's mental states. Based on this "theory of mind," they are impaired in the metarepresentational and metalinguistic capacity that is required for symbolic development and the appropriate use of language in a social context. Considerable controversy still exists with respect to the scope and explanatory power of this cognitive model (Mundy & Sigman, 1989a, b).

LANGUAGE BEHAVIOR IN RELATED DISORDERS: A COMPARISON WITH HIGH-FUNCTIONING AUTISM

A Historical and Current Diagnostic Perspective

The relationship between autism, schizophrenia, and related disorders has been at issue since Kanner's early description of the autistic disorder (Bender, 1971; Cantor *et al.*, 1982; Kanner, 1943, 1949; Kolvin *et al.*, 1971; Rutter, 1972; Rutter &

Schopler, 1987). This concern still exists. Clinically, the issue becomes highly relevant, particularly concerning higher-functioning individuals in later childhood or early adolescence, or where autism, schizophrenia, pervasive developmental disorder not otherwise specified, or schizotypal personality disorder are under consideration as possible diagnoses. The first might include situations where an earlier diagnosis of autism must be reconsidered in later childhood or adolescence due to changing symptomatology. The latter may involve instances where a diagnosis was never made, has been inadequate, or a restricted symptom picture has been considered. The issue of dual diagnosis or of changing diagnosis then might also arise, and will be discussed further below.

Kanner initially thought that autism was an early manifestation of schizophrenia, but later changed his thinking. The most extensive clinical study defining the current diagnostic separation of autism from the other disorders mentioned above is provided by the work of Kolvin and his colleagues (Kolvin, 1971; Kolvin *et al.*, 1971). They associated diagnostic differences with age of onset as well as family characteristics. Autism or *infantile psychosis* (IP) had an earlier onset (before the age of 3) and a less weighted family pedigree for psychosis. The other disorders, labeled *late-onset psychosis* (LOP) had a later onset (after the age of 5), with a heavier family incidence of psychosis. It is interesting to note that almost 90% of the LOP children were described as odd by parents or mental health professionals prior to the clear onset of their psychosis.

Within the current diagnostic framework (DSM-III-R; American Psychiatric Association, 1987), disorders in the LOP group of children would include schizophrenia, schizotypal personality disorder (SPD), and childhood-onset pervasive developmental disorder not otherwise specified (PDDNOS). Schizoid disorder and Asperger syndrome are additional terms used that are more closely associated with European investigations. Schizotypal personality disorder and pervasive developmental disorder NOS are diagnoses that have only been defined relatively recently (in DSM-III and DSM-III-R). They were introduced to categorize patients with lesser degrees of psychopathology involving social communication. A diagnosis of SPD is frequently used for the higher-functioning individual who, by symptomatology, appears to fall between autism and schizophrenia. The diagnosis is generally made in early adolescence when language is reasonably well developed (Nagy & Szatmari, 1986). With respect to PDDNOS the criteria appear somewhat less specific than for autism. This diagnosis is generally made in childhood, often in cases where the diagnosis of autism does not quite fit. Schizophrenia, an adult diagnosis, also refers to children when they fit the diagnostic picture.

Thus, from a historical perspective, all of these disorders appear to be linked by a close symptom picture. As this chapter will show, one area in this picture appears to be communication. All these disorders demonstrate considerable similarities in social use of language, in addition to language delay and deviant language function. The analysis of communication behavior therefore becomes particularly relevant with regard to differential diagnosis. Table 11-1 shows those deficits

Table 11-1. Pragmatic and Linguistic Behaviors in Autism, Schizophrenia, Schizotypal Personality Disorder, and Pervasive Developmental Disorders Not Otherwise Specified (DSM-III-R)

Autism	Schizophrenia	Schizotypal Personality Disorder	Pervasive Developmental Disorder Not Otherwise Specified
Qualitative impairment in reciprocal social interaction, verbal and nonverbal communication, and imaginative activity as manifested by the following: • No mode of communication, such as communicative babbling, facial expression, gesture, mime, or spoken language • Markedly abnormal nonverbal communication, as in the use of eye-to-eye gaze, facial expression, body posture, or gestures to initiate or modulate social interaction • Absence of imaginative activity such as playacting of adult roles, fantasy characters, or animals; lack of interest in stories about imaginary events • Marked abnormalities in the production of speech, includ-	When the onset is in childhood or adolescence, failure to achieve expected level of social development • (Bizarre) delusions • Prominent hallucinations • Incoherence or marked loosening of associations • Catatonic behavior • Flat or grossly inappropriate affect *Prodromal or residual symptoms; marked social isolation or withdrawal* • Marked impairment in role functioning • Marked peculiar behavior (including talking to self) • Blunted or inappropriate affect • Digressive, vague, overelaborate, or circumstantial speech, or poverty of content of speech	Pervasive pattern of deficits in interpersonal relatedness and peculiarities of ideation, appearance, and behavior • Ideas of reference (excluding delusions of reference • Excessive social anxiety, e.g., extreme discomfort in social situations involving unfamiliar people • Odd beliefs or magical thinking (in children and adolescents, bizarre fantasies and preoccupations) • Odd speech (without loosening of associations or incoherence), e.g., speech that is impoverished, digressive, vague, or inappropriately abstract • Inappropriate or constricted affect, e.g., silly, aloof, rarely reciprocates gestures or facial expressions, such as	Qualitative impairment in the development of reciprocal social interaction and of verbal and nonverbal communication skills *but the criteria are not met for autistic disorder, schizophrenia, or schizotypal personality disorder*

ing volume, pitch, stress, rate rhythm, and intonation • Marked abnormalities in the form or content of speech, including stereotyped and repetitive use of speech; idiosyncratic use of words or phrases; or frequent irrelevant remarks • Marked impairment in the ability to initiate or sustain a conversation with others, despite adequate speech • Markedly restricted range of interests and preoccupation with one narrow interest	• Odd beliefs or magical thinking including overvalued ideas of reference • Marked lack of initiative, interests, or energy (may affect speech) *Catatonic type* • Catatonic stupor or mutism *Disorganized type* • Incoherence, marked loosening of associations • Flat or grossly inappropriate affect *Paranoid type* • Preoccupation with one or more systematized delusions or with frequent auditory hallucinations related to a single theme • None of the following: incoherence, marked loosening of associations, flat or grossly inappropriate affect, catatonic behavior, grossly disorganized behavior *Undifferentiated type* • Prominent delusions, hallucinations, incoherence, grossly disorganized behavior	smiles and nods • Suspiciousness or paranoid ideation • *Occurrence not exclusively during the course of schizophrenia or pervasive developmental disorder*

that appear related to the social use of language, as well as other deficiencies in language function currently part of the diagnostic criteria for these different disorders (DSM-III-R).

It is evident from this table that many of these criteria appear to overlap among the four diagnostic categories. While the social use of language has been studied extensively in autism, few such studies are available for children and adolescents diagnosed with these other disorders. With few exceptions, available studies on the symptom picture in these disorders have largely ignored specific communication characteristics. It seems likely that, following a more detailed pragmatic and linguistic analysis, many similarities but also differences would become more evident when compared to communication in the high-functioning autistic individual. For example, in the current diagnostic framework (DSM-III-R), language in schizophrenia is described as *incoherent* or *with marked loosening of associations*. Prodromal and residual symptoms include language as *digressive, vague, overelaborate, circumstantial,* and as *impoverished in content as well as in output*. The communication characteristics for *schizotypal personality disorder* include *odd speech, without loosening of associations or incoherence, e.g., speech that is impoverished, digressive, vague, or inappropriately abstract*. The communication characteristics for *pervasive developmental disorder not otherwise specified (PDD-NOS)* are only described as *qualitative impairment in the development of reciprocal social interaction and of verbal and nonverbal skills*.

Many of the descriptors for these three disorders that are shown in Table 11-1 can be restated as deficits in pragmatics such as those seen in the higher-functioning autistic individual. Others may reflect abnormalities in the form (grammatical structure) and content (semantics) of language, also described for autism. Still others, relating to affect, may be reflected in the prosody of speech (volume, pitch, rate, rhythm, and intonation), and in nonverbal interaction (eye gaze, facial expression, and body posture), which are also deviant in the autistic individual. In addition, a pervasive pattern of deficits in interpersonal relatedness, social isolation, and withdrawal are seen as diagnostic characteristics in schizophrenia and schizotypal personality disorder. Taken together, these verbal and nonverbal characteristics appear quite similar to the deficit patterns seen in the higher-functioning autistic individual.

Developmental Language Histories

In both schizophrenia and schizotypal personality disorder, the focus has generally been on behavior and thought, while language development and early manifestations of communication have largely been overlooked or merely commented on (Harrison, Hess, & Zrull, 1963; Jordan & Prugh, 1971; Potter, 1933). However, it appears that early communication skills play an important role. The information gleaned from various studies will be presented in some detail below.

Lack or delay of language development, loss of acquired language, or peculiarities of language behavior are among the earliest characteristics that generally bring the child with autism to medical attention. What is not so well-known is that children with schizophrenia, schizotypal personality disorder, or related disorders also have a high incidence of early communication problems. The possibility of such problems has been overlooked by some investigators and merely commented on by others without detailed analysis. Kolvin *et al.* (1971) found that close to half (16 of 33) of the children ages 5 to 13, with late-onset psychosis showed a developmental delay. This was confined to language in almost all of the affected children (15 of 16). *Delay* was defined as an "incapacity for three word phrases by the age of three years" (p. 388). The authors noted, however, that this delay was never as extensive as in their autistic (IP) group. The linguistic deficits further described for the late-onset psychosis group included "spoke like younger child," "meaningless words or phrases (at any time)," "echolalia," "partial answers," and "jerky speech." Personality oddities were also noted in more than three-quarters of the late-onset psychosis group. Personality abnormalities can at least in part be conceptualized as involving pragmatics. When the autistic group was compared, all showed early language delay ($n = 47$). Their linguistic deficits were described as "pronoun reversal," "spoke like a younger child," "meaningless words or phrases at any time," "echolalia," "partial answers," and "jerky speech." The incidence of partial answers and jerky speech was not significantly different between the groups.

While the incidence of schizophrenia prior to the age of 10 was rare in the late-onset psychosis group, onset was described as slow and insidious. This made pinpointing the actual age of occurrence difficult to determine. However, when the communication characteristics of the late-onset psychosis children were examined, evidence of the development of the disorder can be seen. Features pertaining to language were described as emotional blunting with abnormalities in the form, stream, and content of thought. Several individual categories relating to thought and expressed in language behaviors were seen. These categories existed to varying degrees in this group and included disorder of association, autistic thinking, derailment of thought, talking past the point, thought blocking, thought deprivation, thought insertion, and thought broadcast. Delusions of different types were also present.

Disorders in the form and stream of thought were also seen in the autistic (IP) group. These consisted of disorder of association, autistic thinking, derailment of thought, talking past the point, and thought blocking.

Since not every child in the late-onset psychosis group or in the autism group had all of these disorders, the communication characteristics pertaining to thought disorder may also not differentiate between any given individual in the late-onset psychosis and the autistic groups.

Bender and Faretra (1972) examined 100 children with symptoms of a major psychiatric disorder. Fifty were diagnosed with childhood schizophrenia, onset after 3½ to 4 years; 50 children were diagnosed with autism, onset in the first 2 years of age. The childhood-schizophrenic group included 12 with an onset of psychosis between 3½ and 4 years, 16 between the ages of 5 and 6 years, and 13 with an onset between 9 and 10 years. There were nine additional children with a symbiotic syndrome, with an onset of psychosis between ages 2 and 3 years. The autistic group consisted of 5 children with symptoms noted before age 2, 18 of whom had a symbiotic syndrome appearing between the age of 2 and 3 years.

The authors noted that normal language development did not occur in any of the children with infantile autism with or without symbiosis. None of the children whose psychotic episode was initiated by symbiosis, and none seen at the age of 3½ to 4 years, had normal language development. Only one-fourth of the children with onset between ages 5 and 6 years, and one-half with onset of psychosis between 9 and 10 years had normal language development.

When the pattern of communication deviance in all the children was examined, slow development with "retarded" use was the most common picture seen in almost one-third of the total sample. This pattern was seen in close to a third of the 50 children in the childhood-schizophrenic group, and was the only deviation seen at age 5 in those children with onset between 9 and 10 years of age. The language deficits seen in the rest of the total sample appeared in many different forms. These included mutism in the presence of good comprehension, or with a total lack of comprehension; failure to use the first person pronoun; neologisms; mumbling, incoherent language, often used egocentrically; explosive obscenities; private language; echolalia; and repetitive questions without waiting for an answer. Often the language was variable from day to day over periods of months. This study again shows the close similarities in language behavior between the two diagnostic groups.

Cantor *et al.* (1982) studied 19 children and 11 adolescents with IQ scores in the normal range who met DSM-III criteria for schizophrenia. With respect to language, delay was the most common finding, seen in nearly two-thirds of the children's group and close to one-third of the adolescents' group. Language delay was present in all but two children seen before the age of 5. A history of deviant language in the form of "incoherence [jargon] and echolalia" was also common in both groups. Only 16% of the younger group and 30% of the older group had a history of normal language development. In the younger group, symptoms were first noted between 2 and 8 years, and in the older group between 2 and 12 years. Seven of the total group showed symptoms prior to the age of 30 months. Even though they showed "autisticlike" symptoms, they were not diagnosed as autistic, because at the time of diagnosis they also had thought disorders.

A symptoms checklist that relates to communication and was developed by the authors showed the following symptoms, which varied to some degree: constricted or inappropriate affect, perseveration, fragmentation of thought, monotonous voice, loose associations, neologisms, echolalia, illogicality, autism, clanging, incoherence, poverty of speech, and poverty of content of speech. Examining these symptoms in greater detail linguistically, it becomes evident that most of these symptoms have also been reported for higher-functioning autistic individuals, often using slightly different terminology (Baltaxe, 1977; Simmons & Baltaxe, 1975).

Communication deficits as seen in autism were also noted in a follow-up study on patients with schizophrenic symptoms. Eggers (1978) presented follow-up data on 57 patients between the ages of 7 to 13 with clear schizophrenic symptoms. This study made brief reference to linguistic disturbances, including "echolalia, phonographism, and neologisms" leading to disintegration of speech prior to the age of 10. In addition, 90% of all patients had early premorbid symptoms including difficulties in making contact, which clearly represents a pragmatic problem.

Wolff and Barlow (1979) compared schizoid, autistic, and normal children.* The schizoid group showed preoccupation with idiosyncratic and rigid ideas and interests, poor social adjustment, and frequent school failure in the presence of an IQ within the normal range. Some were "strikingly original in their verbal and material productions," while the mothers of these children saw them as "remote," "lacking in feeling," and "strange," with general difficulties in adapting to changing circumstances and difficulties since the preschool years. Other common features included emotional detachment and solitariness, rigidity, occasional suspiciousness and paranoid ideation, lack of empathy for the feelings of others, and odd ideation, often with metaphorical use of language. This clinical picture was identical to the autistic psychopathology described by Asperger (1944). Wolff and Barlow found that autistic and schizoid children were similar on their verbal/performance score discrepancies. On verbal subtests, schizoid children were more like normal than autistic children, but differed from normal and autistic children in their low scores on digit span. In all cognitive, language, and memory tests the schizoid children were more distractable than the normal group. In language function they resembled the autistic group, although language disabilities were less severe. When affect was considered, the schizoid group used fewer emotional constructs than the autistic group when describing people. Again, this study shows more similarities than differences among the groups.

Garralda (1985) studied 20 children and adolescents between the ages of 8 and 16 years with onset of psychosis occurring after 5 years of age.† Significantly more abnormalities in expressive language were seen in the psychotic group than in a comparison group of 20 children with behavioral or emotional disorders. These abnormalities consisted of "incoherence, mutism, laconism [poverty of speech], and repetitive speech." Additional behaviors relating to language included "stopping in the middle of a sentence" and "starting to sing." The psychotic group also suffered from delusions and displayed inappropriate affect, hypoactivity, and bizarre behavior, as well as social withdrawal. Flat affect was uncommon, but over one-half of the subjects had incongruous affect and a possible formal thought disorder, as indicated by incoherence of speech. It is not clear from the study whether these language characteristics emerged with onset of the psychosis and to what extent they existed prior to the diagnosis.

*The diagnostic system used by Wolff and Barlow is somewhat different from the system used in the United States, and the diagnostic categories of 'Asperger syndrome" may simply be included in the broader autism category under DSM-III-R, while "schizoid' may fall somewhere between autism and schizotypal personality

†Psychosis is schizophreniclike, but without the observed prodromal period necessary for a diagnosis of schizophrenia.

Kydd and Werry (1982) reviewed the medical data on all of the schizophrenic children admitted as inpatients to a child psychiatric unit over a 10-year period. The diagnoses had been based on clinical symptomatology and DSM-III criteria. Ten children who had been first seen at least one year earlier were followed up with a reassessment of clinical status and level of adaptive functioning. Of these 10, 6 had unequivocal prodromal symptoms, seen as problems in academic functioning, social withdrawal, and magical thinking. Although problems in school performance often also imply problems in language, it is not clear from the report how long these problems had predated diagnosis, nor to what extent language was involved.

Green *et al.* (1984) compared schizophrenic, autistic, and conduct-disordered children between the ages of 5.2 and 12.10 years who had been diagnosed using DSM-III criteria. Although language was not addressed in the developmental histories, the authors noted that for the schizophrenic group, Verbal IQ was somewhat lower than Performance IQ, and symptoms of a formal thought disorder were present. These included incoherence, marked loosening of associations, markedly illogical thinking or marked poverty of content of speech, and blunted, flat, or inappropriate affect. Again, although all of these symptoms involve verbal and nonverbal communication, they were not studied from a communication perspective.

Watkins, Asarnow, and Tanguay (1987) analyzed the developmental histories of 18 children with schizophrenia meeting the DSM-III criteria. Onset was prior to 10 years of age. The children were rated at each of four age levels using the Achenbach Child Behavior Checklist (Achenbach & Edelbrock, 1983). Watkins *et al.* found a gradual developmental unfolding of a broad spectrum of symptoms affecting social, cognitive, sensory, and motor functioning that began many years prior to the appearance of schizophrenic symptoms. In 13 children, severe language deficits and motor problems were found before the age of 6. Symptomatic differences among all 18 patients faded in the 9- to 11-year-old group. Seven had onset prior to 30 months and met the criteria for infantile autism. Eight had onset after 8 years and were diagnosed as schizophrenic without a prior history of autism. Three met the criteria of childhood-onset pervasive developmental disorder, with onset after 31 months but before 9 years of age. These latter 11 patients constituted the authors' schizophrenic group.

The majority of the children in the schizophrenic group had significant developmental delays beginning in infancy. Language deficits appeared in 55% in the period of 0–30 months, but diminished to 27% in the 31 months–5 years period and to 18% in the 6–8 years period. After age 9, no further deficits were reported.

In the autistic group, language deficits were seen in all seven of the children through age 5, in six through age 8, and in two through age 11. Echolalia earlier in development was reported for only one of the schizophrenic children without an earlier history of autism, but for all seven of the children with a history of autism. The study showed that the onset of schizophrenia was earliest in those children with autistic symptoms, but did not occur before the age of 3.

This study is important because it shows an apparent developmental sequence in the expression of communication-related schizophrenic symptoms. The presence of a formal thought disorder was seen in 8 of the 11 schizophrenic children with no history of autism, and was first seen in two children between the ages of 6 and 8, and in a total of eight children (72%) between the ages of 9 and 11. In the seven children with a history of autism, five had a formal thought disorder, first noted between the ages of 6 and 8. In only three, it was noted between the ages of 9 and 11. Flat or inappropriate affect was found in two of the schizophrenic children between 6 and 8 years of age, and in a total of seven children between 9 and 11 years. Of those with a history of autism, six showed flat or inappropriate affect between 6 and 8 years, but only four between 9 and 11 years. Delusions and hallucinations were found in one schizophrenic child between the ages of 6 and 8 years, and in seven children between ages 9 and 11. In the autistic group, two showed delusions and hallucinations between 6 and 8 years, and four between 9 and 11 years. This study emphasizes a significant language delay in schizophrenic children and highlights overlapping symptomatology between autism and schizophrenia.

Baltaxe, Russell, Simmons, and Bott (1987) studied 10 schizophrenic and 10 schizotypal children between the ages of 7 and 14 years and with IQ scores in the normal range. They found developmental historics for language delay and disturbance in 9 of the 10 schizophrenic children and 8 of the 10 schizotypal children. For the schizophrenic group, developmental descriptions included "poor auditory memory," "hard to follow," "trouble expressing self," "gibberish," "trouble with word comprehension," "cannot remember instructions while talking," "difficulty sequencing information," "pronoun reversals," "poor articulation and syntax," "does not have meaningful speech," "incoherent," "speech arrest for many weeks," and "word approximations."

For the schizotypal group, developmental descriptions included "difficulty pronouncing words," "difficult to understand," "comprehension problem," "perseveration," "immature language," "inability to process auditory information," "perseverative," "submucous cleft," "articulation problems," "nonsensical words," and "poor auditory memory."

In the schizophrenic group, four showed Verbal IQ scores significantly poorer than Performance IQ scores. For two additional subjects, the reverse was true. For the schizotypal group, three were lower in Verbal IQ, and two in Performance IQ.

Thirteen of the 20 received formal language tests. Disturbances were as follows: 61% had problems on receptive vocabulary, and 38% on receptive syntax. Expressive impairment was also seen (38% vocabulary, 46% syntax, 38% articulation, fluency 61%, voice 23%). Auditory processing was deficient in 85% of the subjects tested.

Nagy and Szatmari (1986) described the early development of 20 children with schizotypal personality disorder whose IQ scores were in the normal range. Twelve (60%) of their subjects had a speech delay, defined as "not speaking one word by age one year, and not being able to speak in two-word phrases by the age of two." A number of these also showed deviant language development, which consisted of delayed echolalia, problems seen in receptive dysphasia, neologisms, and overly metaphorical speech. Two-thirds of the 18 children had discrepancies between Verbal and Performance IQ, equally distributed between deficits in Verbal and deficits in Performance IQs. All of those with a lower Verbal than Performance IQ also showed evidence of an earlier speech delay. Academic problems existed in the majority of the children, with 14 attending special education classes full time.

Based on the details in language behavior, it is clear that similarities outweigh differences in the developmental language histories of the diagnostic groups described above.

Perspectives from High-Risk Studies

Studies of children and adolescents identified as being at risk for psychopathology because of major psychiatric disorders in one or both parents may provide additional insight into the relationship among the above disorders through communication characteristics and developmental language histories. For the purpose of this chapter, the at-risk population is defined as the offspring of schizophrenic parents. Of concern here is that language may be an early indicator of developing psychopathology.

Moldin, Gottesman, and Erlenmeyer-Kimling (1987) in the New York High Risk studies noted that children of a schizophrenic parent were 10 to 15 times more likely to develop the disorder than children in the general population. The offspring of two schizophrenic parents were 40 times more likely to become affected than children of normal parents.

Sameroff, Seifer, Zax, and Barocas (1987) reported on early indicators of developmental risk from the Rochester Longitudinal study, utilizing cognitive, psychomotor, social, and emotional assessments at birth and at 4, 12, 30, and 48 months of age. Children with high multiple environmental risk scores had worse outcomes than children with low multiple scores.

In the Israeli High Risk Study of 50 preadolescent children born to at least one schizophrenic parent, followed at various ages, 13 showed poor motor and sensorimotor performance during the first year of life, although their overall developmental functioning was often in the normal range (Marcus *et al.*, 1987). The group also showed impaired psychosocial functioning, poor school adjustment, attention difficulties, deficits in perceptual motor skills, and learning disabilities with a lower proficiency in arithmetic, and "a basic distortion in cognitive integration" (Kaffman, 1986, p. 15). At ages 11 and 16, the high-risk group was uniformly rated as more impaired than a control group of 50 children with nonimpaired parents. Statistically significant differences were found in severity of psychopathology, quality of social and school adjustment, and presence of neurological "soft" signs. Communication and language were not specifically described. However, it can be assumed that deficits in these areas occurred in combination with the problems described.

The Stony Brook High Risk Project studied 80 offspring of schizophrenic parents in a three-year follow-up. These children showed multiple and extensive cognitive, attentional, and social impairments (Weintraub, 1987). By school age, more than 35% of the children with one schizophrenic parent had some significant clinical findings, compared to 9.8% of a normal control group. These children showed deficits in the ability to maintain attention and to ignore irrelevant input, and also evidenced patterns of cognitive slippage. They differed from control children across the entire battery of attentional and cognitive measures. An analysis of tape-recorded speech samples of these children showed considerable structural deviance (Harvey, Weintraub, & Neale, 1982). They also evidenced low verbal productivity, inadequate patterns of cohesion between ideas, and unclear and ambiguous references to previously mentioned ideas. The pattern of speech was quite similar to that found in adult schizophrenic patients, but did not meet clinical criteria for thought disorder (Rochester & Martin, 1979); it more closely resembled cognitive slippage described by Meehl (1962). These children were also rated by teachers and peers as being different, using descriptors such as "abrasive," "withdrawn," and "low in social competence." At the age of 18 years or older, 23% were assigned a DSM-III diagnosis, compared to 9.6% of normal controls.

The Copenhagen High Risk Project studied 207 children considered at high risk for schizophrenia because of schizophrenic mothers (Mednick, Parnas, & Schulsinger, 1987). At initial assessment, the children ranged between 10 and 20 years of age (mean age 15.1). When compared to controls, this group showed more disturbing behavior in school, as well as more deviant performance on a word association task (Mednick & Schulsinger, 1965). At follow-up, when the children were about 20 years of age, 42% of the high-risk individuals were given a schizophrenia spectrum diagnosis. Those children who became schizophrenic had experienced more traumatic births than any other diagnostic subgroup in the study. Children who were psychotic or seriously mentally disturbed when they were first interviewed in 1962 were excluded from the sample. Parnas, Schulsinger, Schulsinger, Mednick, and Teasdale (1982) examined premorbid behavioral data on those individuals who had received a schizophrenia spectrum diagnosis (schizophrenia and schizotypal personality disorder). They reported that, in addition to being passive babies, these individuals also had short attention spans and interpersonal difficulties in school. In adolescence, they showed comparable and significantly higher levels of formal thought disorder and defective emotional rapport than did high-risk controls. This study raises an important question regarding the relative contributions of biology and environment on the development of communication in the high-risk group of children.

Fish (1987) tested the hypothesis that "specific neurointegrative disorders in infancy predict vulnerability to later schizophrenia and schizotypal personality disorder" (p. 395). Twelve offspring of schizophrenic mothers were compared with 12 controls from similar backgrounds. They were assessed with regard to physical growth measures and the analysis of Gesell tests, which include separate quotients for gross motor, visual motor, and language development skills. Her findings could not be interpreted with respect to possible language dysfunction. However, on follow-up between the ages of 10 and 15 years and based on the Wechsler Comprehension subtest, comprehension had dropped by 2 to 7 points in half of the at-risk group, and in 7 of 10 at-risk subjects, vocabulary subtest scores dropped 3 to 6 points. Fish also noted a high incidence of dyslexia and poor interpersonal relationships (the latter implying pragmatic deficits) in this group of children. All seven showed pandysmaturation, and six had been disturbed since early infancy. One had a subsequent diagnosis of schizophrenia, five had schizotypal personality disorder, and one had paranoid personality disorder. Fish (1987) did not specifically focus on language and communication, although it appears evident that the subjects who developed psychopathology also had deficient language characteristics.

The above group of studies seems to show that language is an early, sensitive indicator of future psychopathology. However, further research is needed to see whether language can be differentiated in this group of disorders.

Specific Language Studies Pertaining to Adolescence and Adulthood

Most language studies of autistic children and adolescents have used a descriptive linguistic framework. There have been few attempts to describe language behavior in schizophrenia using a similar framework. Also, schizophrenic language has been studied primarily in adults. Two major methodological approaches dominate these studies. The first is a psychiatric approach, best characterized in the work of Holzman and Andreason (Andreason 1979a, b; Holzman, 1978, 1986; Rumsey *et al.*, 1986). Both Holzman and Andreason attempt to objectify the characteristics of a thought disorder; Holzman's descriptions are primarily cognitive, whereas Andreason attempts to include more linguistic descriptions. The latter has developed a rating scale through which thought, language, and communication in schizophrenia are identified and measured (Andreason, 1979a, b). Her approach assumes that thought is expressed in language. The rating scale then identifies specific characteristics of a thought disorder as seen in expressive language through poverty of speech, tangentiality, derailment, illogicality, incoherence, neologisms, and blocking. Most of these characteristics are assumed to measure deviations in thinking. By listening for them as they are expressed in language behavior, the diagnosis of a thought disorder in schizophrenia can be made.

Using the Andreason rating scale, Rumsey *et al.* (1986) compared the language of 14 adults with a DSM-III diagnosis of autism, residual state, with that of adult schizophrenics. Videotaped psychiatric interviews were analyzed for subtypes of thought disorder and affective flattening. The autistic group showed a high incidence as well as severity in the following: poverty of speech, perseveration, poverty of content of speech, echolalia, and incoherence, as well as affective flattening. They also showed pressure of speech, tangentiality, derailment, and circumstantiality. The schizophrenic group showed all of these characteristics, but in addition also had stilted speech, self-reference, blocking, illogicality, and loss of goal. More intensive comparisons revealed that the autistic group showed more poverty of speech, while the schizophrenic group had more derailment, illogicality, and loss of goal. However, the two groups did not differ on a scale of affective flattening, which included facial expression, spontaneous movement, expressive gestures, eye contact, affective responsivity, affect, vocal inflection, rhythm, and response latency. These results indicate that not only verbal but also nonverbal characteristics are very similar among the two groups.

The second approach to the analysis of schizophrenic language is a linguistic one. This approach is characterized by discourse analysis as well as the analysis of the grammatical structure. Discourse analysis examines linguistic markers in connected speech that are used by speakers to make their discourse more coherent and understandable to the listener (Halliday & Hasan, 1976). Rochester and colleagues were able to identify specific deficits in the discourse of schizophrenics that differentiated them from normal and manic adults (Rochester & Martin, 1979; Rochester, Martin, & Thurston, 1977). In their initial study, they showed that it was possible to identify reliably thought-disordered speech on the basis of lay judges' evaluations of coherence in language transcripts and linguistic variables measuring coherence. The linguistic measures that best predicted judges' evaluations were those that showed that the schizophrenic speaker made the listener's task difficult by asking the listener to search for information that he had never clearly given and by providing relatively few conjunctive links between clauses. Thought-disordered speakers differed in that they had proportionately fewer conjunctions and more lexical cohesions than normal subjects. They also used more situational references outside the discourse. The results were interpreted as an interpersonal failure on the part of the thought-disordered speaker to take into account the point of view of the listener.

No comparable studies on the discourse of high-functioning autistic adolescents or adults are currently available. However, pragmatic studies on the communication of autistic adolescents and adults have led to a similar conclusion: The high-functioning autistic speaker fails to take into account the point of view of the listener (Baltaxe, 1977; Baltaxe & Simmons, 1977). Formal discourse analysis may be a promising approach to compare the language of schizophrenic and high-functioning autistic individuals, since it takes into consideration morphosyntactic form in the expression of pragmatic function.

In a linguistic study, but focusing on grammar, Morice and Ingram (1982) distinguished a group of schizophrenic patients from normal subjects. The language of schizophrenics was syntactically less complex, more dysfluent, and contained more semantic and syntactic errors. Using a more refined computer analysis, Morice and McNicol (1986) studied the diagnostic utility of language criteria in schizophrenia. The spoken language of normal-IQ schizophrenic subjects was compared with that of normal subjects. Impairment identified in the schizophrenic group included reduced syntactic complexity, with less depth of clausal embedding and fewer reduced relative clauses, in addition to more semantically deviant sentences and greater dysfluency. The language characteristics in both these studies parallel those seen in high-functioning autistic individuals (Baltaxe & Simmons, 1977, 1983; Simmons & Baltaxe, 1975).

Fraser, King, Thomas, and Kendell (1986) replicated the results of Morice and Ingram (1982) in 77 schizophrenic and 50 normal subjects, aged 16 to 65 years. They were able to classify subjects back into their diagnostic group with more than 75% accuracy. Using the same method, King, Fraser, and Thomas (1987) analyzed the language samples of a high-functioning autistic female at ages 17 and 22. Despite similarities, their results also suggested some differences in the profile of the autistic individual. The authors concluded that autistic and schizophrenic language could be confused. Also, both conditions could coexist, and both conditions could produce grammatical abnormalities, neologisms, echolalia, and abnormal prosody. Language could also seem incoherent in either condition, with major problems in pragmatics.

According to these authors, one characteristic that distinguishes the two conditions is the greater linguistic versatility in schizophrenia, with the patient asking questions and making statements. In contrast, the high-functioning autistic individual remains closed to the listener's needs. The authors base their conclusion on the lack of questions and an abundance of statements and declarations in the autistic individual. Their autistic subject also produced more syntactic and semantic errors than did normal or schizophrenic individuals. Interestingly, based on a five-year follow-up, the autistic individual's language continued to improve, as demonstrated by the greater number of well-formed utterances, more nondeclarative sentences, fewer errors, and less densely complex sentences. In contrast, the schizophrenics' speech appeared to deteriorate. These results must be regarded as highly tentative, since only one autistic subject was analyzed.

Coming from a slightly different perspective, Paul and Cohen (1984) examined communication characteristics in a group of 18 subjects, initially diagnosed as childhood "aphasic" and followed through adolescence. A slow and steady growth in language, with expression progressing more rapidly than comprehension, was seen in these subjects. Their analysis showed that about one-half could not be distinguished from adolescents who had been diagnosed as autistic in childhood. At the time of the study, these subjects showed the oddities of communication, language deficits, and social behavior generally associated with residual autism in adolescence. Because these subjects also showed social deficits early on, the authors concluded that social deficits were important prognostic indicators of later social and communicative development, which required the earliest possible intensive intervention in the pragmatic area. This study also suggests that the outcomes for children with various degrees of pathology, but with normal IQ, did not seem to differ greatly, regardless of whether the child was diagnosed with clear infantile autism, childhood onset of pervasive development disorder not otherwise specified, or a form of the disorder that was too mild to be considered either of the two.

As all of the above studies appear to show, and despite the limited number of comparison studies using the same measures, the similarities in communication profiles in high-functioning autistic individuals and those with related disorders far outweigh their differences.

Language Changes in Autistic Children Who Become Schizophrenic

Several recent reports have focused on a possible longitudinal relationship between autism and schizophrenia. Because a schizophrenia diagnosis generally requires the presence of a thought disorder, such a crossover or second diagnosis has significant implications with regard to the communication characteristics seen in these children. In a review of patients with infantile psychosis (autism), Dahl (1976) noted that more than half had become schizophrenic later in life. Petty, Ornitz, Michelman, and Zimmerman (1984) provided a detailed description of three children who initially had met the criteria for autism with onset prior to 30 months of age. All three showed higher Verbal than Performance IQ on the WISC-R. Linguistically, they fitted the profile of infantile autism early in life. In the first case, diagnosed at age 12, the subsequent schizophrenia diagnosis was supported by auditory hallucinations and "incoherent muttering and whispering" (Petty *et al.*, 1984, p. 130). In the second case, diagnosed at age 8, early linguistic autistic symptomatology was followed by preoccupations with bizarre and fearful thoughts in middle childhood and the gradual emergence of bizarre, loosely associated, and illogical ideas. In the third case, diagnosed at age 17, deterioration was seen by age 7, despite evidence of an unusually good memory for vocabulary at age 6. Language behavior was characterized by clanging, loose associations, ungrammatical statements, illogical speech, perseveration, and incoherence. All three of these children had communicative language, despite severe disturbances in initial language development. Also, all three had close to normal IQ scores, with Verbal IQ being higher than Performance IQ.

The authors concluded that the children had the cognitive as well as communicative ability to express a schizophrenic thought disorder linguistically. Petty *et al.* (1984) suggested that schizophrenia and autism were unlikely to co-occur by chance; common, underlying mechanisms must be considered in these disorders. Cantor *et al.* (1982) had also noted that some of their schizophrenic children, with an onset of psychosis prior to 30 months, had autistic symptoms during the first several years of life. Similarly, Watkins *et al.* (1987) found that more than one-third of their schizophrenic children had earlier symptoms that met the diagnosis of autism. Again, their sample was nonretarded. These authors suggested that symptoms of schizophrenia and autism each appeared "to serve as final common pathways for a variety of causal factors and pathophysiologic processes" and that "there is no reason to believe that some risk factors might not contribute to the development of both disorders" (Watkins *et al.*, 1987, p. 875).

The above studies appear to suggest that communicative, social, and cognitive development all present variables that need to be considered carefully when examining the relationship among the above disorders.

CONCLUSION

In most of the studies comparing autism, schizophrenia, and related disorders, language has received limited consideration. The focus has been on age of onset and family characteristics; these have supported separate diagnostic groups. This chapter is an attempt to highlight communication characteristics in related disorders with onset in childhood and adolescence, and to compare them to those seen in high-functioning autistic individuals. The intent is not to provide definitive answers, but rather to show that language may be a fruitful parameter for comparison in future research. Communication characteristics in these related disorders were examined from a number of different perspectives. These included the current diagnostic criteria used for these disorders (DSM-III-R), developmental language histories, language considerations from high-risk studies, specific language studies pertaining to older individuals with these disorders, and consideration of the language characteristics of autistic children who become schizophrenic in childhood or adolescence. Pragmatics, or the social use of language, was an area where major disturbances and parallels were seen in all of these disorders. However, similarities in other areas of communication emerged as well, including early developmental delays. Early language delay has long been known and associated with autism. However, this chapter clearly shows that a very significant number of children and adolescents with a diagnosis of schizophrenia and these other disorders also have a history of developmental language delay. Evidence from high-risk studies further supports these early developmental lags in communication.

Peculiarities of language performance—such as echolalia, dysfluencies, problems in semantics and syntax, and prosody—are known to exist in high-functioning autistic individuals. As this review shows, these problems are also seen in these related disorders. The similarities in nonverbal communication also become evident.

From the evidence presented, it must be concluded that early language delay or deficits may not be as benign as sometimes assumed. This is particularly true when coupled with problems in social development. Language delay or deficits often seem to be the first concerns that bring the child to psychiatric attention. The above results lead us to conclude that language abilities may be a most sensitive early indicator of neurodevelopmental function and later severe psychopathology.

The present study suggests that when general cognitive level is taken into consideration, many of the differences in language behavior among the above disorders seem to disappear, and that some of the language characteristics seen in schizophrenia and schizotypal personality disorders appear to depend on a more advanced level of language. These characteristics may only become apparent in the higher-functioning autistic individual and not be obvious when autism is coupled with mental retardation. Changes in the diagnosis of autism to schizophrenia or the addition of a diagnosis of schizophrenia to autism in the same individual, at least in the earlier years, may therefore also depend on a relatively high level of communicative functioning.

From a diagnostic point of view, an interesting way of conceptualizing these diagnoses has recently been suggested by Tanguay (1990), who proposed to unify them in a larger, more inclusive diagnostic category of a *social communication spectrum disorder*. From a theoretical perspective, the communicative behaviors in these related disorders may lead us to hypothesize that impairment in metarepresentational capacity, of a similar nature as in autism, may also underlie these disorders, resulting in a wide range of problems in the social use of language.

Future research, with interdisciplinary cooperation between communication specialists and psychiatrists, is needed in order to provide some of the more specific answers to the issues raised here.

REFERENCES

Achenbach, T. M., & Edelbrock, C. S. (1983). *Manual for Child Behavior Checklist and Revised Behavior Profile*. Burlington: University of Vermont, Department of Psychiatry.

American Psychiatric Association (1987). *Diagnostic and statistical manual of mental disorders* (rev. 3rd ed.). Washington, DC: Author.

Andreason, N. (1979a). The clinical assessment of thought, language and communication disorders: I. The definition of terms and their reliability. *Archives of General Psychiatry, 36,* 1315–1321.

Andreason, N. (1979b). Thought, language, and communication disorders: II. Diagnostic significance. *Archives of General Psychiatry, 36,* 1325–1330.

Asperger, H. (1944). Die "autistischen Psychopathen" im Kindesalter. *Archiv fur Psychiatrie und Nervenkrankheiten, 117,* 76–136.

Baltaxe, C. (1977). Pragmatic deficits in the language of autistic adolescents. *Journal of Pediatric Psychology, 2*(4), 176–180.

Baltaxe, C., Russell, A., Simmons, J. Q., & Bott, L. (1987). *Thought, language, and communication disorders in prepubertal onset of schizophrenia and schizotypal personality disorders*. Paper presented at the Academy of Child and Adolescent Psychiatry, Washington, DC.

Baltaxe, C., & Simmons, J. Q. (1977). Language patterns of German and English autistic adolescents. In P. Mittler (Ed.), *Proceedings of the International Association for the Scientific Study of Mental Deficiency* (pp. 267–278). New York: University Park Press.

Baltaxe, C., & Simmons, J. Q. (1981). Disorders of language in childhood psychosis: Current concepts and approaches. In J. Darby (Ed.), *Speech evaluation in psychiatry* (pp. 285–328). New York: Grune & Stratton.

Baltaxe, C., & Simmons, J. Q. (1983). Communication deficits in the adolescent and adult autistic. *Seminars in Speech and Language, 4,* 27–42.

Baltaxe, C., & Simmons, J. Q. (1985). Prosodic development in normal and autistic children. In E. Schopler & G. Mesibov (Eds.), *Communication problems in autism* (pp. 95–123). New York: Plenum.

Baltaxe, C., & Simmons, J. Q. (1987). Communication deficits in the adolescent with autism, schizophrenia, and language-learning disabilities. In T. L. Layton (Ed.), *Language and treatment of autistic and developmentally disordered children* (pp. 155–180). New York: Charles C Thomas.

Baltaxe, C., & Simmons, J. Q. (1988). Pragmatic deficits in emotionally disturbed children and adolescents. In R. Schiefelbush & L. Lloyd (Eds.), *Language perspectives: Acquisition, retardation and intervention* (2nd ed., pp. 223–253). Austin, TX: Pro-Ed.

Baltaxe, C., Simmons, J. Q., & Zee, E. (1984). Intonation patterns in normal, autistic, and aphasic children. In *Proceedings of the Tenth International Congress of Phonetic Sciences* (pp. 713–718). Dordrecht, The Netherlands: Foris.

Baron-Cohen, S. (1988). Social and pragmatic deficits in autism: Cognitive or affective? *Journal of Autism and Developmental Disorders, 18*(3), 379–403.

Baron-Cohen, S. (1989a). Perceptual role-taking and protodeclarative pointing in autism. *British Journal of Developmental Psychology, 7,* 113–127.

Baron-Cohen, S. (1989b). The autistic child's theory of mind: A case of specific developmental delay. *Journal of Child Psychology and Psychiatry, 30,* 285–297.

Baron-Cohen, Leslie, A., & Frith, U. (1985). Does the autistic child have a "theory of mind"? *Cognition, 21,* 37–46.

Bartolucci, G., Pierce, S., & Streiner, D. (1980). Cross-sectional studies of grammatical morphemes in autism and mentally retarded children. *Journal of Autism and Developmental Disorders, 10*(1), 39–50.

Beitchman, J. (1983). Childhood schizophrenia: A review and comparison with adult onset schizophrenia. *Psychiatric Journal of the University of Ottawa, 8*(2), 25–37.

Bender, L. (1971). Childhood schizophrenia. *American Journal of Orthopsychiatry, 17,* 40–56.

Bender, L., & Faretra, G. (1972). The relationship between childhood and adult schizophrenia. In A. Kaplan (Ed.), *Genetic factors in schizophrenia* (pp. 28–64). Springfield, IL: Charles C Thomas.

Bettes, B., & Walker, E. (1987). Positive and negative symptoms in psychotic and other psychiatrically disturbed children. *Journal of Child Psychology and Psychiatry, 28*(4), 555–568.

Bradley, C., & Bowen, M. (1941). Behavior characteristics of schizophrenic children. *Psychiatric Quarterly, 15,* 296–313.

Cantor, S., Evans, J., Pearce, J., & Pezzot-Pearce, T. (1982). Childhood schizophrenia present but not accounted for. *American Journal of Psychiatry, 139,* 758–762.

Cantor, S., Pearce, J., Pezzot-Pearce, T., & Evans, J. (1981). The group of hypotonic schizophrenics. *Schizophrenia Bulletin, 7*(1), 1–11.

Dahl, V. (1976). A follow-up study of a child psychiatric clientele with special regard to the diagnosis of psychosis. *Acta Psychiatrica Scandinavica, 54,* 106–112.

Eggers, C. (1978). Course and prognosis of childhood schizophrenia. *Journal of Autism and Childhood Schizophrenia, 8*(1), 21–36.

Fillmore, C. (1981). Pragmatics and the description of discourse. In P. Cole (Ed.), *Radical pragmatics* (pp. 143–166). New York: Academic Press.

Fish, B. (1987). Infant predictors of the longitudinal course of schizophrenic development. *Schizophrenia Bulletin, 13*(3), 395–409.

Fraser, W., King, K., Thomas, P., & Kendell, R. (1986). The diagnosis of schizophrenia by language analysis. *British Journal of Psychiatry, 148,* 275–278.

Garralda, M. (1985). Characteristics of the psychoses of late onset in children and adolescents (a comparative study of hallucinating children). *Journal of Adolescence, 8,* 195–208.

Green, W., Campbell, M., Hardesty, A., Grega, D., Padron-Gayoil, M., Shell, M., & Erlenmeyer-Kimling, L. (1984). A comparison of schizophrenic and autistic children. *Journal of the American Academy of Child Psychiatry, 23*(4), 399–409.

Halliday, M., & Hasan, R. (1976). *Cohesion in English.* London: Longman.

Harrison, S., Hess, J., & Zrull, J. (1963). Paranoid reactions in children. *Journal of the American Academy of Child Psychiatry, 112,* 819–825.

Harvey, P., Weintraub, S., & Neale, J. (1982). Speech competence in children vulnerable to psychopathology. *Journal of Abnormal Child Psychology, 10*(3), 373–388.

Hobson, R. P. (1986). The autistic child's appraisal of expressions of emotion. *Journal of Child Psychology and Psychiatry, 27,* 671–680.

Holzman, P. (1978). Cognitive impairment and cognitive stability: Towards a theory of thought disorder. In G. Serban (Ed.), *Cognitive defects in the development of mental illness* (pp. 361–376). New York: Brunner/Mazel.

Holzman, P. (1986). Thought disorder in schizophrenia: Editor's introduction. *Schizophrenia Bulletin, 12*(3), 342–346.

Jordan, K., & Prugh, D. (1971). Schizophreniform psychosis of childhood. *American Journal of Psychiatry, 128,* 323–331.

Kaffman, M. (1986). Review of the NIMH Israeli Kibbutz–City Study and the Jerusalem Infant Development Study. *Schizophrenia Bulletin, 12*(2), 151–157.

Kanner, L. (1943). Autistic disturbances of affective contact. *Nervous Child, 2,* 217–250.

Kanner, L. (1949). Problems of nosology and psychodynamics of early infantile autism. *American Journal of Orthopsychiatry, 19,* 416–429.

King, K., Fraser, W., & Thomas, P. (1987). Computer-assisted linguistic analysis of an autistic adolescent's language: Implications for the diagnosis of Asperger's syndrome and atypical psychosis. *Journal of Mental Deficiency Research, 31,* 279–286.

Kolvin, I. (1971). Studies in the childhood psychoses: I. Diagnostic criteria and classification. *British Journal of Psychiatry, 118,* 381–384.

Kolvin, I., Ounsted, C., Humphrey, M., & McNay, A. (1971). Studies in the childhood psychoses: II. The phenomenology of childhood psychoses. *British Journal of Psychiatry, 118,* 385–395.

Kydd, R., & Werry, J. (1982). Schizophrenia in children under 16 years. *Journal of Autism and Developmental Disorders, 12*(4), 343–357.

Leslie, A. (1987). Pretense and representation: The origins of "theory of mind." *Psychological Review, 94,* 412–426.

Leslie, A., & Frith, U. (1987). Metarepresentation and autism: How not to lose one's marbles. *Cognition, 27,* 291–294.

Leslie, A., & Frith, U. (1988). Autistic children's understanding of seeing, knowing, and believing. *British Journal of Developmental Psychology, 6,* 315–324.

Lord, C. (1985). Autism and the comprehension of language. In E. Schopler & G. B. Mesibov (Eds.), *Communication problems in autism* (pp. 257–279). New York: Plenum.

Marcus, J., Hans, S., Nagler, S. Auerbach, J., Mirsky, A., & Aubrey, A. (1987). Review of the NIMH Israeli Kibbutz–City Study and the Jerusalem Infant Development Study, *Schizophrenia Bulletin, 13*(3), 425–438.

Mednick, S., Parnas, J., & Schulsinger, F. (1987). The Copenhagen High-Risk project, 1962–86. *Schizophrenia Bulletin, 13*(3), 485–495.

Mednick, S. A., & Schulsinger, F. (1965). A longitudinal study of children with a high risk for schizophrenia: A preliminary report. In S. Vandenberg (Ed.), *Methods and goals in human behavior genetics* (pp. 255–296). New York: Academic Press.

Meehl, P. E. (1962). Schizotaxia, schizotypy, schizophrenia. *American Psychologist, 17,* 827–838.

Menyuk, P., & Quill, K. (1985). Semantic problems in autistic children. In E. Schopler & G. B. Mesibov (Eds.), *Communication problems in autism* (pp. 127–144). New York: Plenum.

Moldin, S., Gottesman, I., & Erlenmeyer-Kimling, L. (1987). Psychometric validation of psychiatric diagnoses in the New York high-risk study. *Psychiatry Research, 22,* 159–177.

Morice, R., & Ingram, J. (1982). Language analysis in schizophrenia: Diagnostic implications. *Australian and New Zealand Journal of Psychiatry, 16,* 11–21.

Morice, R., & McNicol, D. (1986). Language changes in schizophrenia: A limited replication. *Schizophrenia Bulletin, 12*(2), 239–251.

Mundy, P., & Sigman, M. (1989a). The theoretical implications of joint attention deficits in autism. In D. Cicchetti (Ed.), *Development and Psychopathology, 1*(3), 173–183.

Mundy, P., & Sigman, M. (1989b). Second thoughts on the nature of autism. In D. Cicchetti (Ed.), *Development and Psychopathology, 1*(3), 213–218.

Nagy, J., & Szatmari, P. (1986). A chart review of schizotypal personality disorders in children. *Journal of Autism and Developmental Disorders, 16*(3), 351–367.

Parnas, P., Schulsinger, F., Schulsinger, M., Mednick, S., & Teasdale, T. (1982, June). Behavioral precursors of schizophrenia spectrum. *Archives of General Psychiatry, 39,* 658–664.

Paul, R., & Cohen, D. (1984). Outcomes of severe disability of language acquisition. *Journal of Autism and Developmental Disorders, 14*(4), 405–421.

Petty, L., Ornitz, E., Michelman, J., & Zimmerman, E. (1984, February). Autistic children who become schizophrenic. *Archives of General Psychiatry, 41,* 129–135.

Potter, H. (1933). Schizophrenia in children. *American Journal of Psychiatry, 12,* 1253–1268.

Prizant, B. (1983). Language acquisition and communicative behavior: Toward an understanding of the "whole of it." *Journal of Speech and Hearing Disorders, 43*(3), 296–307.

Prizant, B., & Duchan, J. (1981). The functions of immediate echolalia in autistic children. *Journal of Speech and Hearing Disorders, 46,* 241–249.

Prizant, B., & Rydell, P. (1984). Analysis of functions of delayed echolalia in autistic children. *Journal of Speech and Hearing Research, 27,* 183–192.

Prutting, C. (1982). Pragmatics as social competence. *Journal of Speech and Hearing Disorders, 47,* 123–134.

Rees, N. (1978). Pragmatics of language: Applications to normal and disordered language development. In R. Schiefelbusch (Ed.), *Bases of Language Intervention* (pp. 191–269). Baltimore: University Park Press.

Ricks, D., & Wing, L. (1975). Language, communication, and the use of symbols in normal and autistic children. *Journal of Autism and Childhood Schizophrenia, 5,* 191–221.

Rochester, S., & Martin, J. (1979): *Crazy talk: A study in the discourse of schizophrenic speakers.* New York: Plenum.

Rochester, S., Martin, J., & Thurston, S. (1977). Thought-process disorder in schizophrenia: The listener's task. *Brain and Language, 4,* 95–114.

Rumsey, J., Andreason, N., & Rappaport, J. (1986). Thought, language, communication, and affective flattening in autistic adults. *Archives of General Psychiatry, 43,* 771–777.

Rutter, M. (1972). Childhood schizophrenia reconsidered. *Journal of Autism and Childhood Schizophrenia, 2*(4), 315–337.

Rutter, M., & Schopler, E. (1987). Autism and pervasive developmental disorders: Concepts and diagnostic issues. *Journal of Autism and Developmental Disorders, 17*(2), 159–187.

Sameroff, A., Seifer, R., Zax, M., & Barocas, R. (1987). Early indicators of developmental risk: Rochester longitudinal study. *Schizophrenia Bulletin, 13*(3), 384–394.

Schuler, A., (1979). Echolalia: Issues and clinical application. *Journal of Speech and Hearing Disorders, 44,* 411–434.

Schulsinger, F., & Mednick, S. (1975). Nature–nurture aspects of schizophrenia. In M. Lader (Ed.), *Studies of schizophrenia.* Ashford, Kent: Headley Brothers.

Sigman, M., Mundy, P., Sherman, T., & Ungerer, J. (1986). Social interactions of autistic, mentally retarded and normal children and their caregivers. *Journal of Child Psychology and Psychiatry, 27,* 647–656.

Simmons, J. Q., & Baltaxe, C. (1975). Language patterns of adolescent autistics. *Journal of Autism and Childhood Schizophrenia, 5,* 333–351.

Snyder, L., & Silverstein, J. (1988). Pragmatics and child language disorders. In R. L. Schiefelbusch & L. L. Lloyd (Eds.), *Language perspectives: Acquisition, retardation and intervention* (pp. 189–222). Austin, TX: Pro-Ed.

Swisher, L., & Demetras, M. (1985). The expressive language characteristics of autistic children compared with mentally retarded or specific language-impaired children. In E. Schopler & G. B. Mesibov (Eds.), *Communication problems in autism* (pp. 147–162). New York: Plenum.

Tager-Flusberg, H. (1981a). Sentence comprehension in autistic children. *Applied Psycholinguistics, 2,* 5–24.

Tager-Flusberg, H. (1981b). On the nature of linguistic functioning in early infantile autism. *Journal of Autism and Developmental Disorders, 11*(1), 45–56.

Tanguay, P. (1990). Infantile autism and social communication spectrum disorders (Editor's note). *Journal of the American Academy of Child and Adolescent Psychiatry, 29,* 54.

Ungerer, J., & Sigman, M. (1981). Symbolic play and language comprehension in autistic children. *Journal of the American Academy of Child Psychiatry, 20,* 318–337.

Watkins, J., Asarnow, R., & Tanguay, P. (1987). Symptom development in childhood onset schizophrenia. *Journal of Child Psychology and Psychiatry, 29*(6), 865–878.

Watson, L. (1988). Pragmatic abilities and disabilities of autistic children. In T. L. Layton (Ed.), *Language and treatment of autistic and developmentally disordered children* (pp. 89–127). Springfield IL: Charles C Thomas.

Weintraub, S. (1987). Risk factors in schizophrenia: The Stony Brook High-Risk Project. *Schizophrenia Bulletin, 13*(3), 439–450.

Wolff, S., & Barlow, A. (1979). Schizoid personality in childhood: A comparative study of schizoid, autistic, and normal children. *Journal of Child Psychology and Psychiatry, 20,* 29–46.

12

Vocational Possibilities for High-Functioning Adults with Autism

MARY E. VAN BOURGONDIEN and AMY V. WOODS

A continuum of vocational options is needed to meet the wide variety of vocational needs of adults with autism. Just as various educational settings are needed, from the highly structured and specialized to complete mainstreaming, vocational settings follow the same continuum. Sheltered workshops that serve as training and work sites for many developmentally disabled adults represent the most specialized option. Competitive employment in regular jobs in the community is at the other end of the continuum. Given the nature of autism, the most successful options are likely to be ones developed with the autistic individual in mind and where there is some degree of continuous support. The purpose of this chapter is to describe the factors critical to successful employment and two vocational options being developed in North Carolina—supported employment, and the integrated vocational and residential program of the Carolina Living and Learning Center. The vocational models described include the job coach, enclave, mobile crew, and small-business models of supported employment, as well as a model where the vocational program is physically and programmatically integrated with the residential program. Each of these programs will be discussed in terms of the critical elements, and relative strengths and weaknesses, of the model.

KEY FACTORS IN SUCCESSFUL VOCATIONAL PLACEMENT

Vocational planning and programming in the TEACCH (*T*reatment and *E*ducation of *A*utistic and related *C*ommunication handicapped *CH*ildren) system are

MARY E. VAN BOURGONDIEN and AMY V. WOODS • Division TEACCH, Department of Psychiatry, The University of North Carolina at Chapel Hill, Chapel Hill, North Carolina 27599-7180.

High-Functioning Individuals with Autism, edited by Eric Schopler and Gary B. Mesibov. Plenum Press, New York, 1992.

based on the same basic concepts and philosophy that have guided the work with families and teachers of autistic children throughout the years (Mesibov, Schopler, & Sloan, 1983). The functional elements used in this program include collaboration, professionals as generalists, an individualized approach to treatment based on a careful assessment, and a two-factor approach to treatment.

Collaborative Approach

The involvement of parents as collaborators or cotherapists in the treatment of their children has always been central to the TEACCH approach (Schopler, 1987). This collaboration between parents and professionals has four basic components (Schopler, Mesibov, Shigley, & Bashford, 1984): Families provide information to the professional about their child, the professional shares information about autism and treatment strategies, each provides the other with mutual support, and together they advocate for the individual with autism in the community. This collaboration is extended to include teachers, vocational specialists, and residential care providers as the individual enters these professionals' care. Within the area of vocational planning, the parents and other caregivers provide the staff with their priorities, concerns, and general knowledge of the adult with autism at this stage of development. The staff member, in turn, provides information on vocational training and placement opportunities to the parents and others who are involved in the client's care. The professionals and parents communicate with one another, solve problems together, and support each other—as well as the adult with autism—during the job placement, training, and long-term support phases. Regardless of the type of vocational placement, the collaboration extends to all aspects of the client's life. For an individual with autism to be successful in a work setting, there needs to be continuous communication among the parents and any other caregivers, work supervisors, and other professionals involved in the client's day-to-day program.

Generalist Model

A second component of the TEACCH approach is the premise that the professionals who work with autistic individuals and their families should be trained as generalists. Early on, the founders of the TEACCH program became convinced that teachers, caretakers, and other professionals working with autistic children must take a holistic approach to the children, thereby becoming accountable for the treatment of the whole child (Schopler, 1987). These workers need to cope with the whole range of problems presented by the child with autism, just as do the parents.

Unfortunately, for families seeking help for their handicapped child, specialization structures professionals to be interested in, or accountable for, primarily their own area of specialization. This approach increases the likelihood that parents receive inconsistent or contradictory opinions on diagnosis and treatment. Moreover, it makes it difficult for anyone to take professional responsibility for the entire child. The generalist model reduces these undesirable consequences of specialization. It enables the treatment-staff members to see the child from the parents' perspective and to work collaboratively with them. It increases staff responsibility, makes the job more interesting, and improves the staff members' ability to use consultation from specialists (Schopler *et al.*, 1984).

The professional who facilitates vocational planning and placement (whether a vocational specialist, job coach, or employer) also needs to be a generalist who is aware of all aspects of the life of the adult with autism. Frequently, changes in an adult's living situation will cause stress that results in an increase in unusual or problematic behaviors at the work site. The job trainer needs to be cognizant of these changes and to collaborate with those in the home and work settings in order to help the autistic individual cope in *all* settings. By taking a holistic approach to the individual, the chances of a successful vocational placement are greatly increased.

Individualized Approach Based on Assessment

Given the heterogeneity of individuals with autism, and the tremendous variation in skills within the same individual, an individualized approach to placement and training based on a careful assessment of the client's skills is essential.

The first step in the assessment process is frequently a direct assessment of the individual's skills, interests, and behaviors. The *Adolescent and Adult Psychoeducational Profile* (AAPEP) (Mesibov, Schopler, Schaffer, & Landrus, 1988) was designed specifically to assess the needs of adolescents and adults with autism. Information is obtained in six basic areas: independent functioning, vocational skills, vocational behaviors, functional communication, leisure skills, and interpersonal behaviors. In addition to a direct observation scale, the AAPEP has both a home observation scale and a school/work observation scale that are completed based on interviews with knowledgeable individuals in those settings.

The AAPEP employs a "pass–emerge–fail" scoring system. Emerging skills are those where the individual has a partial understanding or ability to complete a task but does not yet have complete mastery. The emerging skills are the areas that are most likely to improve with instruction from the vocational instructor. By comparing this assessment of the person's strengths, emerging skills, interests, and deficits with the requirements of the work setting, teachers and vocational planners can make a preliminary determination of the appropriateness of the job placement and possible treatment strategies.

In the vocational placement process, this formal assessment and an assessment at the job site are both essential. The functional assessment in the actual work site examines work skills and behaviors specific to that job. These skills are evaluated on a daily basis using the same pass–emerge–fail system to determine progress, need for instruction around emerging skills, or restructuring of the task around deficit areas. Given the uneven pattern of skills and the problem of generalization of skills common to autism (Carr, 1981), these assessments are a critical part of the vocational placement process. Professionals working with clients with severe handicaps have found that taking individual preferences and interests into account is essential in maintaining morale in leisure activities (Favell & Cannon, 1976). Fitting jobs to peoples' interests and strengths is also likely to increase their morale, regardless of whether or not they happen to have a handicap.

Two-Factor Approach to Treatment

The maximum adaptation of children or adults with autism is generally accomplished by doing two things (Schopler *et al.*, 1984): directly improving the skills and adaptive behaviors of each individual, and structuring the environment in order to compensate for areas of deficit. Both of these approaches can improve an individual's ability to function independently in the environment. Given the severity and extent of the deficits of most individuals with autism, successful placement usually requires both the acquisition of skills and environmental accommodation.

VOCATIONAL OPTIONS

Supported Employment

Supported employment was included in Title VII(c) of the Rehabilitation Act Amendments of 1986. *Supported employment* has been defined as an individual with a severe disability working in a regular job in business or industry in the community at least 20 hours a week (Wehman, Moon, Everson, Wood, & Barcus, 1988). The worker receives wages and benefits commensurate with those of non-handicapped employees and receives continuous support services. There are four general models of supported employment: (1) job coach, (2) enclave, (3) mobile crew, and (4) the entrepreneurial or small-business model (Mank, Rhodes, & Bellamy, 1986).

Job Coach

In the job-coach or trainer-advocate model (Levy, 1983), the trainer works directly with an individual client. The job coach locates the job, does a task analysis of it, and trains the individual to do the job. More importantly for employees with autism, the job coach trains the individual in behaviors necessary to work in that setting (e.g., getting along with coworkers, arriving at work on time, or asking for help). The job coach is gradually faded out so that the client takes all directions from the employer. However, there continues to be a trained support person who checks in with the client, employer, and caregiver on a regular basis and provides assistance and coordination as needed.

Since 1988, 37 adults with autism in North Carolina have been placed in jobs using the job coach model. Of those placed, 76% remain in employment, working an average of 34 hours a week for an average wage of $4.99 an hour, and are generally higher functioning. Most are able to communicate verbally (receptively and expressively), which enables them to take direction from their employers. Their cognitive skills range from moderate mental retardation to average intelligence. Although they may have behavioral difficulties, rarely are they aggressive towards themselves or others.

For the employer, there are numerous advantages to hiring individuals with autism. They can appreciate the stability of employing an individual with autism in jobs that generally have a high turnover rate. The tendency of individuals with autism to be very precise and exact means that they often will repeat the work routine exactly as taught. Jobs that others find unpleasant, repetitive, or in socially isolated situations are often very appropriate for workers with autism.

Key Factors. An individualized approach has been essential to successful placements. Factors to be taken into consideration in job placement include characteristics and interests of both the individual with autism and his or her family, the approach of the employer, and issues related to the local job market. In general, jobs that involve a minimum amount of required interactions with others are best. Jobs that involve a routine or a predictable schedule, a set of regular duties, and a flexible employer are likely to be good matches.

Two common types of placements include clerk and food-service positions. These jobs use the prevocational, self-care, and domestic skills that parents and teachers have taught the person with autism from an early age. Some individuals work as line servers in cafeterias, others bus tables, and other individuals do best as dishwashers or utility workers, where less social interaction is required and their work station can be somewhat removed from the general flow of traffic and noise.

Clerk positions in libraries, supply stores, office settings, and small businesses can be a good match for individuals with basic clerical skills such as filing, sorting, simple bookkeeping, taking inventories, or data processing. These jobs are often well-suited to individuals who are high functioning and prefer predictability and routines, but not necessarily repetition. Placing an individual in a job that takes advantage of a peak skill or interest can be difficult if the job requires a commensurate level of social interactions or judgment that the autistic employee is not likely to have.

There is a wide variety of other jobs, including animal care technician, packer, and custodian, that have proven to be appropriate depending on the specific skills, interests, and deficits of the person being placed.

The collaboration in this particular job model initially emphasizes the relationship among the parents or caregivers, the job coach and long-term support person, and the worker's direct supervisor and the employer. As the job coach fades, the direct collaboration between the client and the supervisor becomes much more important as the client learns to take direction from the actual employer.

Continued intensive collaboration among TEACCH staff, families or caregivers, employers, and workers, however, remains the stalwart of success in providing supported employment through the TEACCH program.

Regardless of the setting, the job coach and long-term support person need to establish good relationships with the direct supervisor and the employer. These supervisors need help understanding autism and the unusual behaviors that can accompany it. Also, supervisors need encouragement to call about the smallest concern so that potential problems can be addressed before they become entrenched and insoluble. As so often happens for nonhandicapped employees, despite initial agreements regarding the scope of the job, employers frequently expand or change the job once the client begins work. The job coach works with employers to help them understand the importance of maintaining the exact specifics of the job and environment as matched to the individual, because individuals with autism need to be able to predict what their responsibilities will be day to day. The job coach also works with the client to help them adapt to new demands of the job.

Both the job coach and the long-term support person must be aware of all aspects of the worker's current situation. Frequently, changes in other aspects of the resident's life (change in staff members at home, a move, etc.) underlie fluctuations in job performance.

Even in these competitive job settings, it is possible and important to provide autistic workers with the structure that will help them maintain an appropriate level of job performance independent of the presence of the job coach. Physical adaptations based on job-site assessments have usually taken the form of placing the worker's work station away from the busiest section of the job site. For one young man, this meant working in the dishwashing room of a cafeteria rather than busing tables in the main dining room. Picture lists or written lists are used to help workers remember the sequence of their duties and how to perform each task. Although most of the clients in these jobs are verbal, the visual directions in the form of written directions or pictures help them to learn and perform the job independently of both the supervisor and the job coach. Establishing routines and written rules for appropriate work behavior is often a major focus of the job coach. The written contract describes exactly what behaviors (e.g., vocational, social) are expected and what behaviors are not appropriate.

In most cases, the contract includes a reinforcer for maintaining appropriate work behavior. In some cases, our workers were able to learn to monitor their own behavior, while in other cases the employer provides the worker with feedback. The reinforcer or motivator is generally provided by the job coach or someone in the home setting, as opposed to the employer. For many of our clients, the job itself does not provide the same level of reinforcement available to nonhandicapped people. Being able to ride the elevator or going out to eat are often more motivating reasons for obeying the job rules than salary, satisfaction of a job well done, or fear of loss of job.

With assistance, many workers with autism have learned to adapt personal coping strategies used in other settings to the work situation. Relaxation tapes can be played before work or during breaks (using earphones so others are not bothered). Individuals who talk to themselves can be taught to do it only at certain times, such as when the vacuum is running, so it does not bother other people.

In the TEACCH job coach model, direct training first is faded out totally in the job site. If the trainee maintains the skills learned to date, the job coach then begins to gradually fade from the site. This method of fading provides support to employers in solving any problems that develop, so they feel more secure in their ability to solve problems with less help in the future.

Enclaves

An enclave is a group of up to eight people with disabilities and at least one full-time job coach working in a business or industry (McGee, 1975; Rhodes & Valenta, 1985). The individuals in the enclave can be paid directly by the business or industry, or by the nonprofit agency that placed them (Rhodes & Valenta, 1985). At TEACCH, the employees with autism in the enclave model are paid by the employer at a rate commensurate with their nonhandicapped peers based on the quantity and quality of their work. Workers in the enclave can be dispersed throughout the setting—for example, the two enclaves developed by TEACCH are located in cafeterias, where the employees are in jobs scattered throughout the cafeteria. Other enclaves group the handicapped individuals and take over an area or specific job in a business, such as one specific assembly or disassembly job in a factory (Wehman *et al.*, 1988).

Employers benefit not only from a tax credit, but also from getting a steady work force in an area where they have experienced lots of turnover or unreliable help. The reliability of workers with autism can be a selling point to employers.

Key Factors. This model is particularly beneficial for those clients who require greater structure and will always need some degree of supervision from someone trained to work with adults who have autism. This generalist maintains a continual collaboration with the employer, the family, the residential caregiver, and the client. The continuing availability of the job coach provides stability and a readily available person to solve problems and help the individual with autism cope with the demands of both the job and home. The job coach is always there to teach new skills or behaviors, to adapt the environment, and to provide quality control. The degree and type of supervision can be individualized from client to client as the situation requires. For a client who is taking longer to learn the job skills, the job coach emphasizes the acquisition of these skills while ensuring that the job gets done until the worker with autism has learned to complete it alone. For another worker, the emphasis of the supervision may be developing and implementing a behavioral program around specific job-related social skills.

Mobile Crew

A mobile crew is a small group of handicapped workers and a supervisor who complete service jobs at various locations in the community. The administrator of the program finds the jobs, and the clients are paid either by the administrator of the crew or (as at TEACCH) directly by the person for whom they provided the service. Typical work crews do landscaping, yard work, housecleaning, or janitorial work in large businesses. Because of the nature of this work, programs that have run mobile crews have experienced some problems with maintaining a steady supply of work (Mank *et al.*, 1986). This fluctuation in work has been a particular problem for work crews engaged in seasonal tasks such as yard work.

Key Factors. The mobile crew has many of the same advantages as enclaves. The availability of continual supervision permits the participation of individuals whose performance or behaviors are not stable enough to maintain a competitive job. In addition, crews can be developed to capitalize on individuals' strengths or interests. Someone who cleans bathrooms well can specialize in this area, while other members of the crew do the other cleaning jobs. Pairing employees with autism with employees with mental retardation without autism has proven to be a good match. The workers with autism are good at following the list of jobs and can perform most tasks, while the workers with mental retardation without autism often have better judgment and can provide quality control. Given the types of jobs generally involved, members of a mobile crew generally work in isolation, so it is a good option for those who have difficulty in public or are very easily distracted.

Mobile crews also can be used as an intermediate step between a sheltered workshop and other forms of supported employment. At TEACCH, individuals have been engaged in a part-time cleaning service while they still attend the sheltered workshop three days a week. The mobile crew provides an excellent opportunity to assess directly the individual's work skills and behaviors while providing sufficient supervision to ensure that a quality job is performed. The supervisor is able to determine the type of supervision the workers need, how they learn new skills, and how they handle correction. The workers' speed, stamina, and ability to handle transitions can be evaluated. The supervision can be individualized so that each client can receive the type of instruction needed to learn new skills and to complete the job independently. Many of the clients earn more money in the two days they are on the cleaning crew than they do during a full week at a workshop. In addition, the mobile crew has turned into a stepping-stone to part-time and full-time jobs in the larger community.

Small-Business or Entrepreneurial Model

The small-business model involves the establishment of a business in the community where 8 to 10 handicapped individuals are employed along with an equal number of nonhandicapped employees (Bellamy, Horner, & Inman, 1979).

The particular business is developed based on an appreciation for the type of work the employees with autism will be able to perform; baking, printing, and electronics are among the most common options. Generally, the initial work force consists primarily of handicapped workers, and the nonhandicapped workers are added as the business expands. The goal is to reach a point where the workers are paid at least minimum wage, but as the business is being established and the workers trained, a prorated wage based on productivity is often the case.

Key Factors. Collaboration and supervision by someone trained as a generalist are equally important in this model. What makes this model different from the ones previously described is the fact that since the business is being established with the autistic worker in mind, the environment and the tasks can be selected, adapted, and structured to a much greater degree than is typical in most competitive job sites. For this reason, this model is particularly appropriate for individuals who continue to need behavior training and production training (Wehman *et al.*, 1988). Since the employers and direct supervisors are trained as generalists to work with clients with autism, this setting is a more viable option for those individuals who lack the communication and social skills necessary to work for less knowledgeable supervisors.

The Carolina Living and Learning Center

The Carolina Living and Learning Center is an integrated vocational and residential program designed specifically for adults with autism. The purpose of this center is to provide direct training to adults with autism, a site for training professionals to understand and work with adults with autism, and an active research program to further understanding of adults with autism and how best to provide them with treatment.

As with Sommerset Court in England (Van Bourgondien & Elgar, 1990) and Bittersweet Farm in Ohio (Kay, 1990), the CLLC is being developed so that the residential or independent living skill training is integrated physically and programmatically with the vocational training program.

Residents will be accepted from anywhere within the state of North Carolina. The center, designed to serve 30 adults with autism at all intellectual and adaptive levels, will eventually include two 5-bed and two 10-bed homes. Some of the homes will be certified as intermediate care facilities for the mentally retarded (ICF-MR) in order to guarantee a level of support and service to meet the needs of autistic adults at all functioning levels.

The vocational training program will include three primary areas of specialization: agriculture and horticulture, baking, and grounds and lawn maintenance. These areas were selected because training within each area can occur at a wide variety of developmental levels within a TEACCH curriculum that provides contextual cues and can be broken down into discrete steps (Landrus & Mesibov, 1986).

Additional job training areas will be developed based on particular client and staff interest.

Key Factors

The CLLC, designed specifically to serve adults with autism, employs as its primary treatment strategy an extension of the highly successful TEACCH cotherapy model (Schopler, 1987). In this residential program for adults, the collaborative approach is extended to encompass the relationship between the staff members and the residents with autism in their care. As cotherapists, staff members work in an apprenticeship relationship with the residents. By working collaborately with the residents, the staff teach them how to carry out various program functions and how to extend the resulting skills, when possible, to vocational placements in the community.

The treatment model is one in which staff and residents work together toward learning and fulfilling the various functions of the community. To facilitate this, the staff are a combination of individuals with a knowledge and background in autism and individuals with expertise in a particular vocational area (e.g., farmers, bakers, and horticultural experts). The staff are cooperative trainers using an apprenticeship approach to training, as opposed to being caretakers. As we know from our existing program, people with autism learn best through observation, demonstration, and experience. Part of the job responsibility of every employee of the center is to train the adults with autism to do their job, regardless of whether the person is a vocational specialist, a cook, or a bookkeeper. Resident teaching is made possible by an intensive multidisciplinary training program that trains all staff members as generalists. Under this model, all staff are expected to have a working knowledge of all problem areas impinging on autism (Schopler, 1987).

An initial assessment of a resident's vocational skills and behaviors will be used to determine each individual's training program and to establish initial teaching objectives within that program. Programs based on an understanding of the characteristics of autism and how individuals with autism learn best have a number of advantages for these individuals over other types of residential and vocational programs.

In order to address the fact that people with autism are a very heterogeneous group of individuals with great variability in their skills within and across individuals, a vocational curriculum has been chosen that has many different parts and levels, so that people from this heterogeneous group can participate at levels appropriate for them. To decrease the confusion resulting from each individuals' difficulty in understanding the world and his or her role in it, it is essential that vocational activities be concrete and relate directly to their basic needs of food, shelter, and activity. The jobs need to be such that the adults see from the context how their actions relate to the overall process. An agriculturally based community allows for vocational training in a wide variety of meaningful areas where the individual with autism can be involved from beginning to end—from planting the seeds to preparing the meal with the food they have grown. A bakery program has many of the same features. Baking bread can be broken down into simple steps where the relationship of a given step (kneading the dough) to the ultimate goal (eating the bread) is always readily apparent. Increasing the meaningfulness of vocational activities decreases the likelihood that individuals with autism will be confused about what they are doing, and improves the probability that they will understand and be proud of their accomplishments.

This 24-hour-a-day integrated vocational and residential program, while appropriate for the majority of individuals with autism, is seen as being most beneficial for those adults who have difficulty dealing with change and transitions and whose ability to process information and perform tasks is at a different rate than the general population.

Integration of the vocational and residential programs on the same property allows greater continuity of programming than is typical when these services are separated. Unlike many community-based programs, the day and evening programs share a common philosophy. They are administered as a single program with the same consultants and an overlap of staff, as well as a single-goal plan that covers the entire day. As a result, there will be a more consistent approach to developing communication skills and to managing behavior problems. In addition, an individual's program can go at a pace that allows that person to function at an optimal level of independence without affecting the programming of others. That is, a resident who needs additional time in the morning to complete grooming tasks can be given some extra time without keeping other residents from their jobs. Allowing the person with autism to work at her or his own pace by reducing artificial time demands results in decreased stress and fewer behavior problems.

PREPARING A STUDENT FOR WORK

The preparation of autistic children for living and working in their community must begin in the early grades (Landrus & Mesibov, 1986) with a curriculum that emphasizes the acquisition of the vocational, domestic, and functional academic and self-help skills necessary to perform most jobs. Functional communication skills such as how to ask for help or how to follow directions are to be included. In the leisure and social areas, students need to know how to entertain themselves during breaks and how to interact or work in close proximity to peers. What to do if you run out of work, how to move from a completed task to a new one, increasing time on tasks, and stamina are all work behaviors that can be taught from an early age.

The two areas that appear most critical to successful adult placement are the adult's ability to function independently and the ability to maintain behavioral control in a variety of settings. During the elementary school years, the emphasis should be on teaching the children in the classroom to use visual systems and routines in order to do their work independently. As the children get older, the systems need to be made more portable so that the children can use these adaptations in other places within the school and then in the community as a whole. The same process is applied to behavioral control systems (e.g., rules, rewards). As children get older, the techniques used to help them cope with frustration and manage their behaviors need to be flexible enough to be used in a variety of settings.

As individuals with autism make the transition in their lives from school to work, the knowledge of their patterns of learning, the collaborative relationship with the family, and specialized methods of structured teaching continue to play an integral part in their future.

SUMMARY

A continuum of vocational options for adults with autism is currently being developed. Successful placements involve collaboration between the autistic individuals, their family, employers, job coach, and residential caregivers. Individuals responsible for job placements must have an understanding of the characteristics of autism and their impact on job placement. An individualized assessment of the potential worker's skills, behaviors, and interests will help determine the optimal job site and the appropriate treatment balance between skill acquisition and restructuring the environment. The vocational options described vary in terms of the amount of specialized supervision and training provided, the degree to which the environment can be modified to compensate for deficit areas, and the degree to which the work and home environments are integrated. Whether an individual will be served best in an integrated residential and vocational program such as the CLLC, one of the models of supported employment, or yet another vocational alternative will depend on an individualized assessment of that person's skills, interests, and needs.

REFERENCES

Bellamy, C. T., Horner, R., & Inman, D. (1979). *Vocational training of severely retarded adults.* Baltimore: University Park Press.

Carr, E. G. (1981, July). *Analysis and remediation of severe behavior problems.* Paper presented at the meeting of the National Society for Children and Adults with Autism, Boston.

Favell, J. E., & Cannon, P. (1976). Evaluation of entertainment materials for severely retarded persons. *American Journal of Mental Deficiency, 81,* 357–361.

Kay, B. R. (1990). Bittersweet Farms. *Journal of Autism and Developmental Disorders, 20,* 309–321.

Landrus, R., & Mesibov, G. B. (1986). *Preparing autistic students for community living: A functional and sequential approach to training.* Unpublished manuscript, University of North Carolina, Division TEACCH, Chapel Hill.

Levy, S. M. (1983). School doesn't last forever; then what? Some vocational alternatives. In E. Schopler & G. Mesibov (Eds.), *Autism in adolescents and adults* (133–148). New York: Plenum.

Mank, D. M., Rhodes, L. E., & Bellamy, G. T. (1986). Four supported employment alternatives. In W. E. Kiernan & J. A. Stark (Eds.), *Pathways to employment for adults with developmental disabilities* (pp. 139–153). Baltimore: Brookes.

McGee, J. (1975). *Workstations in industry*. Omaha, NE: University of Nebraska.

Mesibov, G. B., Schopler, E., Schaffer, B., & Landrus, R. (1988). *Adolescent and adult psychoeducational profile (AAPEP)*. Austin, TX: Pro-Ed.

Mesibov, G. B., Schopler, E., & Sloan, J. L. (1983). Service development for adolescents and adults in North Carolina's TEACCH program. In E. Schopler & G. B. Mesibov (Eds.), *Autism in adolescents and adults* (pp. 411–432). New York: Plenum.

Rhodes, L. E., & Valenta, L. (1985). Industry based supported employment. *Journal of the Association for Persons with Severe Handicaps, 10,* 12–20.

Schopler, E. (1987). Specific and nonspecific treatment factors in the effectiveness of a treatment system. *American Psychologist, 42,* 379–383.

Schopler, E., Mesibov, G. B., Shigley, R. H., & Bashford, A. (1984). Helping autistic children through their parents: The TEACCH model. In E. Schopler & G. B. Mesibov (Eds.), *The effects of autism on the family* (pp. 65–81). New York: Plenum.

Van Bourgondien, M. E., & Elgar, S. (1990). The relationship between existing residential services and the needs of autistic adults. *Journal of Autism and Developmental Disorders, 20,* 299–308.

Wehman, P., Moon, M. S., Everson, J. M., Wood, W., & Barcus, J. M. (1988). *Transition from school to work*. Baltimore: Brookes.

IV

Parental Issues and Personal Accounts

13

Parent Essays

RAIN MAN AND JOSEPH

Ruth C. Sullivan

"When is Dustin Hoffman going to look at my dead-end streets album?" Joseph, our 30-year-old autistic son, called to me as he sat awkwardly on the foot of a twin bed. Lights, huge cameras, large cables on the floor, and exotic-looking equipment were all over the place. Dozens of people were milling about, some hooked up to headphones, others with heavy belts of dangling instruments. . . . It was Memorial Day weekend, 1988, in Cincinnati and we were on the set of *Rain Man,* a film in which Dustin Hoffman plays the role of Raymond, a high-functioning autistic man who is much like Joseph.

I was surprised at the low-key, informal rehearsal in progress. Barry Levinson, the director, was going over some lines with Tom Cruise, the costar who plays Raymond's brother, Charlie. They were rehearsing the scene where Raymond had innocently wandered into the adjoining motel room where Tom Cruise (Charlie) and his girlfriend were making love until they realized Raymond was sitting on the foot of their bed. Tom was practicing being irate. Dustin was quietly being autistic as his brother angrily scolded him. It occurred to me much later that the fictional Raymond probably sat there much as Joseph did that day—self-absorbed, uneasy in the strange environment, not understanding the nuances of all the activity, waiting stiffly until someone could pay attention to him.

In March of 1988, I had met Dustin through Gail Mutrux, the film's associate

---

RUTH C. SULLIVAN • Autism Services Center, P.O. Box 507, Huntington, West Virginia 25710-0507. CLARA PARK • 29 Hoxsey Street, Williamstown, Massachusetts 02167. CONSTANCE V. TORISKY • 738 Greenleaf Drive, Monroeville, Pennsylvania 15146. MARY S. AKERLEY • 10609 Glenwild Road, Silver Spring, Maryland 20901. NEIL OFFEN • 700 Bolinwood Drive, Chapel Hill, North Carolina 27514. MARGARET A. DEWEY • 2301 Woodside Road, Ann Arbor, Michigan 48104.

High-Functioning Individuals with Autism, edited by Eric Schopler and Gary B. Mesibov. Plenum Press, New York, 1992.

producer. Earlier she had located Joseph and me while searching for information for Dustin on high-functioning autistic adults who have savant skills, often referred to in the autism literature as splinter skills. The character of Raymond is good at math, and that is an important part of the *Rain Man* story. Joseph can multiply 2 four-digit numbers in his head almost as quickly as you can punch the buttons on a calculator. Among his other skills are perfect pitch, an uncanny memory for such things as license or telephone numbers, spatial memory (e.g., puzzles, where things are), and the ability to tell you the day if you give him a date (calendar manipulation). As it turned out, he became one of the two models upon whom Dustin Hoffman based his fictional character.

Joseph's unusual skills manifested themselves early. At 18 months I'd found him putting together a puzzle of the United States. Shortly after that time he was singing (more like "uh-uh-uh-ing," since he had no speech) whole musical phrases of "The Star Spangled Banner," note perfect—including "and the rockets' red glare," which even adults often find difficult.

Before Joseph's third birthday we already knew that our handsome little boy was not like any child we'd ever known. The aloneness, the lack of communication that was more than just a lack of speech, the seeming disinterest in any other human being, the extreme hyperactivity, the lack of sleep, the haunting and inconsolable wailing—all were inexplicable to us. I now know that he was displaying classic symptoms of autism.

One day when he was about 4, we were alone in the station wagon. The almost-always-silent Joseph threw off the blanket he had wrapped around his head, popped his thumb out of his mouth, and said—to no one in particular— "Dangerous Intersection, 21 letters," then went back to his reverie. This from a child whose daily speech might be 2 two-word sentences a day (e.g., "want juice" or "go car").

His savant skills grew as he got older, and we saw that he had a special interest in numbers. One day when he was about 10, he called out a four-digit house number as we drove down the street. "That's a prime number," he said. I had no idea he had any concept of what a prime number was.

When Joseph was about 16, my sister, Fran, and her husband, Jerry Buckingham, were visiting us for the Easter holidays. Jerry was then the administrator of a large hospital in New York City and was full of news about a huge new computer that had been installed only a few days before. One of his staff had shown him some of the marvels of computer technology. Knowing Joseph's affinity and competence with numbers, he told us of being able to ask the computer such questions as what number times what number will give the answer of 1,234,567,890. Just about then Joseph walked into the room.

"Joseph, what number times what number will give you 1, 2, 3, 4, 5, 6, 7, 8, 9, 0?"

As quickly as you could say your own telephone number, Joseph said, "9 times 137,174,210."

Recently at another family gathering, Jerry (now living in Los Angeles) was telling us that he has a prized old photograph of his grandfather sitting at a desk under a bare bulb entering numbers in a ledger. A Calcasieu National Bank calendar is on the wall behind him that clearly shows the date of Monday, January 25. But the year cannot be read. He'd always hoped to find out the year and took this occasion to ask Joseph, "In what years would Monday, January 25 fall?"

Joseph became thoughtful and after a few seconds said, "1982, 1971, 1965, 1954, 1937, 1943, 1926, 1909," in that order. He stopped, then said, "I forgot 1915."

Several years ago I was reading Luria's (1968) *The Mind of a Mnemonist* and was intrigued by his subject's (referred to only as "S.") ability to imprint and then call out from memory a matrix of 50 numbers after studying it for about three minutes (p. 17).

I decided to test Joseph. I wrote these 36 random numbers:

6 2 4 8 4 9
7 3 2 5 0 3
4 8 9 3 4 3
1 3 5 8 9 4
5 7 2 8 4 2
2 4 7 9 0 3

on a piece of paper and said to Joseph, "Study these until you think you have them memorized, then I'll take the paper and will ask you to tell me the numbers." After 43 seconds he handed the paper back to me and said he was ready. With an almost steady cadence he recited them all—by rows, but in no sequence that seemed logical to me. It was the first row, then the third, then the last, then the second, and so forth. Interestingly, he had a much harder time when I asked him later to give me the columns.

It was skills like these that in 1967 had led a University of Oklahoma film team to Voorheesville, New York, right outside Albany where we were living at the time, to put a 7-year-old Joseph and three other autistic children on record for the award-winning documentary *Autism, the Invisible Wall.* Seventeen years later (in 1984) that same team, now at UCLA's Neuropsychiatric Institute Media Lab, came to our home in Huntington, West Virginia, to film a now-adult Joseph. It was that film, *Portrait of an Autistic Young Man,* that Dustin Hoffman had seen before he met us.

When Gail Mutrux learned I was in Los Angeles in March of 1988, she invited me and my daughter, Lydia—just younger than Joseph—to meet Dustin. We were delighted to be asked, of course. He is a famous and admired movie star, but over and above that he has a reputation for carefully studying his roles. Knowing he was to play an autistic man made my meeting with him especially meaningful. Autism is still a mysterious and little-known disorder. Here was an important actor about to play the role of an individual the likes of which I've lived with for 28 years. I suddenly felt an immense responsibility to all autistic people and their families to say the right things, to present autism as accurately, plainly and memorably as possible. *Rain Man* with Dustin Hoffman in the role would give the condition a worldwide forum, heighten awareness, and help pave the long and difficult road to adequate services (now almost always grossly inadequate, if available at all).

Lydia and I were immediately made comfortable by Gail, Dustin, Mark Johnson (the producer), and Barry Levinson (the director). The atmosphere in the modest office was friendly, quiet, even "laid-back." Each was casually dressed. Dustin was in jeans and tennis shoes. It belied, however, the intensity of their interest and attention. They wanted to hear about Joseph and seemed to not get enough of our stories about him. Months later I learned that they had not only seen *Portrait . . .* but *studied* it, spending many hours at the UCLA Media Lab pouring over the "outtakes"—the extensive footage that had been edited out.

About an hour into the visit, Dustin seemed to suddenly withdraw from the conversation. He seemed lost in thought; his face became serious. He shifted slightly on his seat.

"Tragedy," he said, imitating one of Joseph's favorite expressions.

It was as though Joseph were sitting in that chair. The facial expression, the special private smile, the intonation, the pronunciation, the exaggerated pursing of the lips, the sense of great fun, the absolute pleasure in delivering the most exquisitely satisfying sounds—"Tuh-*r-a-a-a-g*-uh-dee"—were all there, just as we had heard it from Joseph thousands of times over the last few years. Drs. Barnett Addis and Daniel Hebert (coproducers of the UCLA documentary) had caught it, and Dustin had reproduced it.

Lydia and I were stunned. Only a few people, mainly his younger sister and brother, Lydia and Richard, have ever been able to produce such a good imitation. Dustin had taken the time and effort to duplicate a small segment of Joseph's behavior.

As an advocate for Joseph and others like him, I have learned over the years that in using the media to spread the word about autism, one must be ready to talk about one's child. You put information about your loved one in the hands of reporters, editors, and other media people with widely varying sensibilities and interests in the subject. You hope they will be accurate and kind in their telling of your story. The cost of going public is the risk that the media will distort, demean, misrepresent, or even hurt the very one(s) you are trying to help.

Seeing Dustin's Joseph, I was moved and relieved. I had come to talk to a stranger about my son. He handled the information caringly, gently, with competence and dignity. Later I read the script, and even before seeing the finished *Rain Man* I trusted it would be well done.

As Lydia and I were preparing to leave, Dustin invited me and Joseph to visit *Rain Man* when production began in Cincinnati, its first location, in late May, 1988. That's how Joseph, his father, and I came to be on the set on that Memorial Day weekend.

The visitation of autism to our home has not all been movie stars and glamour.

In 1962, when our beautiful, agile, strong, impish, 2-year-old Joseph was first diagnosed, even most professionals had not heard of autism. There was almost a total shut-out of the service system for children like him. The few available (many were called "child guidance clinics") were almost all psychoanalytically based—meaning the assumption was made that the condition was environmentally caused. That translated into "Mother did it." I know parents who at every quest for professional help were told there was nothing wrong with their child, that it was the mother who needed help. Those who could afford it often went into psychoanalysis.

Bruno Bettelheim's famous residential school in Chicago would take children only if parents agreed to not come visit for up to two years! They called it a "parentectomy."

Fortunately, new research in such fields as neuroanatomy, biochemistry, and genetics is giving us clues about defects in the brain that may lead to the cause or causes of this bizarre disorder. Though I still occasionally hear from parents that professionals blame them, that theory has largely been put to rest. I know of no authority in the autism field today who still espouses a psychogenic causation.

Though Joseph is now considered high functioning, we did not know that outcome when he was 2. At that age he was not talking, though he'd had several words at 1 year that were all gone by the time he was 18 months old—typical in autism. He was so physically precocious that when I finally entertained the possibility that he might be mentally retarded, the idea was immediately dismissed. How could he be when at age 2 he was singing snatches of the "Star Spangled Banner," could put together a puzzle of the United States, even when all pieces were turned over so the color wouldn't show? He could dismantle a toaster or a door lock or a wall heater with those strong, sure little fingers. He could climb anywhere; we called him our little mountain goat.

At about 2, he began to be extremely hyperactive, as though his idle was stuck at rocket speed. He slept an average of three to four hours a night and screamed the rest. My husband and I took turns staying up with him in the farthest parts of the house so the rest of the family could sleep.

And he ran away. We raised the latches on all the outside screen doors, but he stacked stools on top of chairs to reach them. With so much other child traffic (Joseph is the fifth of seven), it was impossible to lock the doors in a way he couldn't get out.

Once when I discovered him missing, I ran down the street to an intersection and could see him happily trotting down the middle of the street, cars going around him. He had shed his diaper and was naked.

Another time I saw a strange car pull up in front of our house, and the driver reached out her window with her left hand and opened the back car door. Out jumped 3-year-old Joseph. I didn't even know he was missing. No telling *where* she'd found him, but by then the neighborhood knew the yellow house was where the runaway kid belonged. And no telling what was said about his mother.

He seemed not to listen or understand. There was no "connection" with other human beings. I seemed no more important to him than a chair. He used my hand like a tool to pull open the refrigerator door for juice, as though the rest of me was just an unimportant accessory to the hand. He wore an amused little smile, as though his thoughts gave him immense pleasure—pleasure we could not share. When I tried to hold him, he giggled and writhed until he got loose. Family group snapshots of those years show Joseph struggling to be free of whoever was holding him.

He was a loner, never voluntarily participating in group activity. Toys did not interest him, or if he did play with them, it was not in the way they were meant to be used. He would spin a wagon wheel for hours at a time if we didn't intervene, often laughing ecstatically—incomprehensively and eerily entertained.

He would not stay put. He could slip out of any tie we could devise to hold him in his high chair. He scratched mosquito bites until they bled and used the blood to finger paint the curtains, the furniture, his clothes, the bed sheets, the towels.

He had to have constant eyes-on supervision. When we were out of the house, he had to be physically held. One family outing I'll never forget was a trip to Niagara Falls when he was about 4. I momentarily took my eye off him, and he darted to the observation wall above the falls. I snatched him just as he began to climb up.

One summer as a young teenager he pulled out all his hair in a circle four inches in diameter. He pulled out eyelashes, drained tears from his eyes with a Q-Tip. He ruined four houses we lived in by writing on the woodwork with a ballpoint pen. Every side of every door frame had his words indelibly scratched in. When he ran out of door frames, he did the floors, the ceiling, the piano, then the furniture, then our books, the silver chest—anything on which he could find a flat surface.

We gave him plenty of paper. My husband, an English professor, used to bring scrap paper from school so Joseph could use the backs of old tests, syllabi, study sheets. I have kept boxes of his drawings and scribbles from that age. At about 3½ I began to find drawings of maps of the United States and other countries. He had taught himself to read and, with a little help from me and his older sibs, to write. At age 4 he was putting in the names of the countries, including Czechoslovakia, correctly spelled, though the letters were sometimes upside down and backwards. He could enlarge any section of any map at will, it seemed.

I found drawings of other houses we'd lived in, as viewed from high above, which of course he'd never seen. The floor plans were exact. To this day he draws floor plans of our Crow Ridge Road house in Voorheesville, New York, with a different perspective in each drawing. Every detail is accurate. He saw it last at age 8. He is now 30.

On his first day of school he came home and drew the L-shaped three-story building in perspective, with each door and window in place. I took the drawing with me later to check it out.

The running away continued until about age 12. He was skillfully riding a bike, but still did not know or understand the rules of the road. As he got older, it was more likely such a normal-looking but socially unskilled Joseph could get into all kinds of trouble. Finally I found a partial solution. Since he could read, write, and tell time, I asked him to write me a note whenever he left. We practiced the format: the time of departure, the expected route, the time he'd be returning. That didn't eliminate my fear he'd have accidents, but at least it gave me a clue where he might be.

At about that age his older brother, Kit, was driving home one day and saw Joseph riding down the middle of a busy street. He saw a policeman stop Joseph and begin to speak to him in a rough voice. Joseph got highly excited and was unpleasantly talking back to the policeman. Kit got there just in time to rescue him. Without an advocate, Joseph, with very deficient social skills, would quickly have escalated the situation, possibly causing the officer to either chase him, shoot at him, or put him in handcuffs and haul him to jail. This has actually happened to a few autistic people I know.

Joseph now has relatively good speech and language skills. He finished high school, with the help of an excellent teacher/advocate and a school system that worked (sometimes reluctantly) with us. At his high school graduation, he got a standing ovation, and there were more wet eyes than mine as he walked across the stage to get his diploma.

Dustin Hoffman's Raymond is also high functioning with some phenomenal abilities. Since *Rain Man* I've often been asked if the film was accurate, especially in its portrayal of some of the feats with numbers. My response is that nothing in it is inaccurate.

In one scene a waitress drops a box of toothpicks, and Raymond quietly gives the number before they hit the floor. That incident is based on a skill of the well-documented retarded identical twins, George and Charles. In his fascinating book *Extraordinary People,* Darold Treffert (1989) reports that

> when a box of matches fell from a table and scattered on the floor . . . [both] twins cried "111" simultaneously. . . . [They] had not only seen the matches but had factored their number of 111 without any concept of what factoring was and without being able to understand multiplication, division or any other rules of arithmetic. (p. 64)

It is probably the same process by which Joseph at age 4 said "21 letters" when he read "Dangerous Intersection." George's explanation (Treffert, 1989): "It's in my head and I can do it" (p. 65).

Several of Raymond's behaviors are Joseph's, notably eating cheese curls with a toothpick, which was shown in *Portrait.* . . . It wasn't until I'd seen the film the second time that I realized Tom Cruise (as Charlie) was *also* using a toothpick! That was a low-keyed, delicate touch, showing how easy it is to accede to the autistic individual's insistent behaviors and routines.

Raymond's interest in taking pictures with his little camera as they drove across the Ohio River at Cincinnati, his compulsive lining up the salt and pepper shakers on the dinner table, the correct multiplication of two large numbers in his head as the small-town psychiatrist punches them into a calculator and shows a stunned Charlie the answer, the dramatic episode when Raymond burns the toast and his stimulus overload causes him to scream and severely bang his head on the wall—all of these are incidents based on Joseph's life. None are surprises to people who know autism.

A pre-opening benefit screening of *Rain Man* was held in Huntington on December 11, 1988, the night before the premiere in New York City. It was a gala event in our town, and the beautiful old Keith-Albee Theatre was filled to capacity—1500 people. Dustin, his wife, Lisa, Gail Mutrux, and Mark Johnson, Barry Levinson, and their wives sat right behind Joseph. They wanted to see his reaction. Later, when asked what he liked best, Joseph said, "The man eating cheese curls with a toothpick." The story line was lost on him.

Rain Man tells us how Charlie changed as he came to understand and learn some important life lessons from his autistic brother. It strikes a deep chord in those who know how autism has changed lives. With two top film stars playing the leads, autism has had its largest audience ever. Playing to full theaters around the world, and later winning four Academy Awards, the *Rain Man* story has helped thousands of autistic individuals and their families. The film has increased awareness and understanding of this little-known disorder in a measure greater than what all of us together have been able to accomplish in the past 25 years.

A few weekends ago we attended a big family wedding in Pittsburgh for my nephew. Only aunts and uncles were invited to the rehearsal dinner. Joseph was on his own for supper. I'd shown him the McDonald's arches from our hotel window and went downstairs with him as we were leaving. I asked the doorman to walk him to the corner and help him cross the street. I explained that Joseph may not seem to understand.

"He's autistic," I offered.

The man's eyes lit up.

"I saw *Rain Man,*" he said.

As we went around the block I saw the two of them on the corner, one carefully giving instructions, the other looking where the man was pointing.

Before *Rain Man* I would not have felt comfortable that Joseph was safe enough in a strange, large city to be left alone.

One film did that.

Reference

Treffert, D. (1989). Extraordinary people: Understanding "idiot savants." Harper & Row: New York.

AUTISM INTO ART: A HANDICAP TRANSFIGURED

Clara Park

At 31, art is a major part of my daughter's high functioning. Her speech is not; to hear it, its broken syntax and its conceptual simplicity, you would not think she could hold a job, keep her checkbook, assume the responsibility for important household tasks—all of which she does. Her art is important, however, in a different way. It allows her to make something beautiful out of what would otherwise be dismissed as autistic obsessions. It brings her in contact with people. It enhances her communication skills. It gives her a productive way to fill the empty time after work is done. Compared with these advantages, it hardly seems significant that it allows her to make money.

As she looks up at the photographer from her half-finished painting (Figure 13-1) her face shows a bit of tension, but the eye contact is good—very good, anyone would say who's had to do with autistic people. Ten years ago she was indifferent when people praised her paintings; now she smiles in pleasure. She likes it when people come to see her work. She can tolerate the interruption; she can even tolerate making one of the mistakes she calls a "painto," the word she invented on the analogy of *typo* (to be joined immediately by *cooko, bake-o,* and *speako*). She used to wail like a banshee when she made a painto, even if it could be fixed with a stroke of the brush. It's not the ease of repair that counts if you're autistic, it's the

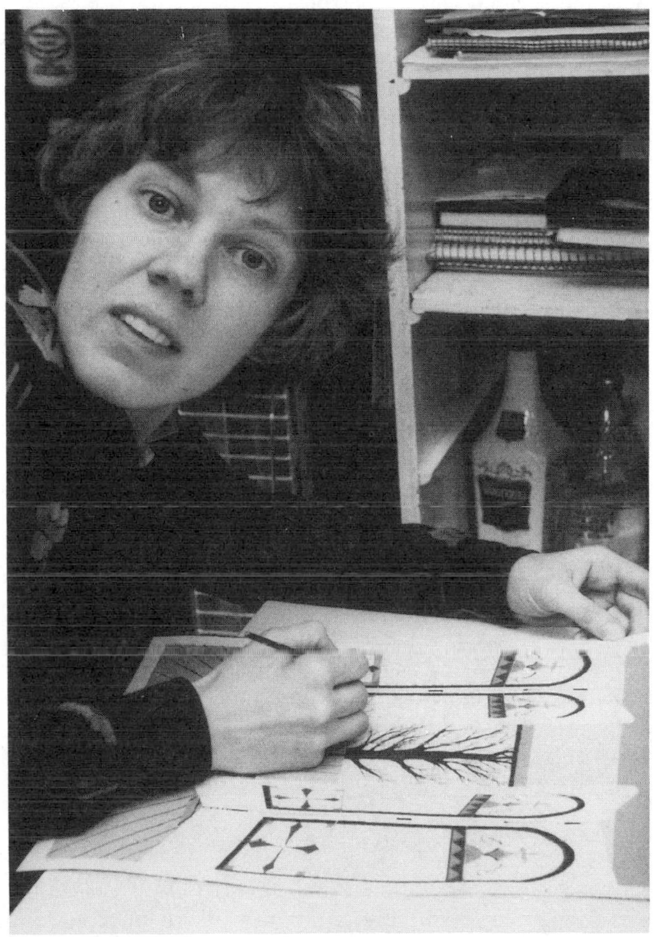

Fig. 13-1. Jessica Park at work on the painting in Fig. 2. (photo: Susan Plageman)

simple fact of error, in a world that seems controllable only when things are done exactly according to rule.

Exactly; that's the word. There is no vagueness in her painting, there are no dashing brushstrokes, no atmospheric washes. It's hard-edge stuff; it always has been. No impressionism for Jessy, and no expressionism either. Even in nursery school she never overlapped one color on another, never scrubbed them together into lovely, messy mud. There were no free splashes, no drips, no finger paint. Her very first paintings were as autistic as these today, repetitive arrangements of shapes and patterns, always controlled, always in balance.

Her art is autistic in other ways, too. Autistic literalism has its visual equivalent: Jessy's eye acts like a camera. The doors of Figures 13-1 and 13-2, even their stained-glass mullions, are rendered in accurate perspective. Should we be surprised? Jessy is the seventh autistic person to come to my attention who drew in perspective before the age of 8. (For the work of three of them, see the references

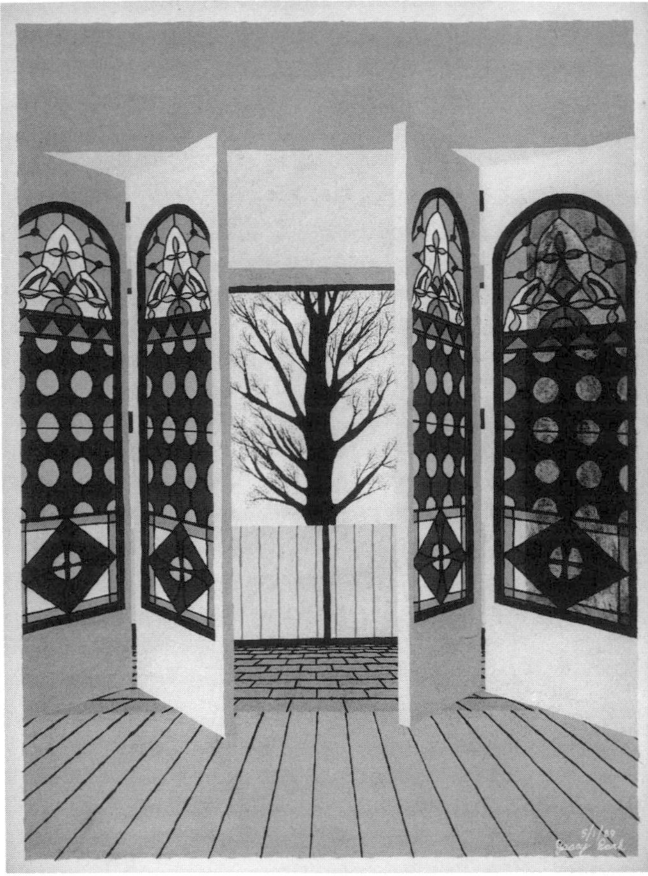

Fig. 13-2. *The Great Stained Glass Doors in Spring at Dawn.* Tiny pale-green buds on the tree mark the season. Note shadow at right.

section.) Perspective seems to us a mark of artistic sophistication; we know that European artists did not master it until the Renaissance. Normal children do not draw in perspective. If we consider, however, E. F. Gombrich's (1960, 1963) insight that the normal child draws not what it sees but what it knows, not its perception of the thing but the idea of the thing, we will not be surprised at the ability of some autistic persons to draw in perspective, even when severely retarded. Cameras do not ponder, they record.

Jessy has always had an extraordinary eye for color. To maintain her hard-won compositional skills, she writes descriptions of her paintings in short, childish sentences: "The sky is purple-black." Twenty-five years ago, when she could barely put two words together, she distinguished two virtually identical Volkswagens as "peacock-green" and "peacock blue"—her first adjectives. Nobody taught her that red mixed with white would make pink, yet she knew how to make pastels. Today, her paintings outdo the rainbow; a typical one may display as many as six different shades of a single color. And yet with all these shades there is no shading; rarely, and only with encouragement, does she try to do what you have to do to make an object look round. The painting she's working on in Figure 13-1, when finished, will show a shadow (Figure 13-2). But a shadow is not shading. This shadow appears in each of the 10 versions she has made of this scene. Why? Anyone who has worked with autistic people will guess why: When she made her original pencil sketch there was something behind the door. The shadow was *there*.

Ten renderings of the same scene, each with no fewer than 27 colors. Everybody who saw the first painting wanted it; it was even stolen from a gallery. She made a replacement, but she balked, quite reasonably, at more copies. But perseveration is part of her handicap, and so is a commitment to order. What can't be changed may sometimes be used. I suggested that she could paint the scene in different seasons, and her whole attitude changed. She painted it in winter, spring, and autumn, dawn and dusk and nighttime, storm and fair weather, altering the colors of each version until the total count was more like 250. However astonishingly she combined them, they always harmonized. And all of them were flat.

No shading. No nuance. Like her speech. Like her simplified comprehension of what people say, of their expressions, their emotions and needs. Barbara Caparulo has reported on the autistic man who, when asked of six test pictures of faces, "How do they feel?" replied, "Soft." No shading in her painting, or in the way she apprehends the world. Nuance *means* shading. Call it a metaphor of her autism, or more than a metaphor.

But if Jessy's paintings bespeak her handicap, it is a handicap not surmounted, but transmuted into something rich and strange. Here is autism in its core characteristics, literal, repetitive, obsessively exact—yet beautiful. In her paintings, reality has been transfigured. Who wouldn't want a painting of their house, recognizable to the last detail, but shimmering in colors no householder could conceive? Especially when (Figure 13-3) they get their favorite constellation thrown in? People pay money for these paintings. They send checks. Jessy deposits them in her account—which is accurate, of course, to the last penny.

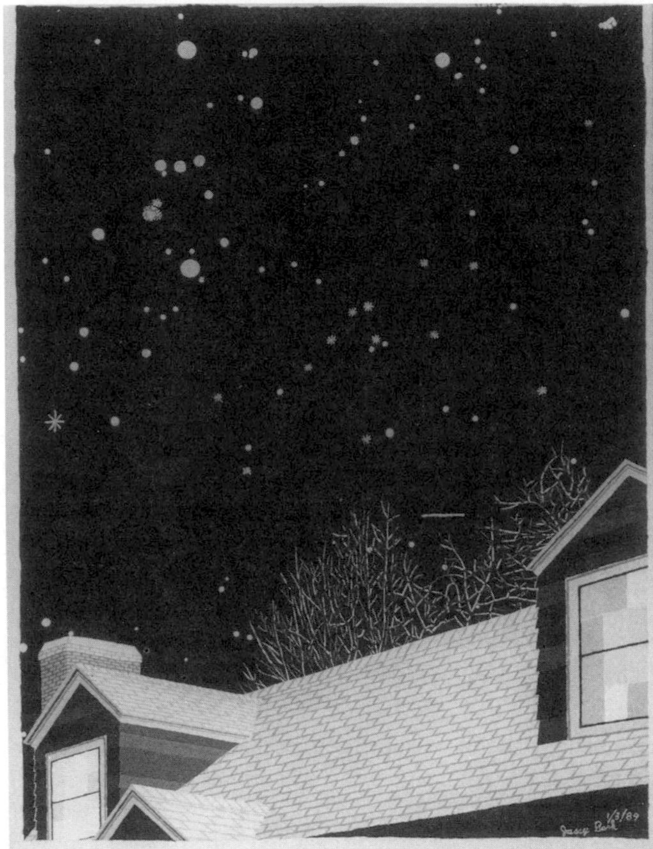

Fig. 13-3. *Barry Prizant's House with Stars and Colored Lights*. According to Jessica's description, visible are "Orion, Taurus, the Pleiades, Lepus, Eridanus, a part of Columba, and a part of Caelum. The tiny dots around the star are Orion's nebula. The yellow line and the color spikes are high-level nocturnal lights."

She paints pictures, they send checks. That's how it works, by the simple principle of reinforcement. It's not free creativity that gave Jessy a rewarding activity to fill the hours when she's back from her mailroom job and the household tasks are done and nobody's home for company. Jessy's art didn't just happen. In autism, development *doesn't* just happen, even the development of a natural talent. Jessy's capacity to paint as she does today was developed as all her capacities were developed, with encouragement and support and shaping, step by slow step. The checks were a stage in that development, unplanned but crucial. I'll return to it in its place.

When Jessy was small, she didn't recognize pictures. She flipped the pages of children's books obsessively, as oblivious to bright pictures as to text. At 2½, though she had no words, she grouped geometric figures by shape and color. But a picture is very different from a circle or a square. At 3½ she could do a child's jigsaw puzzle, but that didn't mean she saw the picture; she could put it together as well upside down. By 4, she could recognize a familiar scene; soon after, she drew her first crude human figure. But there was nothing automatic about the way she had learned; she'd been taught, slowly, over months (C. Park, 1977, 1982). Even today she does not look at a picture without a reason; a trip to a gallery is an exercise in frustration, though if she is painting from a photograph she will reproduce details no one else notices. Back then, at 4, at 5, at 6, at 7, though she *could* draw a figure, or a house, or a tree—the staples of children's art—she hardly ever did. Instead, sheet after sheet of repetitive lines, shapes, zigzags.

All the time, however, I was drawing for her people and places and things she could recognize. Pictures are a major means of communication for a child with rudimentary speech. She would attend to my drawing, perhaps because it was simple and familiar, perhaps because she could watch it gradually take shape. By age 8, as she entered more and more into our human world, she began to draw people more often. Yet when she did it was almost as if she had set out to illustrate her autism. Numbers had become important to her; she would draw human beings as numbers. Zeroes and ones and twos and threes acquired heads and arms and legs; she lined them up in rows, over and over again, number girls and boys, from zero as high as 49 (C. Park, 1982). But other drawings were more socially encouraging, as she began to use her crayon to communicate, or at least to express, the preoccupations of her daily experience. Over and over she drew the dog feces she was learning not to point at when we passed them in the grass; every day for a year and a half she drew her own adaptations of the adventures of *Harold and the Purple Crayon*, inserting her family and herself into the cast of characters, along with the radiator whose noises bothered her and the emergency switches nobody was supposed to touch. She drew her anxieties and compulsions: the shadows she wouldn't walk through, the building where a single light left on would set her screaming (C. Park, 1978).

None of these were artistically impressive; the people were crude stick figures, conventionalized, rapid, unvarying ideograms. Yet among them, unexpectedly, would appear an accurate visual representation: a stick figure cast an eerily realistic stick shadow, a stick Jessy kicked the offending building (rendered in perspective, of course—and from memory). The drawings were inventive, too, in ways I have not space to describe—a weirdly fascinating window into a unique world.

At last, at 13 Jessy entered her regional high school, to be accorded for the first time a full school day (C. Park, 1977). How did she move from such drawings to a point where she might almost be called a professional artist?

As always, she was encouraged and taught. She learned from me; she learned at school; more and more she learned from the "Jessy girls," the wonderful young people we found to live with us and share the continuous process of what Dr. Kiyo Kitahara would later call "daily life therapy." One of them was a painter. After nursery school, Jessy hadn't painted much. For all her fine color discrimination, she rarely switched crayons while drawing. She painted only when it was made easy, and used only the colors set before her. But Valerie had acrylics, and acrylics are easy to use. With her support, Jessy's obsessions bloomed into glory. That summer's recurrent theme was Dutch elm disease, three trees healthy and one afflicted, a background of greens and rich reds, or stars or rainbows, or a shining sun the number of whose rays correlated (Jessy told us later) with the quality of the day—12 for average, fewer for bad, more for good, down to 1 ray and up to 24. Valerie got her to sing, and then to illustrate the songs. Autism was a ticket to instant surrealism; when Jessy illustrated the line "God gave Noah the rainbow sign," the familiar human ideogram appeared with a rainbow indeed—displayed on a flat board on a signpost. But another illustration was anything but naive, as moonlight streaming through a window cast on the floor the exact shadow of the panes.

Valerie only stayed one summer. It was the realism, not the surrealism, that was encouraged after she left. Entering high school, art (like business math and gourmet cooking) was a class Jessy could take with normal children. It didn't take long for the teachers to discover that this bizarre youngster, who screamed at the bells and scratched in the wrong places and could hardly talk, could do any assignment given the normal teenagers. She could do a still life with a flag and a bottle; she could render the same subject cubistically . . . *if* she understood that that was what she was supposed to do. So it was that two new Jessy girls—twins—entered her life. Fascinated by the paradox of a someone nearly their own age who acted like a 4-year old when she wasn't acting worse, yet could draw anything set in front of her, they appointed themselves interpreters between her and the busy teachers. Talented but unsophisticated artists, they didn't go for surrealism or cubism either, and they discouraged weird subject matter they discouraged as "immature." They were among the few who could draw better than she could, and they decided *really* to teach her to draw. Their method was old-fashioned, but exactly right for a person with autism; they made model drawings and had her copy them. There was nothing "creative" about their requirements, nothing expressive. Once or twice people had tried to get Jessy to "draw a happy (sad/angry) picture"; she had no idea what they wanted of her. The twins were concrete and definite; they told her firmly what to do, and she did it. They set her subjects she never would have chosen—flowers, interiors, even portraits. She developed a line of exquisite sureness; a drawing of a girl seated looks almost like Matisse (C. Park, 1982). (The twins knew nothing of Matisse, though; they pressed her to add shading, and the pure line was obscured.) Valerie had tapped her imagination. The twins taught her academic drawing. And year after year, for the nine years she remained in high school, the art teachers taught her too.

But the three didn't come together. Jessy could draw, but the twins followed Valerie off to college, and without them (outside of school) Jessy rarely took up a pencil, let alone a brush. It was years since she had produced the strange and fascinating drawings that recorded her anxieties. But the art of normal children, too, loses its freshness when the demands of realism begin to take over, and few children regain it. Perhaps, we reflected, we should welcome Jessy's academic realism as normal development, not regret it as a sacrifice. After all, we had no plans to make Jessy into an artist.

We couldn't have guessed how luck would bring everything together—luck and the principle of numerical reinforcement. We took Jessy to an autism meeting where I was making a speech; she was already 21, too old for the activities provided, and I suggested she sketch to keep her busy. She made an accurate, ugly drawing of the ugly building we were meeting in, a man who'd heard my speech offered five dollars for it, and that's what started her career as an artist. Once she'd worked for "points" and improved her behavior amazingly (C. Park, 1982, 1983, 1986; D. Park, 1974). Money worked the same way. For years she had had no *reason* to paint or draw. Concepts of creativity or fame, of course, meant nothing to her. Money didn't mean much more. But numbers did, and she liked to see them rise in her checkbook. The staff at the Society for Autistic Children were very kind at first; they gave her a little exhibition, and sketches and school paintings were sold for small sums; one of the old Dutch elm disease paintings was taken for a poster. Eric Schopler and Division TEACCH provided invaluable encouragement with purchases and commissions. The glorious colors began to come back, and then to proliferate. Perhaps she remembered a school exercise from years before: She had been told to paint a snow scene, first in its natural evergreen and white, then in whatever colors fantasy might suggest. At any rate, Jessy was drawing again, not because she was told to but because she wanted to. Once more she was finding her own subject matter, as she had years ago. She drew, then painted, not snow landscapes, still less portraits or even buildings; she drew radio dials, speedometers and mileage gauges, clocks, quartz heaters, and electric blanket controls (Figure 13-4). People with autism are fascinated by such things. Jessy's fascination gave these new paintings the strangeness and intensity that her academic drawings had lacked. Not that these weren't realistic; but a dial is more than a dial when it is realized in apricot and turquoise. Jessy's dials and gauges dazzled; her heaters throbbed with color as in a dream, transfiguring the simple grid her geometrizing eye perceived.

Jessy had reverted to the abstract patterns of her childhood. But now they were abstractions in the true sense of the word, patterns perceived in, drawn from, *abstracted* from the real world. There was a third-story window in a house near us; by some architectural quirk, a chimney was visible inside it, right up against the glass. Jessy was fascinated by the patterns of bricks. She made four versions—first just the chimney; then the chimney and the window; then chimney, window, and roof; finally chimney, window, roof, and the night sky with trees and stars (*Schizophrenia Bulletin,* 1985). People liked the dials and heaters; if we'd lived in New York they would have gone over big, for Jessy is a natural pop artist. But art, for a person with autism, can be a vehicle of social learning: Jessy had already learned, reluctantly, that people won't buy just anything. She had to put time into her work; now she learned that though people like dials and heaters, most of them prefer houses, trees, and stars. She had begun to spend hours poring over the *Field Guide to the Stars;* astronomy was a new obsession. Jessy wanted to paint a starry sky, but

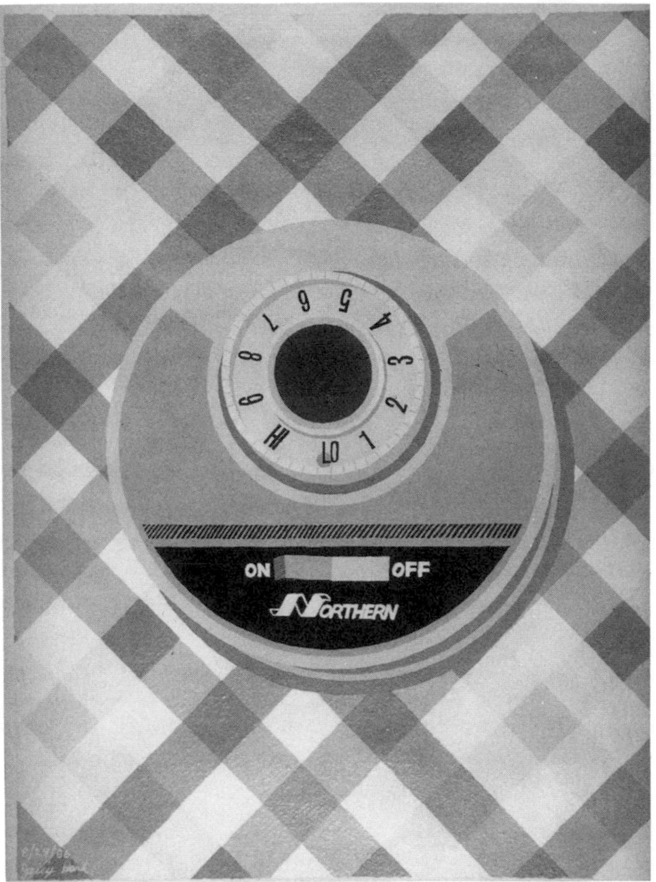

Fig. 13-4. *The Northern Electric Blanket Control.* The settings at "Off" and "Lo" and the multicolored grid pattern are characteristic, as is the beautifully rendered lettering. Compare Jessy's own signature.

she didn't know how she could paint the house and the chimney when everything was dark. She needed the support of tactful suggestion—tactful, for she has grown very sensitive to what she perceives as criticism. Honoring surrealism and strangeness, we suggested that she could paint the house in the daylight yellow of her earlier versions, and *still* have stars above. So she painted the sky "purple-black," and Orion with Betelgeuse and Rigel in their correct colors and magnitudes, and Venus, a planet the very name of which made her shiver with delight. And that is how Jessy came to paint pictures like the one you see (though bereft of its color) in Figure 13-3, pictures that convert autistic perseveration into an artist's exploration of a theme, and how last year she earned a thousand dollars from commissioned paintings to deposit in her bank account.

But money isn't everything. I have mentioned some social side effects; others are even more significant. Not all her painting is paid for. Jessy paints gifts now, for family and special friends. She paints birthday cards, too, and cards for Valentine's Day and Easter and Christmas. For each she chooses subject matter that she deems appropriate to the recipient. What progress! To describe these subjects and the degree to which they really are appropriate would tell a lot about autism, for an autistic person's idea of social appropriateness is sometimes a bit, shall we say, surreal. I could go on for pages, for I have left a great deal out. But I have come to the end of my space.

References

Caparulo, B. (1981, July). Development of communicative competence in autism. In *Proceedings of the 1981 International Conference on Autism* (pp. 232–244). Washington, DC: National Society for Children and Adults with Autism.

Gombrich, E. H. (1960). *Art and illusion*. Princeton, NJ: Princeton University Press.

Gombrich, E. H. (1963). *Meditations on a hobbyhorse*. London: Phaidon.

Paine, Sheila. (Ed.). (1981). *Six children draw*. London: Academic Press.

Park, C. C. (1977). Elly and the right to education. *Phi Theta Kappan, 4*, 534–537. [Reprinted in R. E. Schmid, J. Moneypenny, & R. Johnston (Eds.), *Contemporary issues in special education*. New York: McGraw-Hill, 1977.]

Park, C. C. (1978). Review of *Nadia: A case of extraordinary drawing ability in an autistic child*, by L. Selfe. *Journal of Autism and Childhood Schizophrenia, 8*, 457–472.

Park, C. C. (1982). *The siege* (2nd ed. with epilogue and plates). New York: Atlantic- Little, Brown. (Original work published 1967)

Park, C. C. (1983). Growing out of autism. In E. Schopler & G. B. Mesibov (Eds.), *Autism in adolescents and adults*. New York: Plenum.

Park, C. C. (1986). Social growth in autism: A parent's perspective. In E. Schopler & G. B. Mesibov (Eds.), *Social behavior in autism*. New York: Plenum.

Park, D. (1974). Operant conditioning of a speaking autistic child. *Journal of Autism and Childhood Schizophrenia, 4*, 189–191.

Park, D., & Youderian, P. (1974). Light and number: Ordering principles in the world of an autistic child. *Journal of Autism and Childhood Schizophrenia, 4*, 313–323.

Schizophrenia Bulletin. (1985). [Cover]. *11*(3).

Wiltshire, S. (1987). *Drawings*. London: J. M. Dent.

CRITICISM AND THE AUTISTIC PERSON

Constance V. Torisky

Introduction

In any gathering or in-depth discussion with parents of children or adults with autism, it is only a matter of time before the subject of criticism surfaces. Synonyms are sometimes used, such as *blame, correction*, or even *suggestions* or *advice*, but the basic scenario remains the same: (a) the person with autism (child or adult) is engaged in objectionable behavior; (b) a caregiver intervenes with appropriate correction (verbal, physical, or gesture); and (c) the autistic person responds with anger, rage, or some other variety of negative reaction ranging from inappropriate to catastrophic and bizarre (Autism Society of Pittsburgh, 1978–1990).

What is criticism actually, and why is it such a trigger for emotional responses from autistic people? It generally is defined as a judgment of merits and faults based on opinions and evaluation. A second definition is judging severely, usually finding fault. Our autistic people seem to react to criticism as though this definition were the only definition—but why?

Given the endless variety of disturbances in perceptual, motor, and language skills and in the ability to relate found in autistic individuals, it is understandable that any interruption in their mode of behavior will be traumatic. Regardless of how inappropriate some of their behaviors might be to others, interruption of those behaviors evokes a protective stance on their part. They seem compelled to defend their behavior against all interruptions, and criticism of any kind seems to be perceived as a threateningly negative and unwelcome interruption (Delacato, 1974).

To empathize with this perception, we only need reflect on those times when our own health, energy level, or mental stability was at its lowest, and our sensitivity correspondingly acute. We might recall our receptivity to even the slightest criticism then. If we did not indulge in a catastrophic reaction to it, it is quite probable that we felt that one was justified.

In normal human development, the concept of criticism is perceived as something intended to help us grow—something to help us. This perception does not come easily; in fact, it is almost a marker for increasing levels of maturity of the human psyche. Few people can say honestly that they genuinely welcome or enjoy criticism (Wilps, 1976), but it is a necessary part of the human condition. Although individuals may or may not internalize or even use criticism, most learn various ways to receive, deal with, and eventually return it.

It is against human nature to be constantly on guard. Everyone prefers being in the company of people where they can enjoy a relaxed and friendly exchange of views. We are equally uncomfortable when we are not permitted an occasional outburst due to stress or adversity (Torisky, 1978). We expect our friends and family to understand this. Our autistic family member, however, does not understand this, and it is usually necessary to deliver only soft, measured, and carefully considered criticism unless we are prepared to deal with a violent reaction. Sometimes it is hard to determine which is more stressful, constant vigilance or catastrophic reactions. Those who live or work with autistic people in any monitoring role constantly must weigh the risks and benefits of their interventions to alter behavior, since they most certainly will share in the resulting experiences. It is easy to see how understaffed facilities may compromise the quality of these interventions. They are trying to survive themselves (Blake, 1988).

Understanding Precedes Strategy

In developing guidelines that are considerate of both the autistic person and the one attempting to guide or alter that person's behavior, any information that sheds light on factors that may impede the understanding and perception of either party is essential. A sympathetic understanding will enhance the process, but unfortunately it may be all one-sided in this situation. There is little reciprocity, and a very uneven exchange. But just as allowances are made for a lost foreigner, allowances must be made for the autistic person's shortcomings in social awareness, while at the same time recognizing the almost uncanny ability that many autistic people have in sizing up our intentions and motives (Powers, 1989). This seems a bit incongruous, but it figures prominently in most reports of incidents that describe the scenario of criticism followed by catastrophic reaction (Autism Society of Pittsburgh, 1978–1990).

> I don't know how he knew I was in a hurry. I was really trying to be patient with him. I talked very slowly, and used all the right words, but he just suddenly exploded!
>
> I can't understand how he could be so ungrateful! He must surely know that I was trying to help him tie his shoe! He acted as though I insulted him!
>
> Everything was going along fine. He was responding to my advice, and then suddenly, blooey! I don't know what I did wrong.

And so on. What usually comes through is the utter bewilderment, or at least puzzlement, of the relative or staff person who has been unceremoniously dismissed by an autistic person they were trying to help.

Environmental Inventories

The day is probably not far off when we will have computerized inventories of all environmental factors that can affect our mood, health, and performance. Until we catch up to "Star Trek" technology, we need to be aware of every possible contribution to a negative or positive reception of our effects to help the autistic person learn and get on with life. There are an infinite number of blockages that can exist, permitting only partial perceptions. We know some of them, we suspect others. These factors include sights, sounds, smells, foods, allergens, light sources, barometric pressure and other weather conditions, air flow, noise level, number and identity of people, and any other source of comfort or stress (Montague, 1965). This endless list does not even include internal disturbances that are all too often overlooked, such as minor aches and pains, possible infections, indigestion, headaches, or even physical or neurological anomalies that might interfere with perception or learning.

If this seems like a monumental task, it is. But amazingly, most parents and good teachers seem to tune in to their charges and develop a rather thorough awareness of these factors. However, being human, they also tend to forget these factors while intensely involved in the teaching process, and remember them in retrospect after an incident has occurred and they are searching for some rational explanation for it (Wing, 1985). It would seem eminently worthwhile to develop a written or graphic profile on each child in a school program that records these individual eccentricities that can become huge stumbling blocks when overlooked.

What Does Not Work

Searching through 20 years of phone conversations logged in our chapter office and personal counseling sessions with hundreds of parents, I can state with certainty that the following will not work: impatience, threats, anger, loudness, negative phrasing, forced confrontation, abrupt physical direction, name-calling of any kind, phony concern or patience, too many words at one time, or criticism geared to the convenience of the caregiver rather than the benefit of the autistic person. The higher the functioning level of the child, the more sensitive that child is to the truth of the critic's motive (Wing, 1985). Note that *firmness* is not included in this list. Interestingly, all these modes of criticism are used and do work effectively to modify behavior of normal people more often than not.

What Does Work

Remembering that each autistic person is an individual and reacts in a highly individual way, there is a small menu of physical, psychological, and body-language communication modes that may be effective alone or in combinations (Konstantareas, Blackstock, & Webster, 1991):

1. *Voice:* calm, firm, even, persistent
2. *Manner:* firm, no-nonsense, matter-of-fact, steady
3. *Posture:* nonthreatening, firm, in charge, in close proximity without crowding
4. *Words:* as few as possible (eliminate any unnecessary words), positive, matter-of-fact, concrete, definitive
5. *Phrasing:* speak in the future conditional (e.g., "If you calm down, we will be able to continue the game"), keep it simple and direct (no descriptions of how the behavior is making you feel), do not hark back to previous episodes ("You always do this . . . ")
6. *Tone:* patient (learned patience that is real, even through clenched teeth), concerned, but not solicitous
7. *Projection:* respectful of the child or adult's personhood

Gentle physical restraint using hands while communicating may be possible, helpful, or even necessary (Rimland, 1964). (It could be necessary, for instance, if the intervention is taking place on or near a busy public street and the person is likely to bolt into traffic.) However, as physical proximity and restraint become more tolerable, verbal criticism also becomes more tolerable, almost at the same time.

Interventions that May Soften the Message of Criticism or Have a Calming Effect

Along with the necessity of ruling out physical and neurological interferences, modifying environmental impediments, and programming effective verbal and body-language postures, there are some supplementary measures available that might soften the blow of criticism when you anticipate its need, or help to neutralize the blow after the fact. These are highly individual in effectiveness and only worth consideration as an adjunct to carefully considered criticism-delivery techniques. They represent parents' successful techniques for calming down an acting-out autistic son or daughter, either before or after an incident that requires criticism as an intervention. These activities that may have a calming effect include a warm bath in a tub or whirlpool, 10 minutes of brisk exercise (swimming, walking, riding a stationary bicycle, walking or running on a treadmill, using weight-lifting machines), massage or sitting in a vibrating recliner chair, a guided imagery session (if verbal), and using headphones to listen to music.

Openness and Proximity

Some parents have reported to us that the most opportune time to discuss anything with their autistic child occurs when there is an illness that produces a high fever. In this state, the autistic person's normal defenses are down, and the receptivity to real help of any kind often is enhanced to a point where near-normal conversations may take place (Delacato, 1974).

As the autistic person matures and becomes more in tune with the primary caregiver, gentle physical restraining while communicating may be possible and even helpful. (This is not to be confused with holding therapy, which has a different developmental timetable and purpose.) Proximity and touching convey a different message at this point and even may be initiated by the autistic person as a means of getting your undivided attention (Montague, 1971). For instance, my son Eddie has progressed from total gaze aversion to putting his face and head against the front of my face when he wants to communicate something that is important to him.

With Real Conversation Comes the Opportunity to Exchange

Parents of nonverbal autistic children will understand the great barrier that is broken once a real conversation happens. Ask any parent who has engaged successfully in facilitated communication techniques. The ability to verbalize or communicate about criticism, to define its use and necessity in daily life, and to talk with an autistic person about why it is necessary is light years ahead of the days of frustration, anger, screaming, and rejection of any form of admonition. It is also a time to instruct the autistic person about ways they themselves can deliver verbal criticism to others.

When my son Edward, now 33, is moved to give his litany of improvements to a visitor or family member, he always lists the fact that he can now accept criticism. He has the concept internalized and equates it with suggestion, advice, or correction. He also can deal better with us when we lose our cool now and then, during which time he retires to a nearby room and loudly proclaims that the argument between family members "has nothing to do with me! I'm not a part of that!" We quickly agree with him, that our spats are not criticism of his presence among us.

If a family argument does not subside quickly, our son pulls out his ultimate weapon. He begins to pray aloud—very loudly—that "everyone will get along." This usually works. He holds up a mirror of sorts—his way of criticizing us.

The Fragile Balance

Once criticism is an intellectual and verbal concept, even though the language is elementary and simple, the concern with environmental inventories becomes even more important. You have finally gotten to a point where you are communicating with your autistic offspring. You do not want to spoil this opportunity and have it degenerate with the ingestion of food allergens, excessive fatigue, or overstimulation from environmental noise.

You can never be sure, for instance, about crowded places such as county fairs, where people, noise, and food are in abundance. With our son Eddie, the wrong combination of food allergens (in his case, corn, milk, and chocolate), sustained loud noise, or oppressive crowding can wear his stability down with alarming suddenness and precipitate an incident or a full-scale blowup. On the other hand, I have known him to tune out much of the activity, revel in the loud music and eat his way through several food booths, finally wear down and become pleasantly tired, and then suddenly react violently to even the mildest suggestion. There are obviously many variables for him that are still indiscernible (Montague, 1965) or not quantified, such as fatigue, barometric pressure or other weather influences, undiagnosed medical problems, drug withdrawal, or airborne allergies. Still, we feel we are gaining on identifying and understanding these, and outings are certainly more predictable than in times past.

Sensitivity Is the Key

The traditional and obligatory role of parents as critics and modifiers of social behavior must be renegotiated with new ground rules and a very lopsided contract to accommodate the autistic person's ability to perceive the concept of contract (Rimland, 1964). Sensitivity becomes the key in assessing and reacting to subtle changes in circumstances that alter the responsibility quotient of the autistic person, and in adjusting criticism to reflect those changes.

A very clear example of the sensitivity that is required occurred recently at a Pittsburgh chapter board meeting. A couple new to Pittsburgh began attending our meetings right away, bringing their autistic daughter with them until we could make arrangements for respite and child care. We wanted them at the meeting, so we all attempted to adjust. However, during a heated discussion about local services, the previously contented child picked up our distress and agitation without understanding that it was aimed at an absent party. She reacted as though we had aimed angry criticism at her. Internalizing the group's agitation and anger and clearly unable to differentiate herself from others, she reacted with anxiety, confusion, and disorganizing distress. We immediately scaled down our discussion and were reminded of the reason that we normally restrict our meetings to parents only.

The sensitivity required to maintain a noncritical atmosphere that will not upset an autistic person is one that is not possible to maintain when the demands of reality are superimposed and a task must be accomplished that requires our normal mode of behavior. This artificial atmosphere—one maintained at great emotional, mental, and physical cost to the adults who are caring for, and teaching, autistic people—cannot be maintained simultaneously with the performance of any other equally important task. You must either compromise the task at hand or the nonthreatening atmosphere necessary to maintain the equilibrium of the autistic person.

As the functioning level of the autistic person increases, this sensitivity becomes more subtle and more complex, but the responsibility for it may be shared somewhat with the higher-functioning autistic person. Their higher ranges of abilities tend to involve them in more complex social situations, but with an increased capacity to develop some strategies to cope with these situations. They are still autistic, however, and the coping strategies need to be preprogrammed in anticipation of situations that would be handled more intuitively by a person without autism (Konstantareas *et al.*, 1991). Since the social deficits in a higher-functioning autistic person are usually offset by some rather formidable skills in other areas, they can often get by with the assistance of programmed social responses, or they are simply excused out of deference to their contributions in their higher skill areas (Wilps, 1976).

How Are Parents, Teachers, and Caregivers Affected?

If you survive the years of personal adjustment and self-training required to deliver criticism appropriately to an autistic person, what has this discipline done to you as a person? Have you totally lost your spontaneity? Obviously, you cannot remain the same carefree and happy-go-lucky student you were when *autism* was only a word in a psychology magazine or book. While the autistic person in our lives is slowly internalizing the concept of criticism, what are we internalizing?

By holding yourself constantly in check, measuring every word, weighing in advance all aspects of your every communication, walking on eggs much of the time and visualizing the consequences of not doing so while hoping always for the best, you will have internalized self-control that you never dreamed possible. If you survive, it will be with a hide so tough that little can ever hurt you—a very big *if*. The field of autism is littered with people who gave up, could not cope, or decided that the cost to them as a person was too high to pay.

What does this say about criticism itself? Criticism has always existed. From the Bible on down to modern manuals on etiquette, criticism has been a part of human discourse wherein one human being expresses a difference of opinion and value to another human being (Wilps, 1976).

After experiencing these extreme reactions to criticism, there is a gradual awareness that you do not have to be autistic to be distressed by criticism! Autistic people are just better equipped to neutralize criticism by making the criticizer more uncomfortable than the one being criticized. (When we are the recipients of criticism, we may long for the status of autistic for just a few moments in order to indulge in the luxury of screaming our rejection of the criticism. But nonhandicapped people are supposed to play by those "other" rules.)

As in nearly every aspect of human interaction, the autistic person holds up a mirror to us, forcing us to examine the components of our criticism—the motives, the urgencies, the level of respect, the actual personal price we are willing to pay to convey it successfully. They allow us to criticize ourselves (in the most positive definition of the word), and they challenge us to grow as far as we can. The irony of it is, after all, the fact that this is what we are asking of them!

References

Autism Society of Pittsburgh. (1978–1990). Unpublished telephone log books.

Blake, A. (1988). Aversives: Are they needed? Are they ethical? *Autism Research Review, 2*(3).

Delacato, C. (1974). *The ultimate stranger: The autistic child.* Navato, CA: Arena.

Konstantareas, M., Blackstock, G., & Webster, C. (1991). *Autism: A primer.* Quebec: Quebec Society for Autistic Children.

Montague, A. (1965). *Life before birth.* New York: Signet.

Montague, A. (1971). *Touching: The human significance of the skin.* New York: Columbia University Press.

Powers, M. (1989). *Children with autism: A parents' guide.* Warwick, RI: Woodbine House.

Rimland, B. (1964). *Infantile autism.* Englewood Cliffs, NJ: Appleton-Century-Crofts.

Torisky, C. (1978). The hostage parent: A life-style or a challenge? *Journal of Autism and Childhood Schizophrenia, 8,* 234–240.

Wilps, R. (1976). *Irresponsible behavior in autistic children, its impact on the parental caring impulse, and overcorrection strategies for its reversal.* Paper presented at the ASA Conference, Orlando, FL.

Wing, L. (1985). *Autistic children: A guide for parents and professionals* (2nd ed.). New York: Brunner/Mazel.

THE LAST BIRD

Mary S. Akerley

But now he walks the streets
And he looks at all he meets
Sad and wan,
And he shakes his feeble head.
That it seems as if he said,
"They are gone."

The mossy marbles rest
On the lips that he has pressed
In their bloom,

And the names he loved to hear
Have been carved for many a year
On the tomb.

And if I should live to be
The last leaf upon the tree
In the spring,
Let them smile, as I do now,
At the old forsaked bough
Where I cling.

from *The Last Leaf,* by Oliver Wendell Holmes

Someone has to be it—the last leaf, or in a family, the last bird to leave the nest. The poet depicts the last leaf as lonely, the symbol for an old person whose friends have all died, leaving him alone on the earth. Nonetheless, there is an implied positive element in "The Last Leaf": There *are* friends to be missed.

The last bird, if it has autism, may not be so fortunate. Its loneliness is not about to end; it is actually just beginning.

Our "last bird" is our son Ed, the youngest of four children and the only one still at home. Even if he were not the youngest, he would probably still be the last bird because he has autism. Like most sane, middle-aged folk, my husband and I would like our nest to be empty. We are looking forward to having our home and our lives to ourselves and to having our adult children as friends, not dependents. Ed is now 25, and it's time for him to be out and on his own. This will be (I think) the last major transition in our parent–child relationship, and probably the most difficult. Of course, none have been easy by any standard.

I am going to digress here just a little to make a distinction between what I'll call obvious or explicit transition points (such as starting school) and those that may not be so apparent. The latter are functions of the child's internal developmental level. They are not marked by discrete events or points in time, but they are just as significant as are their more easily recognized counterparts. Explicit transition points occur irrespective of the child's developmental level (e.g., in our society, children must start school by a certain age whether or not they are ready); internal transitions take place only when initiated by the developing child. However, there are usually expectations as to when these internal events should occur; when the expectations and the reality don't coincide, life can get harder than it needs to.

I believe the difficulty in this area can cut two ways for parents of children with disabilities. For example, under normal circumstances, we expect our children to begin playing interactively with their peers, at least for short periods, by the time they are 2½ or 3 years old. When this doesn't happen on schedule, the parents may try to force it. When the cause of the delayed social development is autism, no amount of forcing is going to work, as everyone reading this knows. Nevertheless, the temptation to push cooperative play may remain strong for a number of reasons. Conversely, *because* the child has autism, the parents may assume that he will never be able to have any appropriate peer interactions. That assumption may trick them into missing signs that their child is now ready for something new. (Parents of normal kids make the same mistakes, but in general, the effects are less serious because normal youngsters are better able to assert themselves and thus protect and maintain their personal developmental pace.)

What follows are somewhat random reflections on the transitions in Ed's life and ours that I think have been particularly significant, although we may not have been aware of what was really going on at the time.

Getting On: Elevators and Animals, or "What Goes Up Will Come Down," and It Won't Bite You in the Process

Ed, like many children with autism, had some irrational fears when he was very young. Two that are especially memorable are elevators and animals, especially dogs. Both are ubiquitous in modern suburban life, so options for dealing with this panic were limited to whether confrontations with the object of terror were planned or unexpected.

For example, on outings to the store or the park, or during a walk in the neighborhood, we frequently encountered dogs—some leashed, some loose. If I saw the dog first, and if it were leashed, I could usually control Ed's reaction. I would say to him, "There's a dog up ahead but it's OK. It's on a leash, so it can't touch you. It won't hurt you." He would tense up and slink along pressed against me (on the non-dog side), whimpering, "No dog." Thus, everyone made it through the situation with a minimum of fuss.

However, if Ed saw the dog first, there was total panic. He shouted out the magic words, "No dog," as he literally climbed up my leg and side much as a cat in similar circumstances would go up the nearest tree. And the whole world naturally turned to watch the show.

Clearly, control was the better way to go, but so long as the control was mine and not Ed's, it did little to solve the overall problem. Similarly with elevators. When possible, we avoided them (as in "Going just one flight? Please use the stairs."). When not possible, I warned him: "We are going to such-and-such a place, and we will have to ride the elevator. I will hold you and you can push the buttons. It will be all right." It wasn't, of course, unless one accepts as "all right" a tense, shaking, sweating child, clutching his mother with a grip of steel, but at least not screaming.

This state of affairs with elevators continued until the issue was forced. We were visiting my mother, who lived on the 16th floor of a luxury high-rise apartment building. The elevators were the kind with automatic timed doors, apparently programmed for an average of two people to get on or off. The six of us, with luggage, did manage to get on, and as the elevator ascended, others joined us. Every time the door opened, Ed thought we were getting out. When we didn't, the screaming started, and it got worse with each subsequent disappointment. The other passengers (well-dressed, middle-aged residents of the upscale high-rise) were bewildered by the intensity of his reaction (and probably by our presence as well—we had just completed an eight-hour drive in the summer heat and most certainly did not look as though we belonged on their elevator).

Fortunately, by the time we reached the 16th floor, the six of us were the elevator's only occupants. The elevator stopped, John and the other kids got out—but before Ed and I could, the door shut and the elevator was on its way down in response to someone else's summons. Ed's screams were now like nothing that should be coming out of the mouth of a human child.

Of course he was in for another heartbreak when the doors opened at the lobby level. The people standing there waiting for the elevator naturally continued to wait for us to get off before getting in, particularly as Ed was howling, "Get off now! Get off now!" I motioned the people on, trying to explain over his screams that we were going up. Ed saw more people getting in and realized it wasn't over. By the time we reached the 16th floor for the second time he was in a complete frenzy, drenched in sweat and tears. John, who had been waiting at the elevator door, said he could hear Ed the whole time!

Then came the miracle. Once we were in my mother's suite, she went to work on Ed with ginger ale and a cold washcloth. He calmed down surprisingly fast and, after he had finished his second glass of ginger ale, said very calmly, "Let's go ride the elevator now!"

There's an epilogue: He developed a fixation (or, as we called it at home, a "hangup") about elevators. He begged to stop and ride the elevator every time we drove past a high-rise building. When he knew we were going somewhere with an elevator, he would grin and—literally—shake with excitement. His fascination was so extreme that his teachers used elevator rides as reinforcers! While his new attitude was certainly an improvement, at least externally, I do not think it represented real progress developmentally.

The dog thing was different. One day I observed Ed crouched at the next-door neighbors' fence, gingerly petting their sheltie through the slats. The dog was sitting quietly, apparently enjoying the attention, and when she'd had enough she got up without barking or jumping to walk away. But even that little bit of unexpected motion was too much for Ed; he jumped up, turned, and ran, obviously scared.

However, he kept trying. He revisited the sheltie almost daily and began making similar overtures toward a pair of dachshunds who lived behind a chain-link fence at the corner house up the street. It got to the point that, when Ed got off the school bus at the corner, the dogs would run toward him, barking and jumping against the fence. Ed seemed to understand this was friendly activity. He didn't run away but stayed and played with the dogs. Of course, the fence was still protecting him.

The dachshunds' owners had been observing all this, and one afternoon they invited Ed to join Duke and Snoopy inside the fence. He accepted, lived through it, and went back for more. He and those dogs got to be such good pals that, on one occasion when the dogs had gotten loose, the owners asked Ed to find them. They knew the dogs would be much more likely to respond to Ed's call than to theirs.

That was a real transition, and I believe it is a perfect illustration of my earlier point. Ed's "love" of elevators was imposed on him before he was ready to deal with his fear. He discovered that nothing terrible happened when he was forced to take a very long elevator ride, and he experienced a truly euphoric relief as a result. So he went back for more thrills, but there wouldn't have been any thrill if fear had not still been present.

On the other hand, his relationship with animals since the events just related has been, in my opinion, entirely normal. He's still a bit skittish around strange dogs (so are a lot of people—it's a sensible reaction), but he's very comfortable around those dogs he knows. He has even helped me "dog sit" for a friend on two occasions.

I think the point of all this is we can condition our children's behavior to make it "acceptable," but there will be no development (i.e., internal transitions) until the kid himself says so. And when he does, he needs sensitive, alert adults around him who know when it's time to invite him to come inside the fence.

Getting Around: Feet and Wheels, or "You Can't Keep a Good Man Down," but You May Knock Him Down When You're Not Looking

The ability of a kid with autism to wander great distances without getting lost is legendary. Ed was no exception, and in spite of my vigilance, he got away a lot. Not surprisingly, we were therefore superstrict about limiting his "free-ranging" space. As he got older, he became very obedient on this score but eventually resentful (and rightly so) of how tightly we were holding the reins.

When he was about 11 he began asking if he could walk to and from church. The walk would require him to cross a six-lane highway, with no traffic signal to assist him, so we said no.

To understand what happened next, the reader needs to know our Sunday routine. John and the kids would go to nine o'clock Mass, after which all four children had Sunday school. While they were in school, I went to Mass; that way we were all ready to come home at the same time. (The routine also gave me a blessed hour of peace and quiet at home on Sunday, in addition to the one I spent in church!)

By the time Ed was 11, the other three were in Catholic junior and senior high schools and no longer going to Sunday school. However, John and I were still doing our relay routine on Sunday mornings because of Ed. It was at this juncture that he began pestering us to let him walk. I got forced into acceding.

One Sunday when I arrived at church for ten o'clock Mass, Ed was waiting for me in the parking lot. "There's no Sunday school today," he announced. "My teacher is sick."

We stood staring at each other like the hero and the bad guy in the final scene of a Western. Each of us knew exactly what the other was thinking. I broke the silence: "Do you want to walk home?" His face lit up the way it used to at the prospect of an elevator ride; and, after eliciting from him promises to look both ways, I went inside to pray. There is a fire station across from the church; throughout Mass, I listened for the sirens. They were blessedly silent, and I did not see my son's squashed body on the way home. That's when I formulated my permission rule: If Ed asks to do something, and if that something is age appropriate, there is no reason for me to say no.

I was able to live by that rule for about 10 years. For example, I applied it to bike riding with very little difficulty. But when it came to cars, I choked. I simply could not believe that Ed would ever be a safe driver. I knew he would learn and obey every rule of the road, including speed limits. The problem as I saw it was that he would never be able to attend to the many simultaneous stimuli and clues to which a driver must react, often without any advance warning. I believed—and still do—that such simultaneous processing of information from several sources, through several senses, is simply more than a brain limited by autism can handle.

Nonetheless, Ed wanted to drive, and he certainly was old enough. I took comfort from the fact that we knew of two other young men, similarly impaired, who were driving successfully. Besides, there wasn't too much I could do to stop him, especially as his father thought the whole thing was a splendid idea.

Ed had taken driver's education in high school, but as any parent knows, that is less than adequate preparation. There is plenty of classroom instruction but only about three hours of total road practice. And that meager amount must be further reduced by time spent on parallel parking, and the time left divided by the number of students sharing the lesson—usually three.

Moreover, that instruction had been so long ago that we were really starting over. The first step was getting a learner's permit, as Ed's had long since expired. To do that in Maryland, where we live, one must pass a written test on the driving laws. Ed began restudying the rule book. He memorized the contents without difficulty, but I do not think he fully understood their meaning and significance. Finally, he announced he was ready to take the test. I am not ashamed to admit I was happy when he flunked, although I do think he should have passed.

The test is administered by computer: A multiple choice question is flashed on the screen, and the applicant has only a few seconds to pick the correct answer. There are a total of 10 questions for the learner's permit; the applicant must get at least seven right. So, to save time, as soon as the fourth wrong answer is entered, the computer turns off—rather like a video game. Ed was in the testing room for such a short time that I am certain he missed the first four. In fact, I suspect he didn't even answer some or even any of the questions, because he is not a fast reader, much less comprehender, and the language of the questions is not verbatim from the rule book.

I considered investigating the possibility of his right to an alternative testing procedure but decided not to for two reasons. First, I would have to justify the request, and I didn't want to raise any doubts in official minds as to his competence to drive. Second, the hurdle presented by the test supported my position that he shouldn't drive (albeit for the wrong reasons) without making me the heavy.

So I hypocritically sympathized with him and equally hypocritically urged him to keep trying. Of course, he needed no such encouragement. Several weeks later, he declared himself ready to try again. Again he flunked, but he was in the testing room much longer—a very bad sign from my perspective. On the third try, he made it.

Now came the hard part: practice driving. Ed wanted me as the tutor because I have a longer fuse than John does. Remembering practice driving with my own parents, I could empathize with his point of view, so I reluctantly agreed. I did not last long; the combination of his inexperience and nervousness, on top of my stark terror and lack of confidence in his ever getting it right, plus a close encounter with a large truck, ended my career as driving instructor. I made a deal with John: If he'd take over completely (he had been sharing tutor duties without stress), I'd let them use my car.

That proved an excellent solution until I got a brand-new bright red convertible. No one was allowed to drive it but me, so that ended the driving lessons, or so I thought.

Ed was too close to his goal to give up. What's more, he had money and, like Donald Trump, he could buy anything he needed. (He'd been working full-time since graduation from high school and, with nothing major on which to spend his paycheck, had saved up a substantial amount.) Ed hired a local driving school to give him double-time private lessons on Saturdays. Their car picked up the young tycoon at his front door and returned him when the lesson was over. And when I refused to let him use my car even to take the test for his permanent license, he simply engaged the school one more time. That was enough; he passed on the first attempt. Moreover, he had enough money to pay cash for a secondhand car. He put over 100 miles on it the day he got it!

So was I wrong? I think not, in spite of the results. He drove without mishap for about two years, but then, while making a right turn, he struck a pedestrian. It happened exactly as I predicted: He *was* being careful, but he couldn't take in everything. He had stopped at a red light and observed that the car facing him in the oncoming lane had its left-turn signal on. He realized that both he and that car would be turning onto the same portion of the road at the same time, so when the light turned green, he continued to keep an eye on the other car. What he failed to do was check the pedestrian signal and the crosswalk right in front of him, where a man was proceeding on a "walk" light. Fortunately, the man was not seriously injured, but he should not have been injured at all.

Ed knows my views about his driving. (Yes, I do ride with him, and yes, he's gotten a lot better and I tell him so—but I still don't like it.) Ed also feels very bad about the accident and hurting another person, but he still drives. Two things matter here: I can't stop him from driving, and he has chosen to drive, knowing the possible consequences. That is a major transition. He has learned that moral decisions are his to make, and he's not afraid to make them even when it means rejecting a point of view that he once considered gospel.

Not too long ago, he was contemplating a vacation trip to a city that we did not think was safe for him to visit, especially alone. When we voiced our concerns, he listened and then said, "It's just advice, right?" He wasn't sure then, but now he is. What we say now *is* "just advice," not a directive. The tough choices are his alone.

Getting Out: Pals and Pads, or "There's No Place Like Home," Except When It's Your Parents' House

Leaving home implies a readiness to be on one's own. There's an implication that the departing adult child has built a life for himself, with his own friends and place in the world (usually defined as—and by—his job).

Ed's not there yet, but he wants to be. And he's working on it. The job was, relatively speaking, the easy part. He graduated from high school as essentially a regular student but with one foot still in special education to preserve his right to vocational rehabilitation services. And it was through these services that he was placed with the federal government as an office clerk in a "Schedule A" slot. Schedule A slots are reserved for persons with disabilities, and do not always provide full employment or benefits. This was the case with Ed.

He was assigned to the Heart and Lung Institute of NIH, where he sorted and delivered mail to several buildings on and off the large central campus. He also had responsibility for photocopying the voluminous documents received and generated at a federal agency. He loved the work and the people, but rightfully resented the lack of benefits. (He was held to a work week of 35 hours, just under the number required for benefit eligibility.) He tried to improve matters within the system but was told his job could not be changed to a regular slot, nor was there an appropriate regular position available. This in spite of the fact that he got excellent performance evaluations.

He recognized the situation as a dead end and shared his frustration with us, but not his solution. He began job hunting on his own by making the rounds of local chain motels, seeking a position as a busboy. (He has always had a desire to become a maître d' and apparently was acting on some "just advice" I had given him in the past as to how one might get started in that career.) He did get two offers, accepted one, quit his job at NIH, and then broke the news to us. Reaction was divided: John and the two oldest kids told him he was crazy (harder work, lower pay, etc.), while his other sister and I were impressed by his initiative. Ed saw only a "real job" (i.e., full-time with benefits).

His career as a busboy lasted two weeks. The dining-room manager at the hotel abolished the position (there were only two busboys at the time), demoted Ed to washing pots and pans, and promoted the other busboy to waiter. Ed was not pleased and was therefore eager to take some advice. I suggested that he go back to the other hotel that had made him an offer and see if they still wanted him. They did, but as a custodian. Ed took the job and quickly came to hate it. (Cleaning up rooms after parties where people have been sick as well as wild is not fun.)

After a year of misery, he swallowed his pride and went back to vocational rehabilitation but made it clear that, this time, he wanted the real thing. He is now, in one sense, back where he started. He is a mail clerk at the Department of Agriculture. The duties are less varied than at NIH, and he's at the bottom of the federal ladder grade-wise, but it is a full-time, fully protected federal job. However, the pay is poverty level: less than $10,000.00 per year—not enough to live on by itself.

But even if it were, there's something else he needs; at least, something I think he does. He needs companions, friends, peers; right now he has none except his siblings.

This is another area where, at least until very recently, my ideas have been relegated to the "just advice" category. For example, there was another young man at NIH who really tried to make friends with Ed. They went out together a few times (mostly to malls on their lunch hour), and Ed seemed to like him. So, when Ed was planning his next vacation, I suggested he see if the new friend might not like to go along. Ed was adamant that my idea was not something he wished to pursue.

We had had similar discussions in the past, but then the focus had been on the undesirability (from my point of view) of solitary vacations. (I was glad that Ed was no longer tagging along with John and me on our vacations, but for many reasons, I hated to see him going off on his own to a strange place.) Now the point of the conversation was developing a friendship, but the result was the same: Ed "vanted to be alone" when he traveled.

Maybe he wants to be alone, period. When he left NIH, the "friend" took him out to lunch and gave him a very nice gift. That's the last they've seen of each other. Ed has ignored my hints that he call the fellow, even though he still calls people he knew in high school, mostly just to chat. (He long ago gave up trying to arrange get-togethers; he was turned down every time.)

I suspect the problem may be that my son is a snob who does not want to hang around with disabled people anymore than normal folks want to hang around with him. I have seen some evidence of this: Ed's married sister has a learning-disabled brother-in-law about Ed's age. Both are solitary, high-functioning, socially inept eccentrics. They see each other at family functions, but nothing has ever "clicked," in spite of the fact that each is an obvious solution to the other's loneliness.

That same sense of snobbery has colored Ed's romantic life. His first major crush (in junior high school) was on the pretty, vivacious head cheerleader. She was very kind but plainly not interested. He's had subsequent crushes on other beauty queens, and I have always dealt with his misery as though he were normal. I've explained that everyone goes through the experience of liking someone who doesn't like him or her back in the same way. I have also told him that the opposite happens, too: Someone you're not interested in will want you for a boyfriend.

It happened. The young lady was disabled, more socially than cognitively, and she really liked Ed. He eventually decided to give her a chance. They dated for three years until he dumped her for being too jealous and possessive. He told me he was going to do it, and I decided the time had come to be blunt: "You don't have anyone else to go out with—not only as a girlfriend but just as a friend your own age. Would you rather have no one at all than Alice?" He would.

But I don't think he wants to be solitary. Now that his siblings have moved out, he does seem to miss their company. In fact, their absence may be helping him move on.

We have within a couple miles of our home Inwood House, an HUD project for disabled adults. It's a very attractive garden-type apartment building, open to persons with any sort of disability. It also is the site for a social program for adults with disabilities who live in the community. I have tried to interest Ed in both offerings, but without success.

In January of 1990, John and I took a two-week vacation. It was the first time Ed had been entirely alone in the house (the prior "bird" had flown just five months before), and I was curious as to how he managed. "How did you like being the only one here?" I asked. "I liked it," he said. "It was like having my own place. I've decided to look into Inwood House. I think I might want to move there."

It will be a while before he moves out, but the last big transition is in sight. I don't believe it will happen successfully until Ed accepts his limitations, but isn't that true for everyone? And I think he is beginning to see that he can't realistically hope to marry a cheerleader or have the secretary of agriculture for his best friend.

Every parent of a disabled child worries about "What will happen after I'm gone?" For parents of high-functioning, near-normal adult children with autism, the "what will happen" may not mean concerns about support and shelter so much as someone for their son or daughter to be with when the family is no longer there. In all probability, my last bird will also be a last leaf. When he is, I hope he has someone to miss besides us.

CULTURAL AND LANGUAGE BARRIERS

Neil Offen

There are, of course, an inordinate number of problems all parents have to deal with when their child is autistic—questions to be answered, situations foreseen, diagnoses made. At best, most things are never totally clear, specifics are hard to come by, and being sure always seems just a bit out of reach.

A high-functioning autistic child, perched precariously on that hazy borderline between normalcy and more disabling dysfunction, fully part of neither world, presents in many senses even more complicated questions. When you add bilingualism and biculturalism to the equations, as we did, not just the answers become more blurred, but even the questions, too. Everything seems more difficult, more confused, harder to pinpoint. The certainties you desperately need—even if you wish to avoid them—are almost completely obscured by what turn out to be red herrings.

Our son, Paul, was born in Paris, France, in 1980. As is common with many autistic children, he was—and remains—an extraordinarily beautiful child, with large, expressive eyes and luxuriously long lashes. He was also, almost from the moment of birth, extremely alert, aware, and interested. When we carried him through the sinewy streets of Paris in his Snugli, or walked through the Place de la

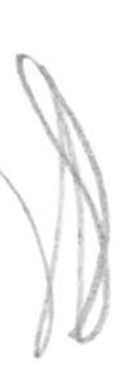

République with him in his stroller, passersby would stop us to admire "this stunning child" and comment on how "*eveillé*" (loosely, "alert") he was.

As an infant, he seemed to smile easily, was interested in everything, and appeared to probe every nuance of our faces with his big, serious, dark eyes. By 2 months, he was already making eye contact and googling away as if he were intent on explaining something. He seemed so gregarious, we were certain he was destined to be an early talker.

When Paul was 7 months old, we moved from Paris to a small, isolated cliffside village in the Luberon region of Provence, in southern France. The population of Bonnieux was not much more than 400 people who, it seemed to us, were either related or had known one another for generations. They probably had.

Like most small French villages, the town had no real children's facilities, no parks, no playground, not even—unusually—any central meeting places. And the rural French, as is their custom, preferred to stay within their families. Consequently, although we were greeted reasonably warmly by the townspeople, it was not easy to have our son play with other little children. Unlike the more child-oriented U.S., with its clubs and groups and organizations, French towns have few social possibilities for the very young. Consequently, Paul, who was our first child, began growing up in a kind of isolation. And without much parenting experience, we had little frame of reference in which to compare and situate his growth.

Yes, we read about all the milestones we were supposed to note, but parents are always cautioned not to take those things too literally. Every child is different, and so on. And not so unusually with an extremely high-functioning autistic child, everything at first did seem within normal parameters.

One day he would be able to turn onto his stomach from a sitting position . . . at 10 months, he got up himself after sleeping in his crib. Amazing! Of course, he did seem to shriek sometimes, rather than simply cry, but that was surely a difficult thing to judge.

When Paul was around 15 months old, we began to suspect there might be a problem. Friends from Paris had come to visit with their child, who was barely 6 weeks older than Paul, and we started to gain some perspective. While Céline romped around the public pool, splashed in the water, and seemed totally uninhibited, Paul was terrified even before nearing the pool's edge. He cried and screamed, resisting all efforts to put him in.

Our surprise at seeing another child play so adventurously made us even more aware of how isolated we all were, and also, perhaps, how overly cautious we had been with Paul. For we'd felt we had had to be protective. We had moved into a 16th-century stone house that, unfortunately, also appeared to have 16th-century wiring and plumbing. It was hardly "childproof." Between the steep stone stairway and the cracked tiles, the old-fashioned heater and the rotting beams, we had gotten into the habit of overseeing Paul's every move. Perhaps we had not let him experiment enough.

In an attempt to give him more independence—and also to reduce his isolation, as well as give us more of a frame of reference—we began bringing Paul to a *garderie* in Apt, the nearest larger town. In France, the social welfare system has supplied *garderies* and *crêches* (public day care centers) throughout the country for many years as an intrinsic part of the social safety net. Together with the government-run pre-kindergarten *maternelle* schools—which children can begin at 2 years of age—it has made private day care practically unnecessary.

The first few times at the *garderie,* which is specifically for part-time, episodic care, went very badly. Paul would cling desperately to us when we wanted to leave, and cry almost continuously when we were not there. The women running the *garderie* said Paul recoiled whenever any of the other children came near him.

They said he was probably just shy.

We said maybe he was just shy.

Paul's doctor, also our doctor, who was, in fact, the only doctor in town, assured us Paul was surely just shy—like *his* daughter had been at that age. Since we were first-time parents, it was understandable, he said, that we were overly concerned and did not realize some children can be extremely shy, yet perfectly normal.

In addition to that natural shyness, there was, of course, the language problem to accentuate it. After all, everybody at the *garderie* was speaking French to Paul, and that could not have been easy for him. In our household, French—although a frequent visitor—was an outsider, still a foreign language. When Paul was a newborn, we decided that we would speak English to him. Living in France—and particularly in an isolated village in the south—he would get his French everywhere: at the store, in the streets, at school, from our friends and acquaintances. But the only way he would get English would be from us. Our goal was for our son to grow up bilingual, as most of the children of other expatriated American friends had.

The difficulty, of course, was that high-functioning autism frequently first manifests itself as a communications problem. But hearing a foreign language can also interfere with one's ability to speak and understand effectively. Growing up bilingual can also cause a lag in the beginnings of spoken language, and limit vocabularies. Early on, children growing up bilingually have vocabularies of about half the size in each language as they would have if there was only one. Together, the total more or less equals that of one tongue.

We were not aware that bilingualism comes rather naturally to children. In our isolation, we considered that Paul might be understandably fearful because he could find French somewhat daunting, and perhaps see it as a foreign interloper in our home. After all, he had not yet heard very much of it. It was understandable, too, that his speech might be delayed, or that—as happened later on—he might speak awkwardly, haltingly. Could that not all simply be a function of having to juggle two languages?

It was more difficult to explain the extreme physical fearfulness, at the *garderie* and elsewhere. Outdoors, he would cling to us almost all the time, shrinking when others came near and refusing to walk without holding someone's hand. He would be terrified of the tiny steps at the entrance of our house. The most striking example was on our walks in town, when we would come to the curb at the end of the one-block-long main street. Paul refused to step up or down without a hand. Having to go an inch or two above or below ground level, he seemed paralyzed. We were not aware, then, of any motor planning problem; we did not even know the term.

With the exception of those moments of paralysis, the problems generally were never extreme. Eventually, for instance, he went back to the *garderie,* at first miserable, then unhappy, finally tolerating it—and, eventually, even loving it. It seemed like the normal progression, if perhaps slow.

But if there was improvement, there was also a cultural confusion that colored the situation much more positive than it really was. When we picked Paul up after a few hours at the *garderie*—or after he had spent time at a babysitter's—we were frequently told that "*c'était bien passé*" ("everything went well"), and he had been *très sage* (very well-behaved). The French are not nearly as child oriented nor fixated on their young as Americans. In most cases, they truly believe that little children should be seen and not heard. They view children as sort of miniature adults, and expect of them the same decorum. To be *sage* is almost the highest of compliments, and usually means the child did not cause any undue problems. What we began to understand later, though, was that everything was *bien passé* and Paul had been *sage* because he had spent the time sitting in the corner, not causing any trouble at all because he wasn't *doing* anything at all. The compliment of *très sage* came to be a terrifying code to us for a child curled up within himself.

When Paul was 2, we took him for his first trip to the U.S., to see family and friends. It was, predictably, a difficult period for us all. After several American stops, by the time we reached Paris on the way home, Paul was reeling. When we took him to a playground in the Luxemburg Gardens, he was almost rigid, refusing to even let go of our hand and petrified of climbing onto the equipment. He cried when we tried to get him to try, and recoiled when other children came near him. Perhaps for the first time, we realized then that something was seriously wrong.

In Paris, we decided to see an English-speaking pediatrician, a Frenchman whom we thought could understand the uniqueness of the bilingual situation. We wanted something more concrete than the theories already offered. The town doctor had said that Paul was *nerveux,* sort of high-strung. The same word had been used by the nurse's assistant who was in charge of the free monthly physicals that were given for infants at the town hall.

The Paris pediatrician told us that Paul had normal intelligence, but also some "personal problems" that were exacerbated by our isolation. He recommended that we consider a different life-style so that Paul would have the chance to play with other kids in small groups—and preferably English-speaking ones. Bilingualism was not the source of Paul's problems, he said, but was an obstacle to a solution.

A pediatrician down south, whom the Paris physician had recommended for a follow-up, suggested after a very cursory examination that we medicate Paul. Perhaps because of their national health system, which reimburses almost the entire price of prescription drugs, French physicians are far more likely than their American counterparts to medicate. It was always the first recourse.

It was not, however, *our* first resort. We never filled the prescription. We had a cranial X-ray done—it showed nothing unusual—and began to "commute" to a sandbox on the other side of the mountain, where children had been spied. We continued with the *garderie*.

At around 2½, Paul began speaking. But the fearfulness remained, and he stopped talking for a while, so we decided, finally, that it was time to investigate some kind of therapy.

The French came late to Freudian ideas. But when they did, they swallowed them whole. Greatly valuing style over substance, the French saw psychotherapy as a fascinating play of ideas and attitudes, a debating field for intellectual theorems. It wasn't necessarily, we were to find out, a practical means to a better life—as it frequently can be here.

The pediatric social services in Apt had a psychologist on staff, whom we began to see. At first we were thrilled—this calm, serious young woman took us seriously, and did not dismiss our concerns as the emotional, exaggerated worries of first-time, isolated parents. But her relationship with Paul was less successful.

The cornerstone of her approach, as it was for most professionals in the field, was language. In French psychotherapy, the word was everything. The word would unlock the psychic trauma—even if there was not one to unlock. Much attention was focused on Paul's "bilingualism," but since he barely spoke English then—and we were not sure how much French he understood—the therapy, if that was what it was, proceeded very slowly.

For months, she simply tried to get to know him. She would see how he would react to toys, what he would play with, if he'd react to her. And she'd listen to our complaints and fears. She gave Paul a number of nonverbal intelligence tests, and he passed with flying colors. We felt reassured. She told us the situation was not "*grave*," and that Paul was progressing. We greedily accepted her judgment.

While she could give us no definitive answers, the problems, she felt, had much to do with Paul's closeness to us, and the bilingualism. He had had to start again from zero in learning to talk, and we should be aware that he had to redo things. We should not judge his progress by his age. When we asked why other children in bilingual situations did not seem to have the same problems, the answers were always, well, each child is different, you know.

As to his fearfulness and difficulties with other kids, why that, she reasoned, could be the legacy of his restricted situation in Bonnieux and our overprotectiveness. It was a question of confidence, she explained in classic Freudian terminology. As he gradually became more self-assured, he would overcome the fears, become more sociable, and could "catch up."

To help him catch up, the psychologist suggested after 6 months of sessions that Paul would benefit from seeing an *éducatrice*. This was a standard procedure; literally, the word translates as "female educator," but neither an equivalent term nor the position exist over here. In fact, she was a sort of psychiatric social worker for children. The idea was for her to form a close, one-to-one relationship with Paul. Through that intense intimacy with someone other than his parents, and the occasional separation from us, went the theory, he would be more open to the world. Implicit, of course, was the view that Paul's problems were tied to that closeness to us.

Paul saw the *éducatrice* for over two years. During that time, the psychologist revised her opinion and admitted that Paul had "serious problems," but did not suggest any specific methods to improve his condition. The *éducatrice* was overseen by a psychiatrist, who concurred that the problems were serious, but they might be remediable as soon as we "unlocked the doors."

The psychiatrist kept talking about psychic trauma, neurosis, and infantile psychosis. Autism was never mentioned. Meanwhile, an American psychiatrist friend 3,000 miles away, who had not seen Paul since infancy, wrote in response to our questions that our child might be autistic. When we questioned the French professional about it, he replied that yes, Paul had "autistic tendencies," but whether he was autistic or not, we still had to unlock the same doors to his "emotional anguish." Until we could get to that anguish, there was no use in trying anything else, no point in attempting to teach Paul how to cope concretely with his problems. When we asked about speech therapy, he appeared bemused, and asked why we would want to waste our time. Occupational therapy was never even mentioned. Waiting to unlock those doors, it became clear to us, meant absolutely no need for any pragmatic services of any kind. The psychiatrist's psychological interpretation of the causes of autism was unshakable, as it was with most French professionals. They saw it very much the way Americans had about 25 years earlier.

Meanwhile, Paul had begun speaking much more, in both languages. But in both, the speech was halting, awkward, with tone and rhythm always a bit off. "Well, of course," French friends insisted, "he has two languages to learn. It's so much harder for him. Don't worry, he'll catch up."

At the *maternelle,* which he began at age 3, he seemed to understand and follow most things, but there were problems. During recess, while the other children ran madly around the playground, Paul sat on the bench with the teachers' assistants. He was always by himself, cut off from the other kids. His teachers attributed that to his biculturalism, the fact he was "different." They told us it would pass.

In the meantime, no one seemed in much of a hurry to do something that would help him *now.* While everyone was waiting, we felt that on a day-to-day basis, he wasn't improving very much. *We* didn't want to wait.

When Paul was a little more than 4, we brought him to the States to see if we could get a complete diagnosis of his condition. The results, as we had suspected, were clear: Paul was high-functioning autistic. He would need to be taught many skills, and would require treatment and support. Could we find in France, our adopted home, the facilities and support services we would need for Paul?

Lee Marcus, of the TEACCH center at The University of North Carolina at

Chapel Hill, put us in touch with Gloria Laxer, the founder of an emerging, parent-oriented French autism society. When we returned to France, Madame Laxer invited us to the organization's annual conference, just about to take place. It would be a way to find out quickly what services were available, and to get an overview of French attitudes toward autism.

For two days in the town of Vichy, we listened. We heard mostly parents and some renegade professionals—and foreign observers, too—complain of the state of things in France. We heard that the French government, always the leader in social planning, had done almost nothing about autism. The medical establishment was adamant that autism was a psychological problem. That left it up to the parents themselves to create schools and services, and they were just beginning to try.

Despite the negativism, we still hoped there might be some program, somewhere in France. After all, it was our home. During a conference break, we talked with Gloria Laxer about what possibilities might still be there for us. We spoke French, and in the middle of the conversation, she suddenly stopped, paused a moment, and then began speaking English, as if to make absolutely sure we would understand.

"Go back to America," she said gently.

We did.

AUTISTIC ECCENTRICITY

Margaret A. Dewey

Some hours since starting my speech, I sit surrounded by old letters, clippings, offprints, and books. As yet, I have not found the parental quotation I was looking for. Words such as *weird, strange, bizarre,* and *eccentric* have come up often. Now I realize that I hardly need to single out one parent for having observed that autistic behavior can go far beyond what one ordinarily associates with the word *eccentric*.

I had planned to open this essay with a quotation I dimly remembered. Some other parent of an autistic son has described the sense of relief she shared with her husband when they first heard the prognosis for their child. He would probably remain somewhat eccentric for the rest of his life, the good doctor had warned. Eccentric? That didn't sound so bad. After all, a lot of successful people are somewhat eccentric. "Little did we know what lay ahead!" was the remark I was looking for.

Is there, then, an essential difference between autistic eccentricity and the garden variety eccentricity that almost any person might display on occasion? How can autistic eccentricity be recognized and related to the basic handicap? What, if anything, is the value of trying to modify eccentric behavior in autistic people? My reflections will be based on many autistic people I have known, as well as the one most intimately known to us. That is our 41-year-old son, Jack, who now lives nearby in his own little house, supporting himself as a piano tuner.

When nonautistic people adopt eccentric behavior, they have made a conscious choice to be different for any of a number of reasons. A strong conviction may be at the root of their decision, as in the example of parents who elect to educate their children outside of schools. Sometimes necessity inspires odd behavior, for which I will offer the example of a traveler washing some soiled clothing in a public restroom. Quite a few individuals seek attention by deliberately doing bizarre things, especially in highly competitive fields such as rock music. In spite of such diverse motives for eccentric behavior, nonautistic people have in common one thing that is generally lacking in autism. They are aware that most people will view their unusual behavior as odd.

I am sure that the motives I have listed for eccentric behavior can also be found in autistic people. They, too, can act from a strong conviction. They can be driven by necessity, and they can seek attention. Beneath the veneer of sameness that autism imposes, one can find a wide range of personality variations and an infinite variety of personal experiences. I will not be concerned with why an autistic person might want to eat health foods, for example, because lots of people make that choice, but why he calls a hostess and tells her exactly how she should prepare his dinner down to the last pinch of seasoning. And why would he have no sense that he had done anything out of the ordinary? Even if challenged to imagine how his hostess might feel about such a request, he would be likely to offer an oblique answer such as "That's the healthy way to cook food." If pressed, he might add, "She should know about it. Somebody should tell her."

Few autistic people would behave in exactly this way. Yet many would unknowingly do something else equally inappropriate in an unfamiliar social situation. The key word is *unknowingly*. They are not at the time aware that other people regard their behavior as unusual.

I believe that the unique quality of autistic eccentricity can be traced to the lack of a theory of mind as described by Leslie and Frith (1987, 1988). *Theory of mind* refers to the fluid, ongoing awareness of mental states in ourselves and other people—that is, knowing what we know and how we know it, while at the same time being able to assess different knowledge, expectations, and emotions in other people.

To understand autistic eccentricity one must go beyond person-to-person knowing and include the social mind of a particular society. By that I mean the "mind" that is implied by the words *most people* in the following sentences:

What would most people think in this situation?
What would most people expect me to do now?
What do most people assume I understand?
What can I assume most people understand without being told?
How would most people interpret my behavior in this situation?

Life can be exceedingly difficult for adults who have a very limited understanding of the social mind. It even can be hazardous, as the following example suggests.

> Jack's employer wants him to tune the store pianos outside of business hours. Usually this means just before opening and just after closing. One night Jack could not sleep, so he decided to go to the store and work. A police officer who happened to glance down an alley saw a man scurrying with a tool box in the darkest hour of night. (You know what most people would think in such a suspicious circumstance.) Luckily for Jack, this officer did not shout, "Freeze! I've got you covered." At that, Jack might well have fled in panic. But he was merely asked to step forward and identify himself, stating his business in the alley. Everything checked out. He had a business card, tuning tools, and a key that fit the exit door of the store nearby. A potential tragedy was averted.

The subject of jumping to conclusions came up once when I was on jury duty. During a break when we could not discuss our case, I mentioned the incident involving Jack in the dark alley. One juror's face lit up. "Oh, I think I know your son," she said. "He must be the Jack Dewey who tuned my piano. We just loved him. But I thought he had some kind of physical handicap. Why does he always hold his head to one side facing down?"

Jack's gaze aversion is pronounced. I invited the jurors to take a simple test: They were to multiply two numbers in their heads (such as 6 times 47) while at the same time looking into the eyes of the next person. A ripple of laughter went around the table as they discovered they were compelled to gaze into space before they could concentrate on such a simple task.

For Jack, listening to people and trying to figure out what they mean is a mind-consuming task. He also needs to focus on his own contribution to a conversation. He tells us that when he looks at people the messages in their eyes confuse him. It would be like trying to figure income tax while listening to a news broadcast.

In yet another category of strangeness, autistic people display distinctive mannerisms. They have ways of walking, rocking, or moving their hands that set them apart. Some of this may be the result of a high level of anxiety. The classic startle posture of a human being resembles the stance of an autistic person with body leaning forward and muscles tense, arms flexed at the elbow. Experience may teach an autistic person always to be alert for the unexpected.

Add to this the anxiety created by dire warnings. Guided by the best of intentions, we burden autistic people with rules and countless variations of rules. Though we sometimes chide them for behaving like robots, we are guilty of programming them for survival in society as if they were, in fact, humanoid computers. It should not be surprising that those who are especially eager to please would take on a mechanical quality occasionally. Unlike robots, they retain the ability to do some unpredictable things on their own initiative.

> In a grocery store where I shop there is a young woman whose behavior, speech, and mannerisms strongly suggest autism. She first worked as a bagger, then moved up to shelving stock. One day I heard her distinctive loud voice in the next aisle. An older employee seemed to be talking to her earnestly about something she was wearing, but I could not make out what that person was

> saying. "Why not?" the girl protested in dismay. "Other people have them. I happen to like mine." When I rounded the corner I saw what the conversation was about—a tiny mustache. The meager amount of fuzz on her upper lip had been darkened with makeup and twirled at the ends. Actually, it was rather cute. Yet most people would think it quite bizarre for a young woman to embellish her lip hair unless she had a reason to want to hide her feminine identity.

Here we have eccentric behavior that was deliberate, but done without awareness of the effect on others. Sometimes an autistic person is painfully aware of certain odd behaviors, but unable to control them. One charming young autistic woman, very high-functioning indeed, is dismayed because she sometimes makes strange noises at inappropriate times. This happens in spite of a great deal of therapy that has been directed at eliminating this unconscious behavior. Attention focused on such a mannerism may actually increase the likelihood that it will recur. I myself had a unique experience with negative suggestion.

> When our junior high school hosted a teachers' conference, I was asked to be a guide. My specific duty was to stand at the foot of a staircase and ask visitors, "May I show you upstairs?" A waggish friend decided to tease me by warning over and over, "Be sure you don't say 'May I throw you upstairs?' " The idea was ludicrous because I was a confident person with facile speech. On the evening of the conference I could hardly believe my ears when I heard my voice ask the first group, "May I throw you upstairs?" In more than half a century since that evening I cannot count the number of times the word *show* has been usurped by *throw*. Just the other day I said to a clerk in a fabric store, "Let me throw you the color."

Some persistent mannerisms may be this much beyond an autistic person's control. If so, they should not be relentlessly pursued. I mention them in this essay only because unusual mannerisms are one noticeable aspect of autistic eccentricity.

Odd mannerisms do not belong exclusively to autism. Lots of people have them. The same can be said of obsessions and compulsions. Sometimes the compulsions of autistic people have a unique quality that does point to autism, however. One man feels compelled to run his hand around the inner frame of every doorway he passes through, as if removing spider webs. Other compulsions of autistic people I know are common in the general population, such as needing to double-check locks and stove burners.

It is often said that autistic people lack empathy. This is certainly the impression when they fail to take accurate account of the emotions of other people. But in cases where the pain or suffering of other people is spelled out clearly—as in a headline, "Children Are Dying From Hunger"—the autistic person can show as much deep concern as any other caring and sensitive person. Those autistic individuals who worry about the welfare of other people, as Jack does, can become quite emotionally involved in the real or imagined sufferings of others. Here is an example of misplaced concern on Jack's part, a reflection of something that matters very much to him. (This was reported by a teacher.)

> The assignment in Jack's civics class in high school was to hand in an original suggestion for a constitutional amendment. Jack turned in the recommendation that the constitution should be amended to require every home to have a piano with 88 keys, and to require that the piano be kept in tune.

Lest you think that Jack was craftily aiming to provide himself with a huge income in the future, be assured that he had no idea that he would earn his living as a tuner when he submitted this item. At that time, he thought he would be a composer. Years later, when he became a tuner, he was so distressed by the need for his services that he donated uncounted hours to teaching other people how to tune. He never worried that this would create competition for jobs, and he did not charge his pupils anything. No, the truth of the matter is that when Jack realized that many homes did not have pianos, and many pianos were painfully out of tune (to his ears), he assumed that other people would feel as bad about this situation as he did. Though he outgrew the notion that it could be corrected by a constitutional amendment, he still takes his work as seriously as a doctor who is dedicated to making sick people healthy.

In case you wonder, Jack gladly gives me permission to tell stories about him. Like many other high-functioning autistic people, he is pleased if he thinks that he has helped other people by being candid about some of his mistaken judgments. Talking about them in the past tense reminds him that he has learned a lot from experience. Here are several short examples of the kind of difficulty Jack has had with assessing our minds.

> About 10 years ago we were watching Beverly Sills perform an operatic selection on TV. When it was finished, Jack said casually, "She liked my tuning." We turned to him in surprise, "Why, Jack, you never told us you had tuned for Beverly Sills!" "I didn't know you knew her," he replied.

Apparently, Beverly had been in Ann Arbor for a performance, and Jack was asked to tune the piano that accompanied her. He has done many concert tunings, so he saw no reason to mention this one to us. Yet, on other occasions, he would enter our house on a Saturday evening with a greeting something like this:

> "Hey, Mother and Father, guess who I tuned for this week!" He is excited, but we can't guess, so he tells us, "Mrs. Hall." That doesn't ring a bell, so we ask, "Who is Mrs. Hall?" "The mother of Ricky Hall. He was in my first grade class."

Jack's keen memory for selected people and events in his early life may be nothing unusual. Everybody has a few vivid memories from early years. The difference with Jack is that he assumes we understand his references without any explanation. Or, conversely, he feels obliged to explain things we would obviously know from context. Not long ago I was puzzled by a reference to someone named Sally. This is the way it happened:

> We were sharing a garden melon with Jack when he commented, "Sally did not like muskmelon. Then she tried some and found out that she liked it after all." I

> pondered this, and asked him to tell me who Sally is. "Dick and Jane's little sister," he replied. After an interlude of 35 years he was making this casual reference to a character in a preprimer.

Although I had forgotten about Sally in intervening years, I still feel a debt of gratitude to the books. Jack approached the usual age for kindergarten without normal speech. He would make his needs known by echoing phrases he had heard earlier. Imagine what the teacher would think if he came to her and asked, "Do you need to use the bathroom?" to indicate that *he* wanted to go. My husband, a language professor, observed that Jack used language as if he were a foreigner with a phrase book. Jack seemed to have a rough idea of what his phrases meant, but he could not handle the components or the nuances. We decided to try to teach Jack basic English as a language teacher does, beginning with reading and writing a simple vocabulary.

This was not a big operation. It was just something that various family members would do with Jack. I doubt that we averaged an hour a day. His older brother and sister were able to get copies of the Dick and Jane books at their school. At first, Jack resisted, wriggling off our laps. I would hold his arms loosely, but tighten my grip if he tried to escape. This way, it was more comfortable for him to stay on my lap and let me talk about words and pictures. The colorful illustrations said a lot without words. I suspect that the word *muskmelon* was not in the preprimer. What Jack would remember is that Sally made a face and pushed her melon away with words such as, "No, no. I do not want to eat this." Maybe the next picture was of Mother looking sternly across the table with the words, "I want you to try it, Sally. It is good." (This is just speculation on my part.) Jack had worn out the books within a year. He learned to read and write with the vocabulary of Dick and Jane. By the age of 6, he talked well enough to start kindergarten.

This digression gave me a chance to point out the symptom of echolalia. It seemed eccentric to us before we learned that it is typical of autistic children. From the beginning, our little boy was different, and words such as *odd* and *peculiar* came often to mind. My mother once remarked, "How strange that Jackie cannot answer a simple yes-or-no question when he can sing any song in the book." Autistic eccentricity is not limited to adults, although it takes different forms at different ages.

In telling the story about Sally, I implied that her mother had urged her to try the melon before condemning it. Perhaps that thought stems from my experience with a young autistic man I call Michael.

> Michael called us from a nearby state to ask whether he could visit our home. I assured him that he would be welcome. His parents are good friends, and we knew they would do the same for Jack. However, I trust that they would treat him somewhat differently from the usual houseguest. I would want them to be outspoken if necessary to guide his behavior in their home. This explains my candor with Michael. When Michael saw the casserole I carried to the table for lunch, he left the table to look in our refrigerator for something more to his liking. I asked, "Does your mother ever tell you to try things she has prepared

> before you decide you do not like them?" "Oh, yes," Michael conceded cheerfully. "She always wants me to do that. In her house I do it. But other people let me get what I want when I am at their house." I told Michael that I happened to feel like his mother. Thereupon he put a generous serving of the casserole on his plate.
>
> Michael next asked for a pepper mill. We watched first in fascination, then in horror, as his steady grinding continued. Finally I said, "That's a lot of pepper, Michael. It will burn your mouth." No problem. He explained that he wanted to hide the taste of the food. His plate resembled a mound of fireplace ashes, completely gray. And he ate it all.

We parents can never take for granted that the social lessons we try to instill at home will be applied elsewhere. An autistic person may assume that parents are a fussy breed whose peculiar demands must be indulged, but only while they are present.

There is another complication in the transfer of social training from the home to other houses. Autistic people are likely to make themselves too much "at home" when they are elsewhere. Over the years, autistic people of many ages have come through our door. With few exceptions, they tend to wander unabashedly through the house. Some have opened cupboards and closets, some have decided without asking to play a record or help themselves to food. One little boy even went to the basement and climbed into our laundry chute to see what kind of detergent we used. No harm was done. We did not mind because we understood all too well.

I am puzzled by a few autistic people whose social awareness seems markedly better than I have come to expect. Aside from obvious variations in the degree of severity of the autistic handicap, there may be some differences in the innate social abilities. Howard Gardner (1983) suggests that the quality of mind that we call intelligence is actually seven distinct and different intelligences that work together. They are: linguistic, musical, mathematical–logical, bodily–kinesthetic, spatial, intrapersonal, and interpersonal.

Gardner offers impressive evidence to support his theory. It is not necessary for me to go into that here, because one can speculate about the implications for autism without requiring absolute proof of the correctness of the theory. My first thought was that autism might be defined as severe impairment of interpersonal intelligence. But on reflection I realized that various handicaps can impair the normal development of individual intelligence. For example, without vision, a baby's spatial intelligence will not develop in the usual way. Yet he or she still has that intelligence and uses it to learn to get around. Some may do better than others.

Or consider the case of a girl severely crippled by cerebral palsy. There is no way that her bodily–kinesthetic intelligence can develop normally. Yet, if she has good innate capacity for using this particular intelligence, it may help her in adapting to her physical limitations.

The same line of reasoning can be applied to autism and interpersonal intelligence. Parents readily admit that their children have different inclinations or talents when it comes to other intelligences (such as musical and mathematical). Why not accept that there can be innate variations among autistic people in their use of interpersonal skills as well?

As for the value of trying to modify eccentric autistic behavior, there can be no pat answer. If we are talking about something that causes harm or acute embarrassment, an extensive effort may be worthwhile. But there comes a point where constant reminders amount to nagging, and nagging begins to take the joy out of living. Do we dare hope that the public can learn to accept some harmless eccentricity in autistic people? After seeing the reaction to *Rain Man,* I believe so.

The behavior of high-functioning autistic adults is often summed up as eccentric. Yet we know that eccentricity is not unique to autism. Normal people as well as autistic individuals may do odd things to attract attention, to make a statement about their individuality, or to uphold a strong conviction.

In general, normal people are aware of their deviations from normal behavior, whereas autistic people are often eccentric without awareness or intention. Their difficulties with interpersonal relationships and preoccupations with special interests can make them seem strange even when they are trying their best to fit in unobtrusively. The cognitive disorder of autism may interfere with their ability to judge appropriate social behavior by taking account of subtle cues in shifting situations.

References

Gardner, H. (1983). *Frames of mind: The theory of multiple intelligences.* New York: Basic Books.

Leslie, A. M., & Frith, U. (1987). Metarepresentation and autism: How not to lose one's marbles. *Cognition, 27,* 291–294.

Leslie, A. M., & Frith, U. (1988). Autistic children's understanding of seeing, knowing, and believing. *British Journal of Developmental Psychology, 6,* 315–324.

14

Personal Essays

AUTISTIC ADULTHOOD: A CHALLENGING JOURNEY

Anne Carpenter

The purpose of this essay is to discuss the problems I have encountered as a high-functioning adult with autism trying to make her way into the world of work, dating, marriage and family, and participation in society as a whole. Because of the many difficulties associated with autism, this has been twice as hard to accomplish, and I am still trying to break through the barriers that have been set before me. I have omitted the term *high-functioning* from the title because once a person is diagnosed as autistic, he or she *remains* autistic for an indefinite period of time. Despite a higher level of functioning, a person like me still has difficulty being a fully participating member of society. Before one can explore the present, it is necessary to go back to where everything originates: childhood and adolescence.

I was born in early 1957 with congenital rubella, as a result of my mother's illness during her first trimester of pregnancy. The resulting problems included cataracted lenses in both eyes, nerve deafness in my right ear, and an open heart valve. Both of my lenses were removed at 2 and 3 months of age, and my heart valve was repaired at 7 months of age.

Unfortunately, a far more serious problem remained. My central nervous system had been wounded by this trauma, and I had a severe developmental delay. I had a weak sucking reflex, did not walk until I was 2, and said one word at 1½, then did not talk again until I was 5. I was placed in a day program at Children's Psychiatric Hospital, where I was first diagnosed as autistic. While I was in the program, I made a great deal of progress; I finally started talking, and I learned how to drink from a cup.

ANNE CARPENTER • 2200 Fuller Road 705-B, Ann Arbor, Michigan 48105. JIM SINCLAIR • P.O. Box 1545, Lawrence, Kansas 66044. THERESE MARIE RONAN • 9307 Slater, Overland Park, Kansas 66212. KATHY LISSNER • 3649 Dunnica, St. Louis, Missouri 63116.

High-Functioning Individuals with Autism, edited by Eric Schopler and Gary B. Mesibov. Plenum Press, New York, 1992.

At the age of 4, I entered a special program for blind and partially sighted children because I was considered to be legally blind. I was not able to talk during the eye examinations, so the ophthalmologist had no way of knowing how to assess my vision correctly. I was given glasses that were based on the best estimate of my visual ability. During the four years that I was in the program, I was mainstreamed into the regular first- and second-grade classrooms. When I was 8, I was prescribed different glasses and was no longer eligible to attend the special program I was in. At the same time, I had serious behavior problems in the second grade because I felt threatened by the teacher. I was assigned to Pattengill School with a black mark on my record.

Nobody understood why I behaved the way I did: jumping out of my seat, interrupting people, making odd noises, throwing temper tantrums. I was placed in Mr. T's room, a classroom of emotionally disturbed boys with whom I did not get along. "What would you like to do during free time?" he had asked. "Read," was my reply. "She's sicker than I am," one of the boys had said. I didn't fit in, and Mr. T. was way too strict. I *hated* that classroom! After a week, Mr. T. realized that I was in the wrong place. "Get her out of here," he said. So, much to my relief, I was put in the regular second and third grade for two years. But I ran into some problems with two girls from very poor families who took advantage of my vulnerability. I was picked on, spat at, and hit on a number of occasions.

In 1967, my mother read a book about minimal brain dysfunction edited by Dr. William Cruikshank and discovered that I had all the symptoms: I was very hyperactive, had difficulties with coordination and motor skills, could not concentrate on any one task for more than a few minutes at a time, and had a serious developmental lag. Dr. Cruikshank was associated with Dr. Sheldon Rapaport, who directed the Pathway School in Pennsylvania, where I went to school for two and a half years. It was there that I learned how to swim, ride a bicycle, write in cursive, and to screen out extraneous stimuli more effectively by sitting in a carrel when I studied.

However, the staff wanted me to stay an extra year to "consolidate my gains"; my social skills were not as well developed, and I did not know *how* to relate comfortably to other people. I did not know when to say something or when not to say something, and I often said and did embarrassing things, such as belching, doing what my grandfather called "coughing in my trousers," and asking questions that were out of context.

Nevertheless, I went to a Quaker-run school in Detroit for four years, until the end of my sophomore year in high school, then went to a Quaker boarding school in Iowa for a year. I spent my last year of high school in Ann Arbor, at an alternative school, then went to Thomas Jefferson College in Allendale, Michigan, for 4 years. I graduated in 1980, then attended graduate school in library science at Western Michigan University, in Kalamazoo. I got my Master of Science in Librarianship in 1982, and thought that the world was my oyster!

But I had a faint, though nagging, feeling that there were rough seas ahead. Because of my lack of social ability, the staff at the library school had reservations about my career choice even though I went on to obtain my degree. After graduation, I was placed in a volunteer library job with the Washtenaw County Library through vocational rehabilitation services. A month later, in early June of 1982, I was asked to leave because of inappropriate behavior. In a conference with my counselor, it was revealed that I had interrupted the supervisor several times because I did not know what to do next, conversed with other staff members at the wrong times, and needed constant help with the IBM Selectric typewriter. I became upset very easily and was never *quite* sure how to handle certain situations. It is very difficult for even a high-functioning autistic adult to know exactly when to say something, when to ask for help, or when to remain quiet. To such a person, life is a game in which the rules are constantly changing without rhyme or reason.

It was thought that Innisfree Village, a community for mentally handicapped adults near Charlottesville, Virginia, would benefit me in a number of ways: I could obtain a library job in Charlottesville, live in a community with a built-in support system, and learn how to change my behavior. At first, I lived in the village itself, a beautiful rural enclave nestled beneath the Blue Ridge mountains, where I wove brightly colored belts and baked rolls with a group of adults with developmental disabilities. Then, I lived in one of the "in town" houses in Charlottesville. There, I lived with a couple who seemed displeased with the fact that I had obtained a master's degree in library science yet behaved so oddly. It was as if I were a different entity altogether.

Despite all the accomplishments I had made, I felt that I was losing ground. Because this particular couple had their own personal problems and because they did not know how to deal with my puzzling behavior, I was yelled at, cajoled, and treated in a demeaning fashion. There was no way of determining how I would fit into the Innisfree program, so I was assigned a number of different jobs as a rough estimate of my abilities was formed. These included volunteer tutoring of handicapped children in an after-school program, a period of work in the new pottery workshop in the basement of my residence, and several months at a sheltered workshop in Charlottesville that I was placed in through vocational rehabilitation services.

In the sheltered workshop, I performed data entry on a computer terminal, but it did not work out. Again, I interrupted the supervisor, got upset when I did not know how to use the computer, and made many errors in my work. After that, I performed other tasks, such as assembling telephone handsets and cleaning circuit boards. All that time, I felt as though I were working below my potential, outside my training and abilities. However, like many autistic people, my skills were uneven. While I had excellent verbal and intellectual skills, my social skills were farther behind. I still talked about myself a great deal without regarding the other person and what he or she was involved in, talked on the same topic repeatedly, and could not make eye contact. I would not have been able to perform such aspects of librarianship as reference or childrens' services because my poor social skills would have been a serious impediment to successful employment.

Because the symptoms of autism are so variable and so little understood, a high-functioning person such as I would be more likely to be placed in an inappropriate work or social situation. Toward the end of 1983, my mother and I realized that there was not any possibility of a library job in Charlottesville and that this particular community was not the right place for me after all.

In January of 1984, I returned to Ann Arbor and lived with my mother in an apartment near town. I renewed my connection with Vocational Rehabilitation Services with the hope of finding a job, but was unable to find work for many months due to the lack of acceptance of people with autism. It was very hard for my counselor to find suitable employment for someone with such uneven abilities.

In August of that year, I started indexing the *Chicago Tribune* at home on a part-time basis for a local company. However, I was never able to deal with the subtle nuances of the work: Which subject heading should I use? Should I index this editorial? I could not figure out the answers. This was a problem that I had had in other jobs as well. I could not generalize from one situation to another and could not deal with the many complexities involved in any one task—a typical problem in autistic people.

I was let go from this job primarily for that reason, although my supervisor greatly admired my work and wanted me to continue. In addition to this, the job was a temporary one and the company was eliminating certain positions. For months after that, I sought employment only to be badly disappointed. My favorite counselor at Michigan Rehabilitation Services moved out of the state and was replaced by several others, all very kind and more than willing to help. However, due to the amorphous nature of autism and the resistance that society feels toward hiring people with disabilities, my counselors and I were, in essence, butting our heads against a brick wall.

In hopes of boosting my job qualifications, I took a number of computer-related courses at the local community college. During that time, I worked as an aide in the microcomputer lab, assisting students in the use of the IBM PCs. I worked there for a few months, and the supervisor was intending to have me stay on through fall. However, another unforeseen problem arose. The lab was reorganized, and there was concern about my ability to read the computer screens from a distance. Although my vision had been 20/40 (20/30 with contact lenses) for quite some time, people often assume that it is much worse than it actually is.

Because autism involves a deficit in sensory processing and because autistic behavior is often very puzzling, people with this syndrome can be mistaken for individuals with vision or hearing impairments when in fact their vision or hearing may be intact or at least less severely affected. This has been a problem that I have encountered many times, because I peer closely at objects and scrutinize what I see. My eyes are very sensitive to light, and I squint as a result. This has been one of my major stumbling blocks.

My course work in computers proved only to be a band-aid solution; there was still no answer as to why I lost one job after another, why I was so inappropriate in social situations, and why I behaved the way I did. Was it some as-yet-unnamed neurological problem that had been lurking in the shadows for years? No one was sure what to do about it. I had been assigned many labels: mentally retarded, emotionally disturbed, borderline personality disorder, aggressive personality disorder. But those labels were only a shot in the dark.

The answer came in late 1987, when my mother and I were trying for a Social Security reconsideration (I had been rejected two times for disability benefits). The financial officer at the local chapter of the Association for Retarded Citizens gave my mother a handout about autism, thinking that this was a possibility that had not yet been explored.

My mother read the handout and then recommended Temple Grandin's book *Emergence: Labelled Autistic*. I read the book, and all the fixations, the repetitive conversations about the same topic, and the weird mannerisms came back to me. It was as if my whole personality were contained in the pages of that book! Upset, but also relieved, I knew that this was it—I was definitely autistic. In October of that year, I was officially diagnosed as having autism by Dr. Andrew Maltz at the Grosse Pointe Center for Individual and Family Therapy in Grosse Pointe Park, Michigan.

That diagnosis was to be the force that would change my life. Now that there was a name to that monstrous problem I had been carrying around for years, maybe I could find ways to eliminate at least some of the odd and socially unappealing behaviors. Over the ensuing months, I became calmer and happier. In May of 1988, I started working as a librarian at the Michigan Society for Autistic Citizens in Lansing. In the process of cataloging the books in the small collection, I was developing better work habits.

I have become very close to the small core staff at MSAC, and through gentle coaching and reminders have attenuated the constant questioning, the strange habits, and the lack of concentration. I can now catch myself in an inappropriate act and stop myself accordingly. I have demonstrated to myself that I *can* work under pressure; when something needs to be done quickly, I can now do it without flying off the handle.

I feel much better about myself now. I like what I have become, and the changes that I have been making in the last two years have been a contributing factor to this improved attitude. A new self-confidence has blossomed, and the old anxiety is losing its grip. I am now living independently in my own apartment.

Because of the changes I have made and am continuing to make, the aspects of adult life that I would like to have happen (a full-time job, marriage, a family, and travel to foreign countries) may be more likely to occur in the new decade that we are entering. Although it is very difficult for a high-functioning autistic adult to navigate in a society that does not understand this curious disorder, I think it is possible. But that person has to really *want* to change abnormal responses to stimuli and to eliminate behavior that is disturbing to people in the outside world. Motivation is the key.

The movie *Rain Man* and the recent research conducted by Eric Courchesne in

San Diego that revealed a cerebellar abnormality in some autistic people has generated new interest in this disease, and may make society more willing to meet the needs of this particular population of developmentally disabled adults.

In concluding, I am reminded of a saying that I have seen on a number of items sold in a religious bookstore: "Please be patient, God is not finished with me yet."

BRIDGING THE GAPS: AN INSIDE-OUT VIEW OF AUTISM (OR, DO YOU KNOW WHAT I DON'T KNOW?)

Jim Sinclair

In May of 1989, I drove 1,200 miles to attend the 10th annual TEACCH conference, where I learned that autistic people can't drive.

No, let's see if I can make that a little less simplistic:

In May of 1989, I drove 1,200 miles to attend the 10th annual TEACCH conference, where I spent two days among people who knew something about what autism means. They didn't think being autistic means being mentally retarded, being emotionally disturbed, or being deliberately obnoxious. They didn't think being spaced out means not paying attention. They didn't think an uneven performance means not trying. They did know about spacing out, and about sensory overload, and about not understanding things other people take for granted. They had a vocabulary for talking about my life.

And almost 10 years after I struggled through driver's training wondering what was wrong with me that I had so much trouble learning to drive, I learned there was an awful lot right with me that I learned to drive at all.

I've been living with autism for 27 years. But I'm just beginning to learn about what that *means*. I grew up hearing the word but never knowing what was behind it. My parents did not attend programs to learn about autism, did not collect literature to educate schools about autism, did not explain—to me or to anyone else—why my world was not the same one that normal people lived in.

(Should parents tell their autistic children that they are autistic? I think so. If the children notice words at all, they already know the word is being used about them. But be sure to tell them what it means. I was told that it meant, among other things, being dumb, crazy, malicious, uncaring, and unmotivated.)

It wasn't so much new facts that I got from this conference. It was new meanings and new perspectives for understanding the facts. I heard professionals describing problems autistic people *have,* not problems autistic people *are*. I heard parents recognizing their children's difficulties, instead of casting themselves as victims of their children's existence. I heard professionals acknowledging their own limitations, without blaming their clients when the help they had to offer was not enough. I heard parents talking about their own frustrations and disappointments, without accusing their children of cheating them by being what they were. Above all, I heard people discussing autism in terms of *not understanding*, rather than *not caring*.

I understand a lot about not understanding. I usually understand when I don't understand something, and I'm beginning to be able to recognize gaps between what I actually understand and what other people *assume* I understand. Some of the missing connections that I can finally name are funny, and some are sad, and some are infuriating. I'm sure there are many that I haven't noticed or that I don't have words for yet. But here are some of the words that I have found, and here are some of the gaps that I hope they can help fill.

Being Autistic Does Not Mean Being Mentally Retarded

Being autistic does not mean being unable to learn. But it does mean there are differences in *how* learning happens. Input–output equipment may work in nonstandard ways. Connections between different sensory modes or different items of stored data may be atypical; processing may be more narrowly or more broadly focused than is considered normal. But what I think is even more basic, and more frequently overlooked, is that autism involves differences in what is known *without* learning.

Simple, basic skills such as recognizing people and things presuppose even simpler, more basic skills such as knowing how to attach meaning to visual stimuli. Understanding speech requires knowing how to process sounds—which first requires recognizing sounds as things that can be processed, and recognizing processing as a way to extract order from chaos. Producing speech (or producing any other kind of motor behavior) requires keeping track of all the body parts involved, and coordinating all their movements. Producing any behavior in response to any perception requires monitoring and coordinating all the inputs and outputs at once, and doing it fast enough to keep up with changing inputs that may call for changing outputs. Do you have to remember to plug in your eyes in order to make sense of what you're seeing? Do you have to find your legs before you can walk? Autistic children may be born not knowing how to eat. Are these normally skills that must be acquired through *learning?*

These are the gaps that I notice most often: gaps between what is expected to be learned and what is assumed to be already understood. Even when I can point to the gap and ask for information about what goes there, my questions are usually ignored, treated as jokes, or met with incredulity, suspicion, or hostility. I'm penalized for my intelligence—people become impatient when I don't understand things they think I'm "smart enough" to know already or to figure out for myself.

Being bright only means I'm good at learning; it doesn't mean I know things without having to learn them first. Figuring things out and finding connections between different parts of a whole are what I do best, and I get a lot of practice because not many of the connections go into place by themselves. But I still have to know what all the parts are before I can find the connections between them.

Assumptions that I know things which in fact I don't understand often lead directly to conclusions that I can't learn things which in fact I already know. Such assumptions nearly led to my being placed in an institution. Because I didn't use speech to communicate until I was 12, there was considerable doubt about whether I would ever be able to learn to function independently. No one guessed how much I understood, because I couldn't say what I knew. And no one guessed the critical thing I *didn't* know, the one missing connection that so much else depended on: I didn't communicate by talking, not because I was incapable of learning to use language, but because I simply didn't know that was what talking was for. Learning *how* to talk follows from knowing *why* to talk—and until I learned that words have meanings, there was no reason to go to the trouble of learning to pronounce them as sounds. Speech therapy was just a lot of meaningless drills in repeating meaningless sounds for incomprehensible reasons. I had no idea that this could be a way to exchange meaning with other minds.

Not all the gaps are caused by my failure to *share* other people's unthinking assumptions. Other people's failure to *question* their assumptions creates at least as many barriers to understanding. The most damaging assumptions—the causes of the most painful misunderstandings—are the same now as they were when I was a child who couldn't talk, a teenager who couldn't drive, and a college student who couldn't get a job: assumptions that I understand what is expected of me, that I know how to do it, and that I fail to perform as expected out of deliberate spite or unconscious hostility.

Other people's assumptions are usually much more resistant to learning than my ignorance. As a graduate student, I encountered these assumptions in employers who had extensive backgrounds in special education. Presumably these people (one of whom was the director of a university-affiliated facility) had access to up-to-date information about developmental disabilities. But they never bothered to apply that information to the things they "knew" without thinking, and the things they expected me to know without learning.

At the same time I had a friend—not a parent driven by love and obligation to want to reach me, not a professional who made a career of studying my condition, but just someone who thought I was interesting enough to want to get to know better—a friend who, with no formal background in psychology or special education, figured out for herself some guidelines for relating to me. She told me what they were: never to assume without asking that I thought, felt, or understood *anything* merely because *she* would have such thoughts, feelings, or understanding in connection with my circumstances or behavior; and never to assume without asking that I *didn't* think, feel, or understand anything merely because I was *not* acting the way she would act in connection with such thoughts, feelings, or understanding. In other words, she learned to *ask* instead of trying to *guess*.

Are these really such difficult ideas to grasp? Are there people who are so certain they know without learning what other people are inside that they *can't* learn to understand anyone who isn't like them? Is that what it means to have "empathy"?

Being Autistic Does Not Mean Being Emotionally Disturbed

Not all the gaps involve facts and ideas. A woman at the conference wondered how she could help her autistic daughter to be able to talk about her feelings. I asked if she had ever tried to teach her daughter what feeling-words mean. Did she talk to her daughter about her own feelings? Did she describe what the feelings felt like, instead of just naming them? There's a difference between *being aware of one's feelings* and *knowing what the feelings are called*. There's also a difference between *having feelings* and *having automatic connections between feelings and expressions*.

When I was growing up, autism was considered an emotional disorder. I spent most of my childhood in one or another type of psychotherapy with therapists who started with the assumption that I knew what the words meant, but didn't know how to monitor my own processing. Their interventions primarily consisted of coaching me to say things I did not feel, and of telling me (and telling my parents) that I was behaving strangely because of various bizarre emotional conflicts that the therapists earnestly wished to work through with me.

If I said that wasn't how I felt, especially if I didn't know words to describe how I *did* feel, I was told (and my parents were told, of course) that I was resisting therapy and did not want to get well. If I obediently repeated the words and remained autistic anyway, I was told that I still wasn't being open enough with my feelings. Occasionally, under extreme circumstances such as the time I broke a bone, I was able to attach words to a subjective experience and make a simple statement such as "my foot hurts." Even when I could find words, no one believed me. I was told that I was only pretending to feel pain, fear, confusion, or whatever I was reporting because I *really* felt whatever the therapist's preferred theory predicted I should feel.

And through all this condescending concern about feelings and emotional issues, no one ever bothered to explain to me what the words meant! No one ever told me that they expected to *see* feelings on my face, or that it confused them when I used words without showing corresponding expressions. No one explained what the signals were or how to use them. They simply assumed that if *they* could not *see* my feelings, *I* could not *feel* them. I think this shows a serious lack of perspective taking!

I finally started learning to talk about feelings when I was 25. I knew someone then who taught me a vocabulary. She didn't know that was what she was doing. She didn't do it because she wanted to help an autistic person learn to "deal with" feelings. She just happened to be someone who talked a lot about her own feelings. She identified what each feeling was called, and where she felt it, and how it felt, and what her face and body were doing about it. When I asked questions about what the words meant, she explained. When she asked questions about my feelings, and I asked for clearer definitions of what she was asking, she clarified the questions until I could answer them. That's all it took to get started; once I realized that words could be used for subjective experiences, too, I took off again the way I did with idea-words when I was 12.

A professional at the conference remarked that therapy with an autistic person is educational therapy, not psychotherapy. Call it educational therapy, interaction therapy, commonsense-explanation therapy—or just call it honest and direct communication. Whatever you call it, a few months of informal, amateur, even accidental nonpsychotherapy did more for my ability to express feelings than decades of professional doubletalk. If professionals are to be more helpful than casual friends, they should be *more* objective than lay people, more willing to explain, less eager to jump to conclusions, more open to questioning their own beliefs.

Assumptions about emotions cause the most impenetrable barriers to understanding, the most devastating damage to relationships, the most harmful interventions, the most irreversible oversights—assumptions that I don't have, don't understand, or can't control my own desires and motivations; that comprehension or communication problems stem from my own conscious or unconscious choices to sabotage functions that would be intact if I truly wanted to use them; that if I fail it's because I don't care enough to succeed; that if I finally succeed, it's because I knew how to do it all along. I've read a lot about how psychodynamic theories blame and harm parents by attributing autism to emotional disturbance. They don't harm the parents nearly as much as they harm the victim when they say a child chooses to be autistic.

The results of these assumptions are often subtle, but they're pervasive and pernicious: I am not taken seriously. My credibility is suspect. My understanding of myself is not considered to be valid, and my perceptions of events are not considered to be based in reality. My rationality is questioned because, regardless of intellect, I still appear odd. My ability to make reasonable decisions, based on my own carefully reasoned priorities, is doubted because I don't make the same decisions that people with different priorities would make. I'm accused of being deliberately obtuse because people who understand the things I don't understand can't understand how anyone can possibly not understand them. (That sentence makes perfect sense. If you have to work a little bit to process it, you may get a slight taste of what it's like to have a language-processing problem.) My greatest difficulties are minimized, and my greatest strengths are invalidated.

I have an *interface* problem, not a core processing problem. I can't always keep track of what's happening outside myself, but I'm never out of touch with my core. Even at worst, when I can't focus and I can't find my body and I can't connect to space or time, I still have my own self. That's how I survive and how I keep growing.

I taught myself to read at 3, and I had to learn it again at 10, and yet again at 17, and at 21, and at 26. The words that it took me 12 years to find have been lost again, and regained, and lost, and still have not come all the way back to where I can be reasonably confident they'll be there when I need them. It wasn't enough to figure out just once how to keep track of my eyes and ears and hands and feet all at the same time; I've lost track of them and had to find them over and over again.

But I *have* found them again. The terror is never complete, and I'm never completely lost in the fog, and I always know that even if it takes forever, I *will* find the connections and put them back together again. I know this because I'm always connected at the core and I never lose track of my own self. This is all I have that I can always count on, all I have that is truly my own. And this is what is denied when I'm told that I bring problems on myself because I'm not stable at the core.

Being Autistic Does Not Mean Being Uncaring

There are other gaps that I'm just beginning to notice, and other assumptions that I'm just beginning to explore. They have to do with interpersonal rather than intrapersonal processing. The assumptions are similar: that I have the same needs for relationships that other people have, that I know how to relate in ways that are considered normal, and that I don't relate normally because I have negative or uncaring attitudes toward other people.

As with other activities I've mentioned, social interactions involve things that most people know without having to learn them. At the conference I met some other autistic people and gained a new insight into how nonautistic people think. During the Thursday-evening workshop sessions, a room was set aside for autistic people to meet informally in an unstructured setting. Four of us were left alone together. Within a few minutes, one person was rambling without enough focus, one was obsessing on a too-narrow focus, and I was having trouble keeping track of both of them at once. The fourth person in the room was invisible. That was interesting to watch; I know I'm invisible sometimes, but I'd never seen how it looks from outside.

After a while some other people came in to see what autistic people talk about, and they started asking questions that gave some structure to the conversation. Then some interesting things came out. I even heard the invisible person talk. While I could guess how odd he must have looked and sounded to people who are always connected to their bodies, it was exciting to *see* him putting his verbal mode on-line, to *hear* how far from his voice he was, and to be able to recognize the kinds of bridges he was building, because they were the same kinds of bridges I build myself. I build them over and over again every day, and no one ever notices unless I slip, but I noticed when I saw someone else building them.

All this happened because some people who weren't autistic came in and asked questions. A computer—or an autistic person—might have predicted what would happen if people who were all impaired in their abilities to communicate and converse were left together with no direction. (This autistic person *did* predict it, and still didn't know what to do about it.) This was a beautiful demonstration of the assumption that human beings, especially human beings who have significant things in common, *will* communicate and converse if given an opportunity, without needing any direction.

I don't know how to do that. I don't even know when I should be trying to do it. People seem to expect me to notice them and relate to them no matter who they are, just because they happen to be there. But if I don't know who people are, I don't know how (or why) to talk to them. I don't have much of a sense of people-in-general as things to be involved with. And I don't know how to have prefabricated relationships; if I happen to be involved with some person-in-particular, I practically have to learn to talk all over again to develop a common language with that person.

That doesn't necessarily mean I don't care. Sometimes I'm not aware of social cues because of the same perceptual problems that affect my understanding of other aspects of the environment. My visual-processing problems are no more the result of indifference than blindness is—are blind people considered insensitive if they fail to recognize people or to respond to others' facial expressions? Sometimes I notice the cues but I don't know what they mean. I have to develop a separate translation code for every person I meet—does it indicate an uncooperative attitude if someone doesn't understand information conveyed in a foreign language? Even if I can tell what the cues mean, I may not know what to do about them. The first time I ever realized that someone needed to be touched was during an encounter with a grief-stricken, hysterically sobbing person who was in no condition to respond to my questions about what I should do to help. I could certainly tell that he was upset. I could even figure out that there was *something* I could do that would be better than doing nothing. But I didn't know what that something was. It's very insulting, and also very discouraging, to be told that if I don't understand someone, it's because I don't care.

Sometimes, though, I'm really not interested. I'm not interested in relationships-in-general, or in people-as-groups. I can be very interested in individuals once I've met them, but I don't feel a need to have relationships in the absence of specific people to relate to. During school breaks I can go for days or weeks without any personal contact with other human beings, and I may get bored, but I don't get lonely. I don't need social contact. And because I don't need it, I have no compelling reason to go out of my way to get it. Mere proximity is no reason for me to become emotionally attached to anyone who isn't interesting to me as a person. Even when someone does attract my interest, when I do become emotionally attached and desire a relationship with that person, I don't become dependent on the relationship or on the person. I don't need them.

But wait. Because I don't *need* other people in my life, I'm free, as nonautistic people can never be free, to *want* other people in my life. Because I don't need relationships with *anyone,* I'm free to choose a relationship with a *someone*—not because I need a relationship, but because I like that person. When I make contact with someone, it's special—and not just because a lot of time and effort have gone into producing a response that's a pale imitation of normal social responses. Pale imitations of normalcy aren't worth any of my time and effort at all. When I make a connection it's special because I don't have to do it, but I choose to do it. It's special because I don't generalize very well from one person to another, so everything I do is intensely focused on just that one person. It's special because, having no idea of what's normal and little talent for imitation, I have created something entirely new for that person and that occasion. It's special because I don't know how to take people for granted, so when I'm relating to someone, that person is the most important thing in my world for the duration of the contact.

But I don't stick. That confuses people sometimes. A friend once asked me for assurance that I really wanted to be together. I answered, "I can leave and be just fine, or I can stay and be even better." Isn't it enough to be just fine on my own, and to be able to choose connections that will make my life even better? I have exactly as many relationships as I want. I relate only as myself, only in ways that are authentic to me. I value people only as themselves, not for their roles or status, and not because I need someone to fill empty spaces in my life. Are these the severe deficits in communicating and relating that I keep reading about?

Actually, there are some pretty serious deficits, but not in my ability to care. There are deficits in my ability to recognize people who aren't able to care, people who aren't authentic, who don't value me as myself, or who aren't connected at their own cores. It's hard for me to tell when someone is lying. It took me a very long time, and a lot of painful experience, just to learn what lying is. And in the social area, as with everything else, I have trouble keeping track of everything that's happening at one time. I have to learn things other people never think about. I have to use cognitive strategies to make up for some basic instincts that I don't have. In the social area, as with everything else, there are a lot of things that I don't understand unless someone explains them to me.

That's a special problem in the social area, because one of the things I need help with is deciding whose explanations and advice to accept. Mentors are supposed to be of critical importance to autistic people's successful functioning. A few years ago, when I was just beginning to explore the idea of making connections with other people, I met someone who offered to teach me what I needed to know. He was a doctoral student in special education who worked with developmentally disabled people in a number of community programs. He was warm and gentle and supportive—at least at first. He said he wanted me to be his little brother. He abused me mentally, emotionally, and sexually. He told me it was my fault. When I told his faculty adviser about it, the professor said that this was friendship, that it was something I needed. What was I supposed to learn from this?

I did learn a lot from it. I learned about lies. I learned about betrayal, almost before I learned about trust. I learned about some feelings that are more typical of child abuse and incest: I was just beginning to be aware of things—about relationships, about touching, about trust—that normal babies are born knowing, and he hurt me in ways I could never be hurt as a child, because I never trusted anyone that way when I was a child. I even learned about friendship, by learning about a lot of things that friendship is *not*.

But probably the most important thing I learned from it was that *I* am capable of making authentic connections, even if he wasn't. That's a good thing to know. Since then I've learned a lot more about how I can make connections, and about what kinds of people I want to make connections with. The future should be interesting.

Being Autistic Will Always Mean Being Different

After reading Temple Grandin's autobiography (Grandin & Scariano, 1986), someone once asked me if I thought a cattle chute would have helped me. I said I didn't need a cattle chute, I needed an orientation manual for extraterrestrials. Being autistic does not mean being inhuman. But it does mean being alien. It means that what is normal for other people is not normal for me, and what is normal for me is not normal for other people. In some ways I am terribly ill-equipped to survive in this world, like an extraterrestrial stranded without an orientation manual.

But my personhood is intact. My selfhood is undamaged. I find great value and meaning in my life, and I have no wish to be cured of being myself. If you would help me, don't try to change me to fit your world. Don't try to confine me to some tiny part of the world that you can change to fit me. Grant me the dignity of meeting me on my own terms—recognize that we are equally alien to each other, that my ways of being are not merely damaged versions of yours. Question your assumptions. Define your terms. Work with me to build more bridges between us.

References

Grandin, T., & Scariano, M. (1986). *Emergence: Labelled autistic*. Novato, CA: Arena.

MY ESSAY

Therese Marie Ronan

When I was born, mother knew that there was something wrong with me from the very beginning. As a child, I was speech delayed and preferred to be alone. I hand-flapped until I was 8, never made any friends, cried often, and was institutionalized for about four years. I had an extremely good memory for dates and was often reminded by my now-deceased father that I had autism.

I was also very easily frightened by the unknown. I hid from people, fearing punishment from them. When the news was on TV, I never looked at the broadcaster's face, bowing my head instead. I loved pictures, especially in magazines, and carefully examined the commercials in my magazines. I would also act aloof by throwing my doll down the clothes hamper. I was especially frightened by the mailman. Throughout my life I have been too sensitive, internalizing everything, especially when people have teased me. I often dwelt on these negative experiences for days at a time.

My schooling was mostly in special education classrooms. As a teenager I took some regular classes: cooking, sewing, gym, and home economics. Throughout my schooling, in regular classes or special education, I was picked on by peers.

My current hobbies are volunteering my time as a Jaycee, going to baseball games, cooking, gardening, Bible study, and active involvement in my community. I do not have a boyfriend. One of my autistic characteristics is poor social skills.

When I am 65, I plan to retire from whatever job I have, and set my sights on selling Mary Kay Cosmetics, using that money to live on. My top priorities are: God first, Autism Society second, job third, Mary Kay Cosmetics fourth, traveling fifth. I have six nephews and one niece. They are wonderful, and I just love them.

My autism has held me back from some things in this life, including close relationships and job advancements. I have never learned how to drive, and some say that I never will. These are unfair limitations that drive me bananas.

Although I love my family, they have never encouraged me to get ahead as far as employment. As far as they are concerned, I have limited vocational potential. I took one typing course about seven years ago.

As a teenager and as an adult, I have had liquor on occasion. I like wine. I seldom ever smoke.

I am very active in my county Autism Society here in Kansas, and I thoroughly enjoy helping them out. I have been through the mental health system, with little luck. I have maintained three friends in recent years, however, thanks to my mental health contacts.

I have been rejected because others view me as so peculiar. I still have a lot of autistic behaviors that are visible to other people. I am still viewed by many as mentally retarded.

I want to help bring autism out of the closet. Many autistic people are in institutions for life. I think that they deserve better treatment. Autism has been in the dark ages for much too long. I plan to help people with autism like myself for the rest of my life.

INSIDER'S POINT OF VIEW

Kathy Lissner

I was born in St. Louis, Missouri, on March 14, 1965, the seventh of eight children in my family. My younger brother, Michael, has just graduated from college, so all eight of us were college graduates by 1989. My story begins during the summer of 1964, when my mother got German measles during the fifth week of her pregnancy with me; in 1964 there was a major German measles epidemic in this country. My mother knew that German measles could give her fetus significant problems. When her doctor verified German measles, he suggested a "D and C," which is an abortion in the first trimester. Mom, being a good Catholic, said no.

When I was born, my parents were relieved because I looked and acted normally. By the time I was 1 year old, they knew that there was something wrong because I didn't grab for toys or react to the confusion and chaos in the house. Mom and Dad had me evaluated at age 2½ to 3 years old, when my IQ was reported as 48.

They were given a grim prognosis, suggesting that I would never learn how to talk, read, or write.

I didn't start talking until I was 4—haven't stopped since. I learned how to talk when dad rounded up all six kids and said, "Spend 15 minutes a day with Kathy. I don't care what you do, just as long as it is 15 minutes a day." Fifteen minutes may not seem like much, but multiply that by 6, 7, 10, or 15 sessions and you get 90, 105, 150, and 225 minutes.

Dad also used Coke to stimulate my language. He placed a Coke on the table in front of me and made me say "Coke" before pouring a drink. His techniques must have worked because soon after that I began talking, and I have been addicted to Coke ever since.

I went to regular schools all of my life, from kindergarten through college. I have had many fixations throughout my life, starting as a little kid interested in numbers. I knew my 12-times tables by the time I was 7. I still daydream a lot about different characters and I remember I used to have number characters that were my size, like 23. I remember names I used to make up: Jinx, Africa, and Louis were my three main characters, and I used to talk about them all of the time. I also remember people moving into the house across the street from ours. I ran up to one of the new kids, and instead of saying, "Hi, you want to play?" I proclaimed, "9 times 9 is equal to 81."

I am no longer as fascinated with numbers, but I am now quite involved with science fiction. Now I combine my interests in numbers and science fiction by making up aliens and giving them unusual names like "49" or "1945^2 minus 19."

Other fixations were Indians and rocks; I still have my rock collection. When I was 9 years old, I went down in the gully to dig up rocks. I still have an arrowhead I found when I was a kid. If you asked me what I wanted to be when I was 9 years old, I would have said a geologist. I was also interested in earthquakes; my biggest wish was to be in a big earthquake like the one that happened in Mexico City a couple of years ago. Four years ago in Missouri, I finally got my wish to be in a tremor.

One of my biggest fixations was on South America, especially Peru and Brazil, a decade ago. Everyone else could be talking about the Philadelphia Phillies and how they won in 14 innings against the St. Louis Cardinals, and I would say, "Lima, Peru." That is all I could think and write about. I was consumed. I remember jumping rope to made-up tunes with the words, "Venezuela, Columbia, Ecuador, Peru, Chile, and Argentina." I have always been fascinated with sounds of words, and at one time it was Peru. The year before, it was Korea and Japan. I remember a house under construction, and I was with my brother, Bobby, and his friends. There were construction men downstairs, and they told us to come and see what they were doing. I saw a big guy eating his lunch and I said, "Peru, Chile, Korea, Japan." The guy rose up and was about to grab me but I ran upstairs. The guy probably thought I was just another little brat.

I remember Girl Scout camp, living in a tent and hearing the whippoorwills. We had to draw pictures of tents, canoes, and redwood trees.

I remember writing *Lima, Peru* all over everything. In my living room I have a map of South America, and I remember the chocolate on Bolivia because I used to kiss it. Now I say to myself, "Gee, how could I have done that as a kid?"

In the seventh grade, my present interest in the Soviet Union and World War II began. To this day, I am fascinated by communist parties and love to read about them. I remember other children thinking about Elvis, rock stars, boys, girls, and partying on Saturday night. Their heros were Shaun Cassidy and Elvis. My heroes were Marshall Tito and Brezhnev.

I come from a big family like on "Eight is Enough" or "The Brady Bunch." People were always in and out. Friends often come over, and there is always something to do. On holidays, especially Easter, Dad would have jelly bean and money hunts. We still have 20 people in their twenties with little pink baskets looking for jelly beans. On Christmas we always have a 20-foot Christmas tree.

Playing spades and other card games has helped me learn how to interact with people. I am very close to my sister, Jenny. Whenever I had a problem, I always went to Jenny. Two and one-half years older than I am, Jenny explained life and the universe to me. My brother, Mike, was the one who forced me to play spades and beat me in every game with the exception of Probe because he cannot spell. Not only did my family help me with all of the chaos and confusion, but also with people and professionals. I was in the learning-disabled class part of the time in elementary school, learning handwriting, spelling, and math.

In May of 1975, my sister Jenny told me to put on a dress for a trip to see a doctor. I cried, and Jenny assured me there would not be any shots. The kind of doctor they had in mind was called a psychiatrist. Mom and Dad couldn't understand why I was intelligent and yet did funny things like talk about South America all of the time. I went to see Dr. Jim Edwards. The main thing I learned from him was how to deal with kids picking on me. He was a good guy.

My mother did not understand autism until 1987. I was diagnosed by age 10, but Mom did not understand much then because of miscommunication between her and the doctor.

Academically I did fine, but some classes like accounting I failed. It was very hard, but when I look back I learned a lot. I always knew I would go to college because everyone else did. I went to Maryville for 3 years and thought college was the promised land, my Israel. I also went to the University of Missouri–Columbia my junior year and then transferred back to Maryville. College was the first time in my life I felt normal, because I met a lot of people from other countries.

I have a friend named Jan who taught me about autism. She told me it affects the way I eat and sleep. I won't go to bed until 1:00 a.m., and I get up at 8:00 a.m. because I work 6 days a week. I have trouble falling asleep at night, but sleep well once I do. I eat the same things over and over again. I have to have Coke everyday. I used to need a daily pizza as well, sometimes for both lunch and dinner. Jan helped. When I got mad in college, I would hit my friends. My family never saw this. I hated every English class I took and once punched my friend, Jan. She had to wrestle me down.

If normal is being selfish, being dishonest, killing, having guns, and waging war, I do not want any of it. If normal is trying to help other people, trying to understand what is going on, and just doing the best you can in every situation, then I'll have it.

If I lived in Germany in 1933 to 1945, I don't think I would want that kind of normalcy. That ain't normal to me!!! It may have been to Hitler but not to me.

Some people have understood me from reading Temple Grandin's book. My little brother, Mike, got a lot out of it. At first he didn't like it, but then he read it again. My sister, Lee, also got a lot out of it.

There are times when I can't let go of something. Mamma and I went to Spain and Portugal last year, and Mom noticed the plants, trees, flowers, birds, and the scenery. I noticed every flag, every communist party poster, and anything in Arabic.

Visualization is very helpful for me. Because I visualize, I often take things literally. Someone once asked me, "Where are you?" and I said, "Massachusetts." She said, "What do you want most out of life?" and I said, "a hamburger." It would have been much better for me if she had said, "Where are you in regard to your personal development in life and the universe?" When you get a literal answer, it may be due to the sentence being misinterpreted or the sentence not being long enough. It makes a difference in how a question is answered if a single adverb or adjective is left out.

I am living in St. Louis by myself in an apartment with my cat Obie and going to Vanderschmidt School to learn medical transcription. I plan to graduate in May and, hopefully, I will find a decent job. (If the economy goes bust, I don't know what I will do. This country is headed for a rough time due to a lack of leadership in Washington.)

I have met other parents, however, whose children are much lower functioning than I am. It is just like a lottery. One week you win nothing, and the next week you hear about someone from Podunk or Center City winning a lottery. It was bum luck that Mom had German measles, but it is good luck that I am here today and doing as well as I am.

Author Index

Subject Index

ty—1500 people. Dustin, his wife, Lisa, Gail Mutrux, and Mark Johnson, Barry Levinson, and their wives sat right behind Joseph. They wanted to see his reaction. Later, when asked what he liked best, Joseph said, "The man eating cheese curls with a toothpick." The story line was lost on him.

Rain Man tells us how Charlie changed as he came to understand and learn some important life lessons from his autistic brother. It strikes a deep chord in those who know how autism has changed lives. With two top film stars playing the leads, autism has had its largest audience ever. Playing to full theaters around the world, and later winning four Academy Awards, the *Rain Man* story has helped thousands of autistic individuals and their families. The film has increased awareness and understanding of this little-known disorder in a measure greater than what all of us together have been able to accomplish in the past 25 years.

A few weekends ago we attended a big family wedding in Pittsburgh for my nephew. Only aunts and uncles were invited to the rehearsal dinner. Joseph was on his own for supper. I'd shown him the McDonald's arches from our hotel window and went downstairs with him as we were leaving. I asked the doorman to walk him to the corner and help him cross the street. I explained that Joseph may not seem to understand.

"He's autistic," I offered.

The man's eyes lit up.

"I saw *Rain Man,*" he said.

As we went around the block I saw the two of them on the corner, one carefully giving instructions, the other looking where the man was pointing.

Before *Rain Man* I would not have felt comfortable that Joseph was safe enough in a strange, large city to be left alone.

One film did that.

Reference

Treffert, D. (1989). Extraordinary people: Understanding "idiot savants." Harper & Row: New York.

AUTISM INTO ART: A HANDICAP TRANSFIGURED

Clara Park

At 31, art is a major part of my daughter's high functioning. Her speech is not; to hear it, its broken syntax and its conceptual simplicity, you would not think she could hold a job, keep her checkbook, assume the responsibility for important household tasks—all of which she does. Her art is important, however, in a different way. It allows her to make something beautiful out of what would otherwise be dismissed as autistic obsessions. It brings her in contact with people. It enhances her communication skills. It gives her a productive way to fill the empty time after work begin to speak to him in a rough voice. Joseph got highly excited and was unpleasantly talking back to the policeman. Kit got there just in time to rescue him. Without an advocate, Joseph, with very deficient social skills, would quickly have escalated the situation, possibly causing the officer to either chase him, shoot at him, or put him in handcuffs and haul him to jail. This has actually happened to a few autistic people I know.

Joseph now has relatively good speech and language skills. He finished high school, with the help of an excellent teacher/advocate and a school system that worked (sometimes reluctantly) with us. At his high school graduation, he got a standing ovation, and there were more wet eyes than mine as he walked across the stage to get his diploma.

Dustin Hoffman's Raymond is also high functioning with some phenomenal abilities. Since *Rain Man* I've often been asked if the film was accurate, especially in its portrayal of some of the feats with numbers. My response is that nothing in it is inaccurate.

In one scene a waitress drops a box of toothpicks, and Raymond quietly gives the number before they hit the floor. That incident is based on a skill of the well-documented retarded identical twins, George and Charles. In his fascinating book *Extraordinary People,* Darold Treffert (1989) reports that

> when a box of matches fell from a table and scattered on the floor . . . [both] twins cried "111" simultaneously. . . . [They] had not only seen the matches but had factored their number of 111 without any concept of what factoring was and without being able to understand multiplication, division or any other rules of arithmetic. (p. 64)

It is probably the same process by which Joseph at age 4 said "21 letters" when he read "Dangerous Intersection." George's explanation (Treffert, 1989): "It's in my head and I can do it" (p. 65).

Several of Raymond's behaviors are Joseph's, notably eating cheese curls with a toothpick, which was shown in *Portrait*. . . . It wasn't until I'd seen the film the second time that I realized Tom Cruise (as Charlie) was *also* using a toothpick! That was a low-keyed, delicate touch, showing how easy it is to accede to the autistic individual's insistent behaviors and routines.

Raymond's interest in taking pictures with his little camera as they drove across the Ohio River at Cincinnati, his compulsive lining up the salt and pepper shakers on the dinner table, the correct multiplication of two large numbers in his head as the small-town psychiatrist punches them into a calculator and shows a stunned Charlie the answer, the dramatic episode when Raymond burns the toast and his stimulus overload causes him to scream and severely bang his head on the wall—all of these are incidents based on Joseph's life. None are surprises to people who know autism.

A pre-opening benefit screening of *Rain Man* was held in Huntington on December 11, 1988, the night before the premiere in New York City. It was a gala event in our town, and the beautiful old Keith-Albee Theatre was filled to capaci-